MEDICAL ETHICS AT THE DAWN OF THE 21ST CENTURY

ANNALS OF THE NEW YORK ACADEMY OF SCIENCES
Volume 913

MEDICAL ETHICS AT THE DAWN OF THE 21ST CENTURY

Edited by Raphael Cohen-Almagor

The New York Academy of Sciences
New York, New York
2000

Copyright © 2000 by the New York Academy of Sciences. All rights reserved. Under the provisions of the United States Copyright Act of 1976, individual readers of the Annals *are permitted to make fair use of the material in them for teaching or research. Permission is granted to quote from the* Annals *provided that the customary acknowledgment is made of the source. Material in the* Annals *may be republished only by permission of the Academy. Address inquiries to the Permissions Department (editorial@nyas.org) at the New York Academy of Sciences.*

Copying fees: *For each copy of an article made beyond the free copying permitted under Section 107 or 108 of the 1976 Copyright Act, a fee should be paid through the Copyright Clearance Center, Inc., 222 Rosewood Drive, Danvers, MA 01923 (www.copyright.com).*

⊗ *The paper used in this publication meets the minimum requirements of the American National Standard for Information Sciences—Permanence of Paper for Printed Library Materials, ANSI Z39.48-1984.*

Library of Congress Cataloging-in-Publication Data

Medical ethics at the dawn of the 21st century / edited by Raphael Cohen-Almagor.
    p. cm. — (Annals of the New York Academy of Sciences ; v. 913)
    Includes bibliographical references and index.
    ISBN 1-57331-299-1 (cloth : alk. paper) . — ISBN 1-57331-300-9 (pbk. : alk. paper)
    1. Medical ethics. 2. Medical ethics—Forecasting. 3. Twenty-first century—Forecasting.
I. Cohen-Almagor, Raphael. II. Series.

Q11.N5 vol. 913
[R724]
500 s—dc21
[174'.2]
                                                                                                                      00-040186

GYAT / B-M Press
Printed in the United States of America
ISBN 1-57331-299-1 (cloth)
ISBN 1-57331-300-9 (paper)
ISSN 0077-8923

ANNALS OF THE NEW YORK ACADEMY OF SCIENCES

Volume 913
September 2000

MEDICAL ETHICS AT THE DAWN OF THE 21ST CENTURY

Editors
RAPHAEL COHEN-ALMAGOR

[This volume is the result of a conference entitled **Medical Ethics at the Dawn of the 21st Century** *held at the Van Leer Jerusalem Institute on January 5–8, 1998 in Jerusalem, Israel.]*

CONTENTS

Preface. *By* RAPHAEL COHEN-ALMAGOR	vii
Introduction. *By* RAPHAEL COHEN-ALMAGOR	1

Part I. Health Care Resources, and the Role of Doctors

Social Values, Socioeconomic Resources, and Effectiveness Coefficients: An Ethical Model for Statistically Based Resource Allocation. *By* EIKE-HENNER W. KLUGE	23
The Ethical Professor of Medicine: Challenges for the Twenty-first Century. *By* FREDERICK H. LOWY	32
Open Heart [*Shiva M'Hodu*]. *By* JOHN LANTOS	41
Truth Telling. *By* ANTONELLA SURBONE	52
The Evolution of a Hospital Ethics Committee *By* G. H. GROWE	63

Part II. Beginning- and End-of-Life Issues

Developments in Abortion Laws: Comparative and International Perspectives. *By* REBECCA J. COOK	74
The Continuing Conflict Between Sanctity of Life and Quality of Life: From Abortion to Medically Assisted Death. *By* BERNARD M. DICKENS	88
Advance Directives and Dementia. *By* RON BERGHMANS	105
The Autonomy Turn in Physician-Assisted Suicide. *By* TOM L. BEAUCHAMP	111
A Circumscribed Plea for Voluntary Physician-Assisted Suicide. *By* RAPHAEL COHEN-ALMAGOR	127

Peter Singer's Theories and their Reception in Germany. *By* JAN C. JOERDEN   150

Problems Involved in the Moral Justification of Medical Assistance in Dying: Coming to Terms with Euthanasia and Physician-Assisted Suicide. *By* EVERT VAN LEEUWEN AND GERRIT KIMSMA   157

Euthanasia: Reflections on the Dutch Discussion. *By* GOVERT DEN HARTOGH   174

Part III. The Age of Biotechnology

Jurisprudence in the Age of Biotechnology: An Israeli Case Analysis. *By* DALIA DORNER   188

Reproductive Liberty and the Right to Clone Human Beings. *By* JOHN A. ROBERTSON   198

Clones, Genes, and Reproductive Autonomy: The Ethics of Human Cloning. *By* JOHN HARRIS   209

Genetic Research: Conversation across Cultures. *By* JOAN MCIVER GIBSON   218

Organ Transplantation without Brain Death. *By* ROBERT D. TRUOG   229

Genetic Testing, Organ Transplantation, and an End to Nondirective Counseling. *By* DENI ELLIOTT   240

Notes on Contributors   249

Index of Contributors   257

Subject Index   259

Financial assistance was received from:

- THE BRITISH COUNCIL
- THE ISRAEL CANCER ASSOCIATION
- THE ISRAELI MINISTRY OF SCIENCE
- LAURA SCHWARZ-KIPP CHAIR OF PROFESSIONAL ETHICS AND PHILOSOPHY OF PRACTICE, TEL AVIV UNIVERSITY
- THE STIFTERVERBAND FÜR DIE DEUTSCHE WISSENSCHAFT
- TEVA PHARMACEUTICAL INDUSTRY
- THE VAN LEER JERUSALEM INSTITUTE

> The New York Academy of Sciences believes it has a responsibility to provide an open forum for discussion of scientific questions. The positions taken by the participants in the reported conferences are their own and not necessarily those of the Academy. The Academy has no intent to influence legislation by providing such forums.

Preface

This volume of the *Annals of the New York Academy of Sciences* contains essays that were presented at an international conference convened at the Van Leer Jerusalem Institute in January 1998. With the support of the Israeli Ministry of Science, we were able to invite seventeen leading scholars from Israel, the United States, Canada, Britain, Germany and the Netherlands. The idea was to bring together scholars from different corners of the world to reflect on the state of the art of medical ethics, and to enable them to enrich one another, and the public at large, with their careful consideration and insights. Indeed, the scholars who were invited examined the way their societies tackle moral decisions in the field of medicine and biotechnology. Justice Dalia Dorner of the Israeli Supreme Court delivered the keynote lecture.

The scholars have produced high-quality papers that will enrich the thinking and knowledge on various issues in the field of medical ethics. They represent the culmination of an idea that was first voiced during a meeting I had in 1995 with Professor Nechemia LevZion, then Executive Director of the Van Leer Jerusalem Institute, in which I suggested establishing a medical ethics think-tank. The objective was to bring together some of the leading scientists in Israel from different disciplines: physicians, philosophers, ethicists, legal theorists, social workers, and religious authorities. In a few months, a group of scholars renowned for their research and scholarship was assembled, and monthly meetings were held for the next two years. Out of these brainstorming sessions, a group of papers were developed and presented at the Van Leer Jerusalem international conference; they will be published in Hebrew sometime next year.

I wish to thank my colleagues at the Van Leer Medical Ethics Think-Tank, and the heads of the Van Leer Jerusalem Institute, Professor Nechemia LevZion and Dr. Shimshon Zelniker, who welcomed the initiative and helped to make it a success. Without their good will, advice, and assistance this volume could never be assembled.

I am most grateful to the Israel Ministry of Science for its generous support and for their trust. Special gratitude is granted to the Director General of the Ministry, Zvi Yanai, and to his successor, Professor Mordechai Bishari. It was the first time that the Ministry supported such a conference outside the realm of "hard science." I am also thankful to the other sponsors of the conference: The Van Leer Jerusalem Institute; the Stifterverband für die Deutsche Wissenschaft; the British Council; TEVA Pharmaceutical Industry; the Israel Cancer Association; and the Laura Schwarz-Kipp Chair of Professional Ethics and Philosophy of Practice, Tel Aviv University.

Finally, I express deep gratitude to Dafna Gold-Melchior for her hard and skillful work in all matters concerning the assembly of this volume and to the Editorial Department of the *Annals* for seeing this book through the press.

—RAPHAEL COHEN-ALMAGOR

—*September 2000*

Introduction

RAPHAEL COHEN-ALMAGOR
The University of Haifa, Mount Carmel, Haifa 31905, Israel

PRELIMINARIES

This book comprises essays that revolve around three main themes: the appropriate roles for doctors, decisions at the beginning and end of life, and medical ethics in the age of biotechnology.

The essays are written from different perspectives, employing different methodologies that enrich the discussion and exhibit a multitude of views. The scholars who contributed to this volume come from the United States, Canada, Israel, Britain, Germany, and the Netherlands. They examine the way their societies tackle moral decisions in the field of medicine and biotechnology. They examine practical questions from theoretical and analytical perspectives, combining theory, law, and scientific knowledge. The result is truly edifying: This volume significantly contributes to the ongoing debate on major issues in medical ethics in liberal societies as we enter the new millennium.

Liberals usually utilize terms of principle in discourse: *liberty* and *tolerance* (Alf Ross,[1] Alexander Meiklejohn,[2] Franklin Haiman,[3] Frederick Schauer,[4] Lee Bollinger[5]), *rights* (Hugo Black,[6] Aryeh Neier[7]), *equality* (Ronald Dworkin[8]), *autonomy* (Martin Hollis, Gerald Dworkin), *truth* (John Stuart Mill), and *justice* (John Rawls[12]). They wish to promote liberty, tolerance and individual autonomy, to seek ways to accommodate different conceptions of the good,[13] and to reach compromises by which the system will respect variety and pluralism and at the same time continue to uphold the rationale of liberal democracy, which may be summarized by the two dicta: do not harm others and promote respect for others.[14]

The liberal ideology places the individual at the center: everything derives from and flows back to the individual. The tradition, evolving from the philosophical thought of John Locke (1632–1704), Thomas Paine (1737–1809), Alexis de Toqueville (1805–1859), John Stuart Mill (1806–1873) and, in our time, John Rawls and Ronald Dworkin, sees the individual—in contrast to the collective—as the basis of the state, and sees the state as a tool meant to serve the interests of the individual. The state is conceptualized as a means of protecting society from external attacks, a framework regulating the implementation of the law for the prosperity of the citizens, a sophisticated tool to ensure individual rights. Therefore, the function of the state is to promote the well being of individuals, including when they are ill. The state has an obligation to preserve individuals' rights; namely, it recognizes that certain demands of individuals are legitimate and must be satisfied within the state's framework. The right to life is recognized as a first-priority right. Followers of John Locke call it a *natural* right in the sense that it is a consequence of nature, a right that comes before the state.[15]

The values of liberalism are enshrined throughout most, if not all the essays of this book. The essays are written from the liberal perspective but from different cultural outlooks.[16] Respect is given to the individual autonomy of patients and physicians; recognition that people are different is granted; and pluralism and variety are cherished throughout. Liberty, tolerance, rights, autonomy, equality, and truth and justice are the common themes that run through these essays. We all yearn to promote these values and strive to find compromises and solutions when we feel that they might come into conflict. For instance, liberty and justice often coincide, but on occasion they might conflict with one another when patients take the liberty to act in ways that physicians find unjustifiable. Physicians do not tolerate harmful behavior, even when patients harm themselves. Respect for autonomy might entail taking actions that some doctors regard as unjust, contradicting their understanding of the medical profession. The principle of *truth* requires physicians to reveal to their patients all relevant medical data, but sometimes doing this might harm the best interests of the patients more than would *not* revealing the entire medical record. We all cherish equality, but often we act upon criteria, deemed relevant and justified, that betray the principle of equality. We also must acknowledge the difference between the "ought" and the "is." Shortage of resources forces us to find the most equitable way to allocate scarce commodities, a way that apparently cannot meet the best interests of *all* people concerned. Indeed, in the United States where more than 40 million people are left without health care insurance, economic considerations outweigh the aspired principles of equality and justice that the U.S. Constitution is said to promote. The age of crude capitalism necessitates a close rereading of the writings of Locke, Paine, de Tocqueville, Mill, Rawls, and Dworkin.

HEALTH CARE RESOURCES AND THE ROLE OF DOCTORS

Throughout the twentieth century, medicine has become more advanced, effective, and technologically based. Doctors, patients, and their families have more information about illnesses, about alternative ways to treat them, and about possible side effects of each treatment. Doctors can save lives that in the past would be lost. People are living longer lives and have advanced medicine at their disposal. Medicine is able to monitor and control endemic diseases that in the past caused rapid death. But the process of dying from diseases such as cancer and AIDS is long, painful, and very costly. Questions arise as to the appropriate deployment and allocation of expensive resources and the criteria we should employ when we limit treatment because society is unable to withstand the cost.

The opening essay proposes a model for allocating resources. Eike Henner Kluge presents two distinct and competing views on the nature of health care. One model sees health care as a right, the other as a commodity. The *rights approach* uses ethical principles to determine the nature and structure of the health care's delivery system and employs economic measures only as tools to effect a just and equitable distribution within the system as ethically structured. The *commodity model* uses economic calculations to determine the nature, range, and distribution of the services it offers and appeals to ethical principles only as socially mandated limits within which all economic activity must be conducted.

Health is a major determinant of people's ability to take advantage of the opportunities that are available within society. Therefore, argues Kluge, a just and equitable society must try to minimize health-based differences so as to create a level playing field for all its citizens. Such a society has an obligation to meet the health care needs of its members so as to minimize health-based interpersonal differences. A publicly funded health care system is society's attempt to meet this obligation. It follows that a publicly funded health care system must start from the premise that health care is a right and not a commodity.

The concept of "rights" speaks of a need that is perceived by those who demand it as legitimate and therefore as the responsibility of the state to meet this need for each and every citizen. Rights are primary moral needs to which every human being should be entitled.[17] In this context, it is possible to differentiate between an individual's rights with reference to the state or government and an individual's rights with reference to fellow individuals. Rights regarding the state that are viewed as legitimate justify political decisions and actions by the government in order to ensure their existence. Rights regarding other individuals justify coercive action's being taken against individuals acting in a nonlegitimate manner.

Kluge discusses rights regarding the state. After establishing the premise that health care is a right and not merely a commodity, he sketches a model for statistically based resource allocation in a publicly funded health care system that integrates fundamental ethical principles, societal values, and effectiveness coefficients in the context of limited resources. His model takes into account the basic liberal principles of equality, justice, and autonomy, while recognizing that society is unable to meet all requirements and needs (Kluge terms this recognition "the principle of impossibility"). Emphasis is placed on the assertion that members of society not only can access the health care services, but also that they fund them. The principle of autonomy therefore assumes that society should have a say in how this funding occurs. This, in turn, means that societal values and preferences should be taken into account when deciding between competing and otherwise equal rights/obligations with respect to those services.

Kluge sets out eleven theorems that constitute his model. These include, *inter alia,* the requirements of equity; the societal obligations to provide health care services to its members in order to remove or minimize health-based differences that might otherwise prevent the members from taking equal advantage of the opportunities that are available within that society; the right of all persons to appropriate palliative care; and societal obligations to provide its members with a basic array of health care services (primary macroallocation), the nature of which is functionally determined by the average health care needs of the members of society. In this context, Kluge explains that a health care intervention is appropriate under primary macroallocation if and only if the intervention has a positive act/effectiveness coefficient, and that if the health status of the affected persons after appropriate primary macroallocation is not equal to or better than it was prior to the allocation—where the retention of or improvement in health status can be traced to the allocatio—then the obligation to provide the macroallocation ceases.

Kluge's model gives precedence to public preferences in the allocation of resources. At the same time, he cautiously states that if the health status of an identifiable group of persons within society is measurably lower than that of the statistical norm for society, and the health care needs of that group are not met by primary macroallocation, then a secondary macroallocation directed at alleviating those needs is *prima facie* mandated, and *vice versa*. But, Kluge maintains, the health status of groups that receive secondary macroallocation must not become greater than the statistically average health status of other members of society.

A relevant notion that relates to the discussion may be termed "the democratic spirit." It is quite a recent development, a product of the last thirty years or so, which is connected to the democratic notion of the public right to know. Doctors must deal with opinions and views that were unknown in the past. These views and opinions are part and parcel of the liberal democratic tradition: many people today ask questions, seek more details, solicit second and third opinions, are aware of the limitations of knowledge, and do not accept the doctor's word as absolute. Many doctors are busy not only with providing treatment, but also with research. Sometimes they might recommend a treatment plan that would serve their own research interests and not necessarily the interests of their patients. Curing and caring might not always be best served when doctors might operate in accordance with such a hidden agenda.

Technological progress enables us to quantify outcomes, define and measure quality, and compare different methods of treatment and different health care systems. Traditional views of the roles, duties, and privileges of doctors are questioned by philosophers, social scientists, social workers, jurists, religious authorities, health care administrators, psychologists, and by doctors themselves. The ensuing discussions and debates often lead to conflicting conclusions. Frederick Lowy, John Lantos, Antonella Surbone, and Gershon Growe discuss pertinent issues relating to the role of doctors in liberal societies.

The behavior of physicians towards patients and health care colleagues, both in their day-to-day relations as well as when faced with ethical dilemmas, is shaped to a large extent by the basic assumptions that contribute to their moral frame of reference. Some of these assumptions originate in the social, religious, and other influences on physicians' personal lives; others can be traced to the important orienting influence of their medical school professors, who serve as the doctors' early medical role models. Frederick Lowy argues that, given the importance of role modeling in shaping human behavior, it is likely that the messages, both intentional and inadvertent, that professors transmit to their students are as influential in determining these future physicians' attitudes and actions as are formal codes of ethics, institutional ethics committees, and even formal ethics courses in medical school curricula. Lowy considers the ethical stance of medical educators, paying particular attention to the challenges that confront the ethical professor of medicine at the turn of the millennium.

Lowy presents two models of ethics: the *traditional beneficence model,* and the *rights-driven model*. In the traditional beneficence model, physicians took responsibility for the welfare of their patients, made decisions on their behalf, and acted as emotional and spiritual mentors. This model is giving way, at least in North America, to a rights-driven model in which, in its extreme form, the physician is merely the technical expert who presents the advantages and disadvantages of various treatment options from which the patient must choose; the technologist physician specialist then executes the choice. In the traditional model the physician's own values have decisive influence, even if lip service is paid to respecting patients' views. In the physician-as-value-neutral-technologist model, the responsibility even for life and death decisions is that of the patient, whose values are determinative.

The problem here, argues Lowy, is that the specialized, technologically focused, positivist utilitarian physician claims the technical ground, but abandons the moral ground. Trained by super-specialist medical professors in tertiary-care institutions, these physicians recognize only a responsibility to diagnose the disease process (as opposed to being concerned with the broader problem of patients' subjective experience of illness) and to provide the patient with the various therapeutic options. What the patient decides to do is not the physician's problem. Within this narrow view of ethical responsibility, physicians undertake only to avoid exploiting the patient by not advocating a treatment that will advance the physicians' financial or career interests.

Lowy shrinks from this model. He advocates an ethical model of medicine according to which doctors take upon themselves responsibilities and apply value judgments in the decision making. He argues that patients and their families need a caring, beneficent, emotionally involved guide. Lowy wishes to reverse the pendulum swing that gained momentum during the past half-century in order to restore the priority of the physician-healer, for whom interpersonal sensitivity and traditional virtues are, again, important means to the therapeutic end. Furthermore, the ethical medical professor has a duty to prepare students for practice in the twenty-first century by presenting, fairly, the range of views on the morally vexing questions of the day, without failing to disclose his or her own ethical position. What the ethical medical professor will **not** do is to model technologically advanced medicine as an end to itself or as a purportedly value-neutral enterprise.

John Lantos is also concerned with the roles and duties of doctors. The debates mentioned above blur the picture as to what we want doctors to be or do or believe or enact. The twentieth century has brought about fundamental changes in biological and epidemiological science. We can do more and understand better whether what we are doing is really helping. These changes, argues Lantos, fundamentally alter the nature of the profession and the assessment of its work. These changes make it pertinent to whether our old-fashioned ideas of what doctors do are still relevant. If we still need doctors, what do we need them *for,* as we move into the twenty-first century?

One place where there is discussion of these issues is in recent fictional and autobiographical literature about doctors and medicine. In this genre, the open-endedness of the format and the relative intellectual unimportance of the medium allow questions to be raised about doctors and medicine, healing and illness, suffering and dying, that cannot be raised in any other discourse. In his paper, Lantos discusses some recent works of literature about doctors and medicine, focusing particularly on A. B. Yehoshua's novel *Open Heart*.[18]

What we learn from Yehoshua's novel is that medicine and doctors are strangely impersonal and amoral. They judge each other, but their judgments seem strangely arbitrary. We are left fearing that the quest for truth will never reach its goal, that the things we discover do not so much add to the total of our knowledge, but instead drop out of the equations, leaving us no closer to solutions. We are better at treating disease and keeping people alive than we have ever been before, but, as a result, there are more people in the processes of dying now then ever before. Somehow, the answer to the question of whether we need doctors or need medicine seems tied to the question of whether we know what makes a good doctor. Yehoshua highlights how difficult it is to know whether there is good medicine, and how, in the end, all we can try to decide is what we have always tried to decide, namely, whether someone is or is not a good doctor.

These questions are reiterated in Antonella Surbone's piece about truth telling in medicine. As mentioned previously, the principle of truth is one of the most celebrated in the liberal tradition: within this tradition the truth principle is more greatly identified with the writings of J.S. Mill more than those of any other thinker.[19] Surbone examines the epistemic, pragmatic, and ethical dimension of truth telling in medicine. Through their variance, complex and differentiated patterns of truth telling emerge in different contexts, and hence the different practices and degrees of truth telling throughout the world.

Surbone argues that truth is something emerging, being discovered and being created, in the patient–doctor relationship, as in any other instance of our lives. Truth is not a static object external to us, awaiting our neutral discovery: rather, truth is a *relational* state that develops in time and space because of dynamic human interaction. Truth is not only something to be *told*; it is also something that we *make*. Both the patient and the doctor contribute to this process of truth making, while the "methodological solipsism" of those who hold that truth can be effectively discerned apart from considerations of social practice is called into question.

Interestingly, Surbone argues that where autonomy is synonymous with "isolation," truth telling as practiced in the "American way" is unlikely to be beneficial to the patient or to foster her dignity.[20] For example, in the American context, objective medical information is sometimes imposed on a patient with a different cultural background or with different beliefs out of a fear of litigation or an abstract belief in the supremacy of Western beliefs (a worrisome and widespread form of cultural hegemony). To avoid this pitfall, different practices of truth telling should be accepted and respected: they should be seen as stemming from differences in the modulation and expression of the same basic principles of human dignity, embedded in different contexts.

Surbone shows deep sensitivity to cultural differences. However, this sensitivity should not lead to subjectivity and relativism. She reiterates that the doctor first has a professional accountability, which is primarily based on her respect for the scientific truth, as well as for the existential truth of the particular patient. This accountability is, at the same time, to the evidence and to the individual and to the community. Surbone is well aware that society cannot be portrayed in simplistic terms as culturally homogeneous and she believes that cultural differences should be acknowledged. Relationships, discussions, opportunities, duties, certain mental states, and a sense of one's own worth cannot be detached from cultural considerations.[21] Indeed, a realistic picture of democracy as we know it consists of a plurality of cultures whose freedoms ought to be ensured by the liberal state. Wars, imperialist inclinations, and conquests, the Industrial Revolution, commercial relationships, and immigration were among the notable factors that made the idea of a culturally homogeneous society obsolete. National, cultural, and ethnic memberships are significant in pursuing our essential interest in leading a good life; therefore taking account of such memberships is an important part of giving equal consideration to the interests of each member of the community.[22]

The concluding essay of the first section addresses the issue of hospitals ethics committees by shedding light on the work of one ethics committee in British Columbia. During the 1970s a body of philosophical literature defining and addressing bioethical concerns started to attract professional and public attention, and hospital ethics committees began to appear. Gershon Growe describes the developments that took place in ethics education, and the steps that were taken to better address the new issues that have arisen in the community, and to reflect the increasing role of other health care personnel and the lay public in defining the health care agenda and its application. Growe then probes the ethics documents that have been devised in response to unfolding concerns and perceptions. He notes that Vancouver has become a much more cosmopolitan community in the last fifteen years and treatment styles are being examined and altered to respond to the cultural needs.

Learning from experience, Growe argues that many of the so-called ethical difficulties on the wards are actually *communications* problems between staff members and patients and their families. Consequently a considerable amount of attention should be given to counseling and conflict resolution.

BEGINNING- AND END-OF-LIFE ISSUES

The issues of abortion and medically assisted death are linked: many participants in the abortion debate confront similar issues regarding assisted suicide and euthanasia, and the reasoning and language heard in the conflict over abortion are employed by legislators, judges, and commentators in their arguments about assisted death. The underlying difference between the participants in both conflicts concerns attitudes toward the inherent sanctity of human life, which would limit human intervention in the natural or divinely mandated processes of life and death, and the issue of the entitlement of human beings to exercise decisive control over these vital processes in order to regulate the quality of human and social experience and achieve a world of their own design.

Rebecca Cook's essay examines recent developments in abortion law reform in courts and legislatures in several countries. She describes the transition from criminal law, which accommodated only limited exceptions from liability to punishment where women's lives or enduring health were at risk, through laws prioritizing women's health, to laws aimed to protect human rights including that of constructing a family according to individuals' goals and aspirations. Criminal-based laws reflect a vision of patriarchal societies in which women's reproductive potential is molded to serve a public or religious agenda, and women's reproductive autonomy is considered threatening to public order and morality. Laws directed to health interests tend to be pragmatic, accepting the separation of the state from religion and addressing the damage to the health of women and families associated with resort to unsafe abortion. Laws serving human rights incorporate but transcend concerns with health, and recognize reproductive autonomy as a significant, but not singular aspect of individual- and family-based self-determination that is a central component of human and family-based dignity.

In his essay, Bernard Dickens addresses the issue of how analysts and commentators approach the relationship between abortion law and laws governing medically assisted death, a discussion that he limits to assisted suicide and voluntary active euthanasia. Attention is given to legal and related analysts and commentators who oppose legalization both of abortion and of medically assisted death, and who resist application of the reasoning that supported decriminalization of abortion to medically assisted death. They represent the so-called pro-life faction in the debate. Furthermore, Dickens discusses the so-called pro-choice position, which favors both liberalized abortion laws and tolerance of medical means by which individuals may end their own lives when they find survival excessively painful, burdensome, or undignified. Consideration is then given to those who oppose liberal abortion laws, perhaps because of fetal vulnerability, but who consider that nonvulnerable, competent persons, such as terminal patients in unrelievable distress, should be legally entitled to assistance in dying. The reverse is then addressed, concerning those who favor women's choice on abortion, but oppose medically assisted death, for instance, because it may be exploitive of disabled patients or it may violate the ethical duties that health care professionals owe their patients. Finally, Dickens proposes that reconciliation of opposing views may be approached through promoting choice, both to continue unplanned pregnancy and burdensome life, through availability of options individuals may be encouraged and supported to adopt.

Indeed, at the heart of Dickens' discussion lies the concept of *choice*. Pro-life and pro-choice approaches to medically induced abortion, suicide, and voluntary euthanasia are in obvious conflict, but Dickens shows that the notion of choice often offers common ground on which to debate. He contends that it is a mistake to believe that adherents to the pro-choice position on abortion are pro-abortion. When choices exist, for instance, through education and access to suitable means to plan pregnancy, and in particular to avoid unplanned pregnancy, the necessity of resorting to abortion can be largely reduced. The choice of childbirth and adoption is no less agreeable in principle to pro-choice than to pro-life advocates, although the issue of children's rights to learn their birth mothers' identities remains contentious. Pro-life advocates may also be sympathetic to women's having options in life in addition to motherhood and they may be able to accept the modern reality in many circumstances that women need to have paid employment outside the home in order to contribute to the well-being of their families.

At the end of life, advocates of different approaches to medically assisted suicide and euthanasia may similarly agree that those considering death should be offered better choices for living in comfort and dignity until the natural cessation of life. And those who sympathize with medical participation in suicide and euthanasia do not oppose options of palliative care.

Choice is also the key issue in Ron Berghmans's and Tom Beauchamp's essays. Berghmans outlines four morally relevant differences between choices in advance directives (prospective autonomy) and contemporaneous choices of competent patients (actual autonomy) which, to his mind, support the view that more confidence should be accorded to the assumption that an individual is the best judge of her own interests in the latter case than in the former. In a number of respects the choices as formulated in a dementia advance directive may fall short of autonomy and are less than fully autonomous decisions. In light of this, Berghmans supports the view that dementia advance directives cannot be given absolute moral authority in the case of nontreatment decisions involving incompetent demented patients.

In turn, Beauchamp argues that law, ethics, and public policy have been poorly served by framing end-of-life issues in terms of killing and letting-die and suggests dismissing this distinction as irrelevant. The problem, argues Beauchamp, is one of authorization rather than causation. If validly authorized, the act is a letting-die; if unauthorized, the same act is a killing. The justification of forgoing the medical technology, not the causal condition of death, is therefore the key condition both in conceptually distinguishing killing and letting-die and in the moral justification of letting-die.

Beauchamp maintains that our moral and legal compass should and will now shift to the moral issue concerning the liberty to choose the means to one's death and the justification, if any, for limiting that liberty. He reviews the recent history of this issue in the United States and then considers how this history reflects the unfolding of a commitment to rights of autonomy. Beauchamp argues that certain acts of assisting persons who request aid-in-dying that are often thought to involve killing are best understood as services for patients, not as acts of killing. He further asserts that concerns about patient autonomy are the most important, but not the sole factors driving current controversies and changes in policy.[23]

In my article emphasis is also placed on the liberal notion of the patient's autonomy. It is conceded that under certain conditions, after satisfying specific preconditions, there is room to consider physician-assisted suicide. Assistance to end the life of a competent and autonomous person at her request may be regarded as a way of showing respect for the person's will and choice. Both of us regard as *bold* (or *gross*) *paternalism* the keeping of a person alive against that person's will. It is our duty to address the needs of patients who have lost their appetite for living and who plead with their doctors for help.

It is reiterated that most patients cling to life; hence the concept of "death with dignity" does not automatically imply a desire to die; it certainly does not mean to put someone to death in a dignified way. In this context I warn against overzealousness and crusades that might promote the concept at the expense of the need for utmost caution. Special attention is given to the controversial role played by Dr. Jack Kevorkian, a role that is resented and condemned. Life should not be seen as a virtue to be preserved at any cost, regardless of the patient's will; at the same time, physician-assisted suicide should not be supported without reservation.

Much of my discussion revolves around terminology. Serious doubts are raised regarding the "quality of life" concept because ethicists who side with mercy killing use the term "quality of life" in a negative sense more often than in a positive one, meaning that they do not seek to improve the patient's life, but to end it. I also express reservations regarding the "double-effect doctrine"[24]; I voice my dissent regarding the term *terminal* (which does not serve the best interests of patients); and I state that terms like *persistent vegetative state* (PVS) and *vegetables* (referring to patients in such a condition) are unethical. Instead, I suggest that the term *post coma unawareness* (PCU) should be in use. The doctors' roles include neither putting a clock over the patients' heads and counting their days, nor dehumanizing them by not considering them as human beings. My discussion strives to use neutral terms that should not be offensive to any of the concerned parties.

Beauchamp and I would like to increase public awareness regarding issues like passive and active euthanasia, assisted suicide and the role of doctors, and to open the discussion to large circles of society. All relevant segments of society should hold serious, open, and frank discussions on these topics. In these discussions medical teams, patients and their beloved people, public leaders and religious figures, ethicists and intellectuals of social and philosophical background, and others who care about end of life issues should take part.

I also support the introduction of specific guidelines for a period of one year during which we will verify whether they are workable. These guidelines would aim at eliminating or narrowing existing "gray zones" by prescribing specific conditions under which physician-assisted suicide should be allowed. We have already been sliding down the slippery slope for some time, and the situation is sufficiently worrisome to call for a change. If society will not take upon itself the urgent responsibility to monitor the policy of mercy medical assistance to terminate life, more "Kevorkian-like" doctors will enter the scene and fill the lacuna by their dangerous presence and unscrupulous activities. Clear and concise medical guidelines would limit the existing dangerous maneuverability of doctors and better serve the interests of all patients: those who wish to live and those who wish to die. Society's answer to these genuine fears should take the form of specifying the roles and duties of doctors and the rights of patients, including their right to ask for a dignified death. This alternative is preferable to leaving the situation as is, where various people around the patient's bed might act in ways that might not be in the best interest of the patient.

Jan Joerden's essay further highlights the importance of sensitivity to terminology. Joerden discusses the Peter Singer debate in Germany. On the one hand, we cherish academic freedom and the basic right to free speech. On the other hand, we need to acknowledge that the German recent history makes it more sensitive and vulnerable to end-of-life issues than other nations.[26] History shapes culture and generations of people. Terms that are used freely around the globe are not tolerated in Germany. For instance, many scholars in Germany refrain from using the term "euthanasia" because of its negative, historical connotations, preferring instead to use the term *Sterbehilfe* [help to die]. Many in Germany feel that Singer should not be allowed to present his views on its soil, because any pronunciations of such views might grant them *legitimacy,* and Germany can not afford to confer legitimacy on such views less than sixty years after the end of Second World War. The anti-Singer campaigners further argue that Singer's positions are murderous, that the right to free speech does not extend to the public propagation of murderous positions, and that for disciplines that study values, the academic *is* the public. Hence free speech in the academy will not be extended to include discussion of murderous positions.[27]

Joerden brings some controversial quotes from Singer's writings[28] to explain why many associations for the handicapped and politically left-wing students in Germany have equated Singer with a national socialist, and have physically stifled his lectures in public forums in Germany. Some of his lectures were canceled; others were not tolerated. As soon as Singer began to speak, a chorus of whistles began and he could not be heard.[29] Joerden reflects on the choice of terminology by Singer, which he finds unjustified. He points out the problematic and inconclusive arguments in Singer's theory. Joerden argues that regardless of all the attacks on Peter Singer's right to freedom of speech, he should be expected to be sensitive and careful when dealing with questions relating to the right to life. Thus, for instance, Joerden thinks that the choice of Singer's book title, *Should the Baby Live?,* was made with an eye more sensitive to considerations of marketing and circulation than to the feelings of concerned people. At the same time, Joerden presents a liberal and tolerant view as to the place of free speech in these controversial circumstances. He is not in favor of excluding Singer *tout court* from Germany; rather he finds some value in his controversial theories that force us to think harder about problematic issues. Joerden would like it to be possible to publicly discuss Singer's theories at universities without being hindered by violent demonstrators. But these discussions should be sensitive to the feelings of the public.[30]

Any deliberation about death with dignity, especially with regard to the legal measures that should be invoked, would be incomplete without paying some consideration to the situation in the Netherlands, which influences the debate on these issues around the globe. The next two essays shed some light on the Dutch experience.

THE DUTCH EXPERIENCE

The Dutch debate on euthanasia began in earnest during the 1960s. The most striking fact about it from the very beginning was the extent to which explicit moral argumentation for the legalization of euthanasia relied on one single principle, the principle of respect for individual self-determination. In 1990, the Dutch government appointed a commission to investigate the medical practice of euthanasia. The Commission, headed by Professor Remmelink, Solicitor General to the Supreme Court, was asked to conduct a comprehensive nation-wide study of medical decisions concerning the end of life (MDEL).[31] The study was repeated in 1995, making it possible to assess for the first time whether there were harmful effects over time that might have been caused by the availability of voluntary euthanasia in the Netherlands.[32] In November 1997, the Ministers of Justice and Healthcare, Well Being and Sports, published their plan to install five regional committees that would supervise the involvement of physicians in the active ending of the lives of their patients. The main goal of installing regional committees is to increase the number of reported cases and thus to make public control effective.

In their paper, Evert van Leeuwen and Gerrit Kimsma review the installation of these regional committees with respect to the legal and moral problems involved. In their opinion, the committees' main goal will be to remove the physicians' objections to the red tape of judicial bureaucracy and to diminish their fear of being involved in the time-consuming process of legal inspection. As a secondary goal, the installation of regional committees would have the effect of decriminalizing voluntary active euthanasia (VAE) and physician-assisted suicide (PAS) to a maximal extent.

Van Leeuwen and Kimsma join Beauchamp and myself in dismissing the distinction between letting-die and actively assisting in dying. They explain under which conditions VAE and PAS are permissible and considered as good medical practice in the Netherlands and the main reason for *not* legalizing VAE and PAS. In their minds, the law has no means to express the intended good in ending the life of someone, and this good is beyond human judgment. Furthermore, the concepts of best interest, health, and well being point to another fundamental difference between law and medical morality. Every general discussion on the question of whether or not death is in the best interest of someone will inevitably end in abstract, general concepts that are not generally applicable in clinical practice. Severe problems will also arise when general categories are developed in which death is considered to be in the best interest of the patient.

Van Leeuwen and Kimsma think that the present legal procedure in the Netherlands establishes a prudent procedural control, first by colleagues, then by judicial authorities. The introduction of regional committees will help to solve the existing problems but, in the end, the gap between the law and medical morality remains.

In turn, Govert den Hartogh emphasizes three themes in his essay: respect for individual autonomy, medical judgment, and *anti*direct paternalism (to be distinguished from *indirect paternalism,* which is permissible). He outlines the main writings in the Dutch medical, ethical, and legal discussions on euthanasia from the 1960s onward and points out that the Dutch people do not seem to be afraid of doctors killing them too early, either intentionally or by mistake. Rather, their primary fear is that their life, mainly as a result of the exercise of medical power, will be lengthened in ways that involve severe suffering and slow decay. den Hartogh argues that the dominant view on the morality of euthanasia has never been accepted by the medical practice or by the law in the Netherlands. As for the medical practice, only one in three patients' requests for euthanasia are finally granted. The denial of patients' requests stems from various reasons, including the absence of unbearable suffering, the availaability if alternative options for treatment, mental disturbance (in particular, the depressive state), defective understanding of diagnosis and prognosis, and undue pressure by third persons. As for the law, the Dutch criminal code has two separate articles that forbid killing someone on his or her earnest request and assisting suicide, and that carry state maximal penalties of 12 and 4 years, respectively. However, den Hartogh reiterates what van Leeuwen and Kimsma explain: the system of penal law contains some general justifying grounds for actions which are covered by its provisions, and one of these grounds is necessity. One of the forms necessity can take is that of a conflict of duties, the one duty being to do what the law requires, and the other duty following from norms that are generally recognized as defining the duties of one's profession.

den Hartogh emphasizes the need for professional medical judgment in deciding on end-of-life issues and contends that only suicide can strictly be a matter of "self-determination." It is generally accepted that competent patients always have the right to refuse any medical treatment, but that does not mean that their refusal is sufficient. On the contrary, this requires an independent and justifiable judgment of the doctor that the treatment will be in the best interests of the patient.

While relying on the work of Joel Feinberg, den Hartogh proceeds with a discussion on paternalism. He holds that if people are treated paternalistically, their grievance is not simply that they have been unnecessarily inconvenienced, but rather that they have been violated, invaded, belittled. They have experienced something analogous to the invasion of their property or the violation of their privacy.[33] Someone who interferes with your way of conducting your own life, and does so for your own good, implicitly presupposes a moral asymmetry between him and you; he does not treat you as an equal and thereby insults you. So the interest in autonomy is not simply one component of your total well-being to be considered as such. For even before aspects of your well-being are to be taken into account, your standing as a full member of the moral community should be established. For that reason the liberal principle of *respect for autonomy* has priority in considerations of well-being.

MEDICAL ETHICS IN THE AGE OF BIOTECHNOLOGY

Advances in biotechnology in recent decades have brought the world revolutionary improvements in health care, new cures and treatments for diseases, and great promises for the future. At the same time, argues Justice Dalia Dorner of the Israeli Supreme Court, these developments have raised both hopes and concerns about the potential uses and abuses of new technology, which affect not only the medical field, but social, political, and legal relations as well. Recent public debates are concerned with biological weapons (Saddam Hussein will remain at the center of world attention as long as he rules, and ruins, Iraq), genetic cloning, and other forms of eugenics. On the political level, there have been great efforts to draft treaties and agreements regulating the use of biotechnology. And in the legal field, which Justice Dorner addresses, we are challenged to apply, adapt, and modify traditional legal doctrines to fit novel issues and conflicts.

Justice Dorner analyzes one case, that of Ruti and Danny Nachmani, which reached the Israeli Supreme Court and which exemplifies the types of challenges to social norms and legal definitions concerning parenthood, gender roles, legal identity, and life itself, posed by new technology.[34] The issue of concern revolved around the right to procreate. The Nachmani case was an unusual one that attracted wide public attention and received unusual attention by the court. In the first instance, the Israeli Supreme Court, hearing the case as a panel of five, reversed the decision of the lower court, and then, because of the novelty of the issue, decided to hear the case again, this time in an unprecedented manner, as a panel of 11 justices. The fact that the President of the Court, Justice Aharon Barak, decided to convene such a wide panel speaks for itself. The *Nachmani* ruling is a milestone decision in Israeli adjudication not just because of the size of the panel, but also because of the detailed reasoning of the justices. Each of the eleven justices on the panel wrote a separate opinion explaining his or her reasoning. Justice Dorner sided with the majority of seven judges in the appeal.

The case was complicated. Because of a malignant disease, Ruti Nachmani had to undergo a hysterectomy. And because the couple still wished to have children of their own, Ruti and Danny Nachmani wanted to use advanced medical technology, and Ruti underwent the arduous medical procedure of having her ova removed in order that later *in vitro* fertilization and implantation in a surrogate mother might occur. At the time, Israeli national health regulations prohibited implantation of ova in surrogate mothers. Ruti and Danny thus appealed to the High Court of Justice, seeking an order allowing the fertilization process to take place at an Israeli hospital. After a legal battle that lasted three years, an agreement was reached, with the Ministry of Health granting the couple's request. Subsequently, Ruti underwent complex medical treatments to remove ova from her body. Eleven ova were then successfully fertilized by Danny's sperm, and were frozen for the purpose of future implantation. At the same time, Danny and Ruti signed a financial agreement with a U.S. surrogacy agency, and made initial payments. However, two months after the signing of the agreement, Danny left Ruti and asked for divorce. Ruti wanted to continue with the implantation process, but Danny refused to grant his consent. Hence the appeal to the courts.

Justice Dorner reviews in detail the conflicting considerations at stake. She explains the logic of the balancing procedure that weighed one right (the right of the husband *not to be* a parent, a right based on his "ownership" of half the genetic material of the embryos) against another (the right of the wife, who provided the remaining half of the genetic material, *to be* a parent). Justice Dorner explains what brought her to decide in favor of Ruti in this Solomon-like decision. She explains that Ruti had relied, to her detriment, on the representations of Danny that he wanted a child with her. Ruti invested considerable amounts of time and money, and underwent painful medical treatments toward the achievement of her goal. The fertilization of her ova with his sperm effectively prevented her from being able to use these ova with another partner. And, more significantly, Ruti was left with no physical alternative to becoming a biological mother. Thus, ruling in favor of Danny would leave Ruti with no other possibility of having children of her own. While relying on John Robertson, Justice Dorner concludes that where the right of one completely destroys the right of the other, it is the latter that should be preferred. Danny could not deny Ruti her last chance to become a biological mother.

Both John Robertson and John Harris use the birth of Dolly, the sheep cloned from the mammary cells of an adult ewe, as their starting point for their discussions on the use of assisted-reproduction technologies. Robertson thinks that we must come to terms with the growing ability to choose, manipulate, or engineer the genome of offspring. He explains that cloning is only the first of several selection techniques that will be available in the relatively near future, and that germline gene therapy, which has a clear therapeutic intent and the benefit of fixing a genetic problem in subsequent offspring, may soon be available. In its wake will come nonmedical genetic enhancement, and even cases of genetic diminishment.

Robertson presents the argument for genetic selection as part of one's procreative liberty. He argues that the right to choose and select offspring characteristics follows from our prevailing conceptions of reproductive and parental freedom. Given the strong commitment to reproductive freedom that exists in ethical, legal, and social practice, a presumptive right to use somatic cell nuclear-transfer human cloning in certain circumstances should follow. Yet that prospect seems unpalatable. Reconciling these two positions is a major challenge for future uses of assisted-reproduction and genetic-selection technology.

Justice Dorner's and Robertson's arguments have much in common: Both think that the moral and legal right to choose whether or not to reproduce is fundamental. Both think that procreative liberty is a *presumptive,* not an absolute, *right.* Therefore, both advocate the *balancing* approach in deciding controversial relevant cases. Robertson explains that courts should presumptively protect actions involving procreative liberty against state interference until the point at which the reproductive choice in question harms or intrudes upon the tangible interests of others. A court deciding such a case, as well as policymakers or professionals confronting those circumstances, would have to analyze the interests served by the interference and the harms and sufferings it tries to prevent. Robertson maintains that the balancing of interest, however, is not made on equal terms. If we resort to terminology from the American free-speech literature, we may say, following Robertson's reasoning, that the right to procreate enjoys a *preferred position*.[36] Only when those seeking to limit procreative choice could show that unrestricted choice would cause compelling, tangible harm to others should interference with procreative choice be permitted.

Robertson concludes that claims of harm must be more carefully scrutinized today than before. Given the variations in how people assign meaning to procreation, and the recognition that reproductive choices are largely reserved to individual choice, no particular view of how reproduction should occur can be imposed. Only tangible harm to others justifies banning or greatly restricting a practice when that practice involves an exercise of fundamental liberty. Whether human cloning poses such harm (or is even a fundamental liberty) remains to be seen. Yet a reasonable argument exists that cloning, while presenting novel variations on kinship relations, causes no more harm than the many forms of assisted reproduction and genetic selection now in use, and therefore should be treated accordingly.

John Harris would probably agree with most, if not all, of Robertson's conclusions. Harris starts his discussion by surveying some of the reactions, which he regards as hasty and panicky, to Dolly's birth. Harris refers, *inter alia,* to the recent resolution of the European Parliament suggesting that cloning violates the principle of equality, "as it permits a eugenic and racist selection of the human race." Well, argues Harris, so does prenatal and preimplantation screening, not to mention egg donation, sperm donation, surrogacy, abortion, and human preference in choice of sexual partner. The fact that a technique could be abused does not constitute an argument against the technique, unless there is no prospect of preventing the abuse or wrongful use. To ban cloning on the grounds that it might be used for racist purposes is tantamount to saying that sexual intercourse should be prohibited because it permits the possibility of rape.

The World Health Organization also objects to cloning on the grounds that the use of cloning for the replication of human individuals would violate the basic principle of respect for the dignity of the human being that governs medically assisted procreation. In response, Harris argues that appeals to human dignity are not only universally attractive, but also comprehensively vague. Furthermore, the notion of human dignity is often linked to Kantian ethics, and Harris explains why he thinks the Kantian principle, invoked without any qualification or gloss, is seldom helpful in medical or bioscience contexts. If we object to cloning on Kantian grounds, then we should also object to blood transfusions (among other reasons because the donor figures in the life of the recipient of blood exclusively as a *means*) and to abortions designed to save the life of the mother. Harris asserts bluntly and conclusively that the Kantian ethics is so vague and so open to selective interpretation, and its scope for application is so limited, that its utility as a fundamental principle in bioethics thought is virtually zero.

Harris thinks that much of the discussion on human cloning is saturated with empty rhetoric, invoking resonant principles with no conceivable or coherent application to the problem at hand. He is pleading for the emergence of bioethical thinking that would seriously address the issue at hand, which obviously is not easy, and for the abandonment of gut feelings and what he terms "nasal reasoning." Addressing the issue without prejudice will reveal that there are powerful arguments in favor of a tolerant attitude to varieties of human reproduction. In Harris's opinion, a *prima facie* case may be made for regarding human cloning as a dimension of procreative autonomy that should not be lightly restricted. Interestingly, in support for his argument, Harris refers to Ronald Dworkin, who uses in his reasoning the same terminology to which Harris formerly objected:

> The right of procreative autonomy has an important place ... in Western political culture more generally. The most important feature of that culture is a belief in *individual human dignity*: that people have the moral right—and the moral responsibility–to confront the most fundamental questions about the meaning and value of their own lives for themselves, answering to their own consciences and convictions ... . The principle of procreative autonomy, in a broad sense, is embedded in any genuinely democratic culture.[38] [*emphasis added.* —ED.]

Here, as in his other writings, Dworkin uses the term "culture" in a broad sense and in a unified manner. It was previously stated that there are some ground rules for liberal democracies, but that we cannot speak of democracies as homogenous entities. Joan McIver Gibson is very sensitive to this issue and explores the need for public conversations and open discussions to make controversial issues intelligible to the public. Gibson claims that reactions to the cloning of Dolly in Scotland and the growing awareness of the international Human Genome Diversity project have served notice that the public does not consider itself to be a full partner in these enterprises. While the scientific community may share a similar level of understanding and enthusiasm for such research, the same cannot be said for many groups and individuals around the world. And, at least in the United States, where the value of autonomy and individual rights is legendary, high hopes are placed on *informed consent* as the mechanism-of-choice for ensuring that potential subjects make free, voluntary, and informed decisions. Generally, however, failure is the result on all counts.

Gibson submits that there is a social franchise that scientists and medical researchers must maintain: they need the public trust and understanding for their research to proceed. Without these, continuing research is jeopardized, as demonstrated by public reaction to recent biotechnological disclosures. Gibson thinks that in our talk and work we fail to appreciate the intrinsically dialogic nature of communication. Society trains its professionals to speak in monologue, thereby foreclosing any possibility that there is a conscious "other," who must be heard, who is a constitutive participant in any consent process, and whose values and context inevitably shape the exchange as much as those of the speaker. We fail to appreciate the contextual nature of the decision-making environment, especially for individuals and cultures where *community* rather than *individual* identity is dominant. Gibson argues that areas of genetic research such as cell line research and the creation of DNA libraries require much greater support from the public than currently is the case. She asserts that we must mount an educational effort that listens as much as it talks, that fosters collaboration across cultures (international, indigenous and intranational, societal, and scientific), and that regularly tests the strength of science's social franchise in the eyes of its public and research subjects.

Robert Truog shares Gibson's call for open discussion and dialogue. He wishes to reopen the debate about the definition of death. Truog provides a historical analysis of what safeguards were used to assure the certainty of the diagnosis of death. He argues that only after the development of mechanical ventilation in the 1950s did a serious discussion arise about the definition of death. For the first time it was possible to separate the cessation of neurological function from the cessation of pulse and respiration.

In the last thirty years or so, a person whose brain stem is dead is considered dead. Truog analyses the concept of "whole brain death" in terms of three distinct levels: the definition ("permanent cessation of functioning of the organism as a whole"); the criteria ("permanent cessation of functioning of the entire brain"); and the tests (specific medical findings). However, he argues that numerous inconsistencies between these levels seriously undermine the coherence of the whole-brain concept. For example, many patients diagnosed as whole-brain-dead on the basis of the required "tests" fail to fulfill the "criteria" because they continue to manifest a variety of brain functions (hormonal regulation, temperature homeostasis, etc.). In addition, patients who meet the "criteria" may fail to meet the "definition" because new technologies for maintaining homeostasis mean that whole-brain death may no longer necessarily imply the cessation of functioning of the organism "as a whole."

Truog suggests two possible options for resolving the inconsistencies: to adopt a "higher brain" standard or to revert to a definition of death based on the traditional cardiopulmonary standard (absence of pulse and respiration). In his opinion, each of these offers a conceptually more appealing and consistent understanding of death. The principal problem with the former standard is the lack of societal willingness to view anyone with adequate respiratory function as "dead." The principal problem with implementing the latter approach would be difficulties in obtaining organs for transplantation.

Indeed, Truog thinks that the concept of brain death was developed in the first place in order to identify a category of persons from whom it is possible to remove greatly needed organs for transplantation. The interesting question is whether the need for conceptual clarity will supersede the pragmatic requirements for both societal "comfort" and transplantable organs. In any event, Truog reiterates, it is necessary to retain the two guiding principles behind transplantation of living organs: consent and nonmaleficence.[39]

The issue of organ transplantation is the focus of Deni Elliott's essay. Elliott argues that rather than looking to organ transplantation as a cure for genetic malady, we ought instead to work toward preventing genetic disease through preconceptual and prenatal testing. To her mind, health-care providers and people who plan to procreate have a moral responsibility to prevent genetic disease where they can. One result of this line of reasoning is that the oxymoron "nondirective counseling" is replaced with an explicit standard-of-care perspective that moves genetic screening into mainstream medical practice.

Transplantation is an expensive, but sometimes available treatment of choice for some genetic diseases, specifically for children, who constitute the overwhelming class of transplant recipients for genetic disease. These transplants are performed to bring about one of the following results: replacement of an organ that did not develop or is irreparably damaged, providing a site for processing or detoxifying bodily substances, or to manufacture a congenitally absent substance or type of cell. However, transplantation does not always offer a cure. In some cases, transplantation restores a damaged organ, but does not resolve the underlying genetic disease. In other cases, transplantation may bring about a delayed or partial cure for genetic disease. Even in cases in which transplantation provides a cure for the manifestations of the disease and something like a normal, albeit complicated or compromised life-span, transplantation does not address the underlying genetic cause of the organ failure and the likelihood of the disease's being passed on to yet another generation by the affected individual or to another child through repeated pregnancy.

Elliott suggests that as we move into the twenty-first century, policymakers, health-care practitioners, and scholars working in the realm of "genethics" should make a concerted effort to promote *prevention* as the treatment of choice for serious genetic disease. Because of the liberal, universal, minimalist moral dictum *First do no harm*, individuals ought not knowingly produce children with serious genetic disease. In addition, those intended to procreate have a role-related responsibility as well. If pregnant women have a responsibility not to cause potential prenatal injury, then they ought not cause avoidable genetic injury as well. New technology not only expand reproductive *choice*; it also expands reproductive *responsibility*.

MEDICAL ETHICS AT THE DAWN OF THE TWENTY-FIRST CENTURY: FUTURE DEVELOPMENTS

Advanced medical technologies present us with the challenge of reconsidering, reapplying, and modifying traditional paradigms to take into account new medical and social realities. As Justice Dorner asserts, we must continue to search for principles of justice and morality to guide us in making decisions about the direction of this new technology, its application, and the resolution of real conflicts. We must try to identify what Dworkin calls a *moral default*, that is, a basic set of convictions that can guide us in the face of the deepest uncertainties. Some have a default conviction for individual freedom, requiring some positive showing of a serious danger to health or safety before they would be ready to endorse legal limits on genetic testing, research, or experimentation. Others have a more conservative instinct, requiring a positive showing that some program of testing or line of research is safe and helpful before they would permit it. Of course, these are only crude paradigms. Dworkin acknowledges that any actual background morality is likely to be more complex, deeply grounded, and harder to articulate. But that kind of critical moral backdrop or default is nevertheless indispensable.[40]

At the dawn of the twenty-first century, liberal democracies must address the major innovations in advanced medicine. These include, according to Frederick Lowy, technological breakthroughs that expand the range of the possible; a recognition of the increasingly pluralistic nature of most societies with respect to culture, ethnicity, religion, and social structures; instant communication, in which new (and at times untested) treatments are described on the Internet and recommended to patients before their physicians have heard of them; funding policies that provide disincentives to optimal care for individual patients; and, in some countries, a litigious public ready to bring suit against health professionals who take too much or too little responsibility in particular cases.

John Lantos articulates two opposing visions of medicine in the twenty-first century: the first is a vision of dreams and ideals; the second is one of limits and frustrated intentions. The optimistic vision is that we are only at the beginning of a biological revolution that will augment and transform medicine's powers exponentially. New drugs, devices, diagnostic tests, and new abilities to manipulate the human genome will allow the elimination or cure of most of the ills from which we now suffer. These interventions will not only be medically effective, but will also be cost-effective, just as polio vaccine was both better and cheaper than the iron lung. It will be a century of cheap health.

The pessimistic view is that medicine will exacerbate our suffering. New discoveries will lead to new problems, new half-way technologies that cannot cure our diseases, but only prolong the end of our lives into a long, drawn-out, expensive technological ritual of suffering. We will create a culture of illness. Medicine will be our nemesis. Time will show which of the two models will predominate, although we can assume that elements of both models will combine and intersect. Let us hope that frequent, open, and public deliberations of ethical concerns will bring society nearer to the optimistic model.

Gibson thinks that medical ethicists in the twenty-first century will pay more attention to the role of family, community, and society in matters of medicine, research, and policy. On the other hand, Beauchamp thinks that a key concept in the twenty-first century, especially with regard to end-of-life issues, will be that of *autonomy*. We will recast autonomy rights to request aid and plan for death using a model analogous to the ways we have used autonomy rights to require informed consent and to allow us to control the dying process through advance directives.

Beauchamp maintains that a wider array of ways to allow competent patients to refuse nutrition and hydration in order to end their lives will be cultivated. The refusal of nutrition and hydration appears to encounter no legal or moral problems in many countries, despite the fact that there is no clear distinction between starving oneself to death and suicide. Another option that is virtually certain to be favored is a dramatically improved and more aggressive use of palliative care. We can expect to see more resources and training in support of this option, and possibly more hospices around the globe.[41]

CONCLUSION

The essays gathered in this volume cover a wide range of practical issues concerning a variety of problems confronted time and again in medicine, ethics, and law. They consider the practical and ethical difficulties that result from the rapid advances being made in technology. They seek to discover how we may learn from our past and how we may promote a better, more ethical, and workable medicine.

This volume will enrich the ongoing professional and public debates about the intricate questions of medical ethics. Its topics and main concerns are timely, significant, very controversial, and hence intellectually compelling. They address issues that bring scholars and students, educators and professionals, doctors, nurses, biologists, social workers, psychologists, philosophers and ethicists, jurists and lawyers, religious authorities, and the general public together, although often not in harmony. The deliberations offered here will draw the attention of people from all walks of life. They will be most useful in medical schools and centers, in classrooms and academic forums, and of benefit to legislatures and judges. Ethics is a social value that must be rooted at the core of professionalism in general, and in medicine in particular, in the coming years.

NOTES AND REFFERENCES

1. Alf Ross, *Why Democracy?* (Cambridge, Mass.: Harvard University Press, 1952).
2. Alexander Meiklejohn, *Political Freedom* (New York: Oxford University Press, 1965).
3. Franklin S. Haiman, *Speech and Law in a Free Society* (Chicago and London: University of Chicago Press, 1981).

4. Frederick Schauer, *Free Speech: A Philosophical Enquiry* (New York: Cambridge University Press, 1982).
5. Lee C. Bollinger, *The Tolerant Society* (Oxford: Clarendon Press, 1986).
6. Hugo L. Black, "The Bill of Rights," *New York University Law Review,* Vol. 35 (1960), pp. 865–881.
7. Aryeh Neier, *Defending My Enemy* (New York: E. P. Dutton, 1979).
8. Ronald M. Dworkin, "In Defence of Equality," *Social Philosophy and Policy,* Vol. I (1983), pp. 24–40; *idem,* "Why Liberals Should Believe in Equality?," *The New York Review of Books,* XXX, No. 1 (1983), pp. 32–34; and *A Matter of Principle* (Oxford: Clarendon Press, 1985).
9. Martin Hollis, *Models of Man* (Cambridge, England: Cambridge University Press, 1977).
10. Gerald Dworkin, *The Theory and Practice of Autonomy* (Cambridge, England: Cambridge University Press, 1988).
11. J. S. Mill, *Utilitarianism, Liberty, and Representative Government* (London: J. M. Dent, 1948, [Everyman edition]).
12. John Rawls, *A Theory of Justice* (Oxford: Oxford University Press, 1971); *idem, Political Liberalism* (New York: Columbia University Press, 1993).
13. "Conception of the good" is a conception that encompasses both personal values and societal circumstances. It consists of a more or less determinate scheme of ends that the doer aspires to carry out for their own sake as well as attachments to other individuals and loyalties to various groups and associations.
14. R. Cohen-Almagor, *The Boundaries of Liberty and Tolerance* (Gainesville, FL: University Press of Florida, 1994); *idem* (Ed.), *Liberal Democracy and the Limits of Tolerance* (Ann Arbor: University of Michigan Press, 2000); Ronald M. Dworkin, *Taking Rights Seriously* (London: Duckworth, 1977); and *A Matter of Principle, op. cit.*
15. See the writings of Locke, http://weber.ucsd.edu/~dmckiern/locke.htm
16. For a communitarian perspective, see Ezekiel J. Emanuel, *The Ends of Human Life* (Cambridge, MA: Harvard University Press, 1991). For general communitarian critiques of liberalism see Daniel Bell, *Communitarianism and Its Critics* (Oxford: Clarendon Press, 1993); Shlomo Avineri and Avner De-Shalit (Eds.), *Communitarianism and Individualism* (Oxford: Oxford University Press, 1992); Will Kymlicka, *Contemporary Political Philosophy* (Oxford: Clarendon Press, 1990), especially 199–237; Michael Sandel, *Liberalism and Its Critics* (Oxford: Basil Blackwell, 1984); Michael Walzer, *Spheres of Justice* (Oxford: Basil Blackwell, 1983); Alasdair MacIntyre, *After Virtue* (London: Duckworth, 1981).
17. For further discussion on the concept of rights, see Ronald Dworkin, *Taking Rights Seriously*; J. Roland Pennock and John W. Chapman (Eds.), *Human Rights* (New York: New York University Press, 1981); L.W. Sumner, *The Moral Foundation of Rights* (Oxford: Clarendon Press, 1989); Michael Freeden, *Rights* (Minneapolis, MN: University of Minnesota Press, 1991); Alan Gewirth, *The Community of Rights* (Chicago: University of Chicago Press, 1996); Hillel Steiner, *An Essay on Rights* (Oxford: Blackwell, 1994); Matthew H. Kramer, N.E. Simmonds and Hillel Steiner, *A Debate over Rights* (Oxford: Clarendon Press, 1998); Michael J. Perry, *The Idea of Human Rights* (New York: Oxford University Press, 1998); John R. Rowan, *Conflicts of Rights* (Boulder, CO: Westview Press, 1999); Jonathan M. Mann, Sofia Gruskin, Michael A. Grodin and George J. Annas (Eds.), *Health and Human Rights* (London: Routledge, 1999).
18. A. B. Yehoshua, *Open Heart* (New York: Doubleday, 1996).
19. Cf. J. S. Mill, *Utilitarianism, Liberty, and Representative Government*, and "Law of Libel and Liberty of the Press," in Geraint L. Williams (Ed.), *John Stuart Mill on Politics and Society* (Glasgow: Fontana, 1976), pp. 143–169, and R. Cohen-Almagor, "Why Tolerate? Reflections on the Millian Truth Principle," *Philosophia,* Vol. 25, Nos. 1–4 (1997), pp. 131–152; *idem,* "Ends and Means in J.S. Mill's *On Liberty*," *The Anglo-American Law Review,* Vol. 26, No. 2 (1997), pp. 141–174. For further discussion, see John Milton, *Areopagitica: A Speech for the Liberty of Unlicensed Printing* (Cambridge: Deighton, Bell & Co., 1973). Milton writes in *Areopagitica* (p. 35): "And though all the winds of doctrine were let loose to play

upon the earth, so Truth be in the field, we do injuriously by licensing and prohibiting to misdoubt her strength. Let her and falsehood grapple; who ever knew Truth put to the worse, in a free and open encounter?."
20. Antonella Surbone, "Truth Telling to the Patient," *JAMA*, No. 268 (1992), pp. 1661–1662.
21. Rawls, Dworkin,and Raz appear to ignore cultural differences in their writings. They speak about pluralism and at the same time depict quite a simplified view of homogenous liberal society. See John Rawls, *A Theory of Justice;* Ronald M. Dworkin, *Taking Rights Seriously; idem, A Matter of Principle,* and Joseph Raz, *The Morality of Freedom* (Oxford: Clarendon Press, 1986).
22. For further deliberation see R. Cohen-Almagor, "Liberalism, and the Limits of Pluralism," *Terrorism and Political Violence,* Vol. 7, No. 2 (1995), pp. 25–48; Will Kymlicka and Raphael Cohen-Almagor, "Democracy and Multiculturalism," in Maria Baghramian and Attracta Ingram (Eds.), *Perspectives on Pluralism* (London: Routledge, forthcoming).
23. For further discussion see James F. Childress, "The Place of Autonomy in Bioethics," *The Hastings Center Report,* Vol. 20, No. 1 (January/February 1990), pp. 12–17.
24. For a critical discussion see Timothy E. Quill, Rebecca Dresser, and Dan W. Brock, "The Rule of Double Effect—A Critique of Its Role in End-of-Live Decision Making," *New England Journal of Medicine,* Vol. 337 (11 December 1997), pp. 1768–1771. See also the correspondence on the rule of double effect in *New England Journal of Medicine,* Vol. 338, No. 19 (7 May 1998), pp. 1389–1390. For a more favorable view of the doctrine see John Finnis, "Intention and Side-Effects," in R.G. Frey and C. Morris (Eds.), *Liability and Responsibility* (Cambridge: Cambridge University Press, 1991), pp. 32–46; *idem,* "A Philosophical Case Against Euthanasia," in J. Keown (Ed.), *Euthanasia Examined* (Cambridge: Cambridge University Press, 1997), pp. 23–35. For general discussion about the doctrine see William E. May, "Double Effect," in Warren T. Reich (Ed.), *Encyclopedia of Bioethics* (New York.: The Free Press, 1978), Vol. 1, pp. 316–319; David Wm. Solomon, "Double Effect," in Lawrence C. Becker (Ed.), *Encyclopedia of Ethics* (New York and London: Garland Publishing, 1992), Vol. I, pp. 268–269; F.M. Kamm, "Physician-Assisted Suicide, the Doctrine of Double Effect, and the Ground of Value," *Ethics,* Vol. 109, No. 3 (1999), esp. pp. 586–591; South Australian Voluntary Euthanasia Society, DID YOU KNOW? The Principle of Double Effect, SAVES, Fact Sheet No. 23 (October 1997), e-mail: metty@ozemail.com.au
25. I prefer to speak of the patients' beloved people rather than of their families. See R. Cohen-Almagor, "The Patients' Right to Die in Dignity and the Role of Their Beloved People," *Annual Review of Law and Ethics,* Vol. 4 (1996), pp. 213–232.
26. Cf. Robert Jay Lifton, *The Nazi Doctors: Medical Killing and the Psychology of Genocide* (New York: Basic Books, 1984); Robert Proctor, *Racial Hygiene: Medicine Under the Nazis* (Cambridge, MA: Harvard University Press, 1988).
27. Cf. Bettina Schöne-Seifert and Klaus-Peter Rippe, "Silencing the Singer: Antibioethics in Germany," *Hastings Center Report,* Vol. 21, No. 6 (November-December 1991), pp. 20–27.
28. Peter Singer (Ed.), *Applied Ethics* (Oxford: Oxford University Press, 1986); Helga Kuhse and Peter Singer, *Should the Baby Live? The Problem of Handicapped Infants* (Oxford: Oxford University Press, 1985).
29. See M.H. Kottow, "Euthanasia after the Holocaust—Is it Possible?," *Bioethics,* Vol. 2, No. 1 (January 1988), pp. 58–69.
30. For further discussion, see Peter Singer, "A German Attack on Applied Ethics: A Statement by Peter Singer," *Journal of Applied Philosophy,* Vol. 9, No. 1 (1992), pp. 85–91; *idem,* "Bioethics and Academic Freedom," *Bioethics,* Vol. 4, No. 1 (January 1990), pp. 33–44; *idem,* "On Being Silenced in Germany," *The New York Review of Books* (August 15, 1991); Hans Johann Glock, "The Euthanasia Debate in Germany - What's the Fuss?," *Journal of Applied Philosophy,* Vol. 11, No. 2 (1994), pp. 213–224; Jenny Teichman, "Freedom of Speech and Public Platform," *Journal of Applied Philosophy,* Vol. 11, No. 1 (1994), pp. 99–105; Anton Leist, "Bioethics in a Low Key: A Report from Germany," *Bioethics,* Vol. 7, No. 2/3 (1993), pp. 271–279; Peter Berkowitz, "Other People's Mothers," *New Republic* (10 January 2000), pp. 27–37;

R. Cohen-Almagor and Merav Shmueli, "Can Life Be Evaluated? The Jewish Halachic Approach vs. the Quality of Life Approach in Medical Ethics: A Critical View," *Theoretical Medicine and Bioethics* (2000).
31. Cf. P.J. van der Maas, J.J.M. van Delden, and L. Pijenborg, *Euthanasia and Other Medical Decisions Concerning the End of Life*, Health Policy Monographs (Amsterdam: Elsevier, 1992).
32. Cf. David Thomasma *et al.* (Eds.), *Asking to Die* (Dordrecht: Kluwer, 1998); John Griffiths *et al.*, *Euthanasia and Law in the Netherlands* (Amsterdam: Amsterdam University Press, 1998); Paul van der Maas and Linda L. Emanuel, "Factual Findings," in L.L. Emanuel (Ed.), *Regulating How We Die* (Cambridge, Mass.: Harvard University Press, 1998), pp. 151–174; J.M. Cuperus-Bosma, "Physician-assisted Death: Policy Making by the Assembly of Prosecutors General in the Netherlands," *European J. of Health Law*, Vol. 4 (1997), pp. 225–238; Paul J. van der Maas *et al.*, "Euthanasia, Physician Assisted Suicide, and Other Medical Practices Involving the End of Life in the Netherlands, 1990–1995," *New England Journal of Medicine*, Vol. 335, No. 22 (1996), pp. 1699–1711; Paul J. van der Maas *et al.*, "Changes in Dutch Opinions on Active Euthanasia, 1966 Through 1991," *JAMA*, Vol. 273, No. 18 (1995), pp. 1411–1414; J.K.M. Gevers, "Physician Assisted Suicide: New Developments in the Netherlands," *Bioethics*, Vol. 9, No. 3/4 (1995), pp. 309–312; Bill Mettyear, "Advocating Legalising Voluntary Euthanasia" (February 1997), http://www.on.net/clients/saves/ South Australian Voluntary Euthanasia Society.
33. Joel Feinberg, *Harm to Self* (New York: Oxford University Press, 1986), p. 27.
34. C.A. 5587/93, *D. Nachmani v. R. Nachmani*, P.D. 49(1) 485; A.H. 2401/95, *R. Nachmani v. D. Nachmani*, D.E. (Dinim Elyon) 44, 98 [not yet published].
35. J. A. Robertson, "Prior Agreements for Disposition of Frozen Embryos," *Ohio State L.J.*, Vol. 51(1990), 407, 420.
36. See Justice Stone's footnote in *United States V. Caroline Products Co.* 304 U.S. 144 (1938), at 152–154. See also Justice Rutledge in *Thomas v Collins* 323 U.S. 516 (1945), 529–530, and Justice Douglas in *Saia v. N.Y.* 334 U.S. 558 (1948), 562. For further deliberation see A. Thomas Mason, *The Supreme Court from Taft to Burger* (Baton Rouge: Louisiana State University Press, 1979), pp. 129–173.
37. For contesting view see R. Cohen-Almagor, "Autonomy, Life as an Intrinsic Value, and Death with Dignity," *Science and Engineering Ethics*, Vol. 1, No. 3 (1995), pp. 261–272.
38. See Ronald Dworkin, *Life's Dominion* (New York: Knopf, 1993), pp. 166–167.
39. For further discussion see Robert D. Truog, "Is It Time to Abandon Brain Death?," *Hastings Center Report*, Vol. 27, No. 1 (Jan.-Feb. 1997); Stuart J. Youngner, C. Seth Landefeld, Claudia J. Coulton, Barbara W. Juknialis, and Mark Leary, "'Brain Death' and Organ Retrieval: A Cross-sectional Survey of Knowledge and Concepts among Health Professionals," *Journal of the American Medical Association*, Vol. 261, No.15 (April 1989), pp. 2205–2210; Daniel Wikler and Alan J. Weisbard, "Appropriate Confusion over 'Brain Death'," *Journal of the American Medical Association*, Vol. 261, No. 15 (April 1989), esp. at 2246.
40. Ronald Dworkin, Report and Summing Up of a 21st Century Trust International Workshop entitled "Genetics, Identity and Justice," Merton College, Oxford (27 March–4 April 1998). See http://www.21stCenturyTrust.org/artlist.html
41. For deliberation on the hospice facility, see Joan K. Harrold and Joanne Lynn (Eds.), *A Good Dying: Shaping Health Care for the Last Months of Life* (New York: Haworth Press, 1998).

Social Values, Socioeconomic Resources, and Effectiveness Coefficients

An Ethical Model for Statistically Based Resource Allocation

EIKE-HENNER W. KLUGE

Department of Philosophy, University of Victoria, Victoria, British Columbia, Canada V8W 3P4

INTRODUCTION

There are two fundamentally distinct and competing views on the nature of health care. One sees health care as a right, the other as a commodity. The two lead to equally distinct approaches to the delivery of health care services. The rights approach uses ethical principles to determine the nature and structure of its delivery system and employs economic measures only as tools to effect a just and equitable distribution within the system as ethically structured. The commodity model uses economic calculations to determine the nature, range, and distribution of the services it offers and appeals to ethical principles only as socially mandated limits within which all economic activity has to be conducted.

As a matter of general principle, the purpose of a publicly funded service is not to generate revenue but to meet a societal need and to respond to a societal right. That is to say, health is a major determinant of someone's ability to take advantage of the opportunities that are available within society. A just and equitable society, therefore, must try to minimize health-based differences so as to create a level playing field for all its citizens. Consequently, a just and equitable society has an obligation to meet the health care needs of its members in order to minimize health-based interpersonal differences. A publicly funded health care system is society's attempt to meet this obligation. It follows that a publicly funded health care system must start from the premise that health care is a right and not a commodity. This entails that for a publicly funded health care system the rights perspective, rather than the commodity perspective, should prevail.

At the same time, such a system cannot ignore outcome and cost/effectiveness considerations since the latter functionally influence the availability of resources, thereby affecting the distribution of the relevant services themselves. Furthermore, population-based differences in health needs should also be a factor in decision-making since social policy should stand the test of equality and justice. However, equality and justice cannot be the only ethical determinants since autonomy is also a fundamental ethical principle. Therefore due importance must be accorded to societal preferences, since society is not only the recipient of these services, but also its ultimate funder.

What follows is a sketch of a model for statistically based resource allocation in a publicly funded health care system that integrates fundamental ethical principles, societal values, and effectiveness coefficients in the context of limited resources.

HYPOTHESIS

Statistically derived health care need indicators, public preferences, and outcome considerations can be combined in an ethically appropriate model of macro-allocation.

ASSUMPTIONS

a. pragmatic

1. The members of society experience various types and degrees of health care needs.
2. The health status of members of society affects their ability to take advantage of the opportunities that are otherwise available within the social context.

b. ethical

3. The Principle of Equality: All persons, considered as persons, are equal to one another.
4. The Principle of Justice: Justice consists in balancing competing rights and obligations and in fulfilling those, which, on balance, are superordinate.
5. The Principle of Autonomy: Everyone has the right to self-determination subject only to the equal and competing rights of others.
6. The Principle of Impossibility: The existence of a duty presupposes the ability to carry out that duty. (Alternatively: All other things being equal,[1] one cannot have a duty to do what is impossible under the circumstances that obtain.)

THE MODEL

The preceding assumptions can then be interrelated into a series of propositions:

THEOREM 1: *The Requirements of Equity*
Equity requires that persons be treated the same except where differential treatment is mandated to allow them to retain or restore their ability to take equal advantage of the opportunities that are available in society.

This general duty follows from assumptions 2, 3 and 4. It can be particularized for the health care setting as the general duty to provide a publicly funded health care system.

THEOREM 2: *General Theorem of Societal Obligation*
A just society has an obligation to provide health care services to its members in order to remove or minimize health-based differences that might otherwise prevent the members from taking equal advantage of the opportunities that are available within that society.

This follows from Assumptions 1, 2, 3 and 4.[2,3]

However, this general obligation cannot be translated into action without adding precise parameters. Specifically, the natures and types of the mandated health care services have to be determined. This can be done by looking at the health status profile of society in general, identifying statistically normal needs, and then translating this into requirements for the health care service itself.

This involves several steps. The initial step focuses on the societal duty to provide primary macro-allocation of health care services to all persons:

THEOREM 3: *Primary Macro-allocation*
A just society has an obligation to provide its members with a basic array of health care services (primary macro-allocation), the nature of which is functionally determined by the average health care needs of the members of society.[4]

EFFECTIVENESS AND NEED

Theorems 1–3 establish a duty for a just society to provide a minimum level of health care services that is functionally determined by the statistical health status profile of society as a whole. This means that contrary to some perceptions,[5] the basic range and extent of these services cannot ethically be determined by societal preferences from some menu since these preferences do not focus on equality and justice, but are a matter of likes and dislikes.

At the same time, the nature of these services cannot be determined by health need alone. Need is a bottomless pit that can swallow up a whole health care budget without discernible effect. In the context of limited resources, what is given to one is taken away from the other. Consequently, the attempt to provide services where no effective treatment exists may undermine the ability of the system to meet the needs–and the corresponding rights–that *can* be met.[6]Therefore some ethically appropriate measure must be introduced to deal with this possibility.

The concept of an act/effectiveness coefficient sets the stage for this:

Definition 1: An act/effectiveness coefficient is the range of effectiveness of a given intervention for a statistically average group of persons having a condition relevant to that intervention.

Definition 2: The act/effectiveness coefficient of a health care modality is positive if that modality either maintains or improves the condition for which it is employed.

With this, one can develop a basic theorem of just and equitable limitation under primary resource allocation in two stages:

THEOREM 4: *Obligatory as opposed to optional services*
a. *Appropriateness of intervention*
A health care intervention is appropriate under primary macro-allocation if and only if the intervention has a positive act/effectiveness coefficient.

If I stands for intervention, ap for appropriate, tn for time and $+$ for positive, then this can be represented schematically as follows:

$$I_{tn}^{ap} \equiv A_{I_{tn}^{+}}$$

But this is not enough. The intervention may be appropriate in the narrow sense defined, but not contribute to the overall health status of the individuals in question. Therefore the preceding has to be combined with another outcome measure that focuses on the effect on the general health status of the relevant parties. The following lemma expresses this condition:

b. *Limitation of primary macro-allocation*
If the health status of the affected persons after appropriate primary macro-allocation is not equal to or better than prior to the allocation, where the retention of or improvement in health status can be traced to the allocation, then the obligation to provide the macro-allocation ceases.[7]

If St^a stands for the health status of the average group, M^p stands for primary macro-allocation, then this can be expressed symbolically as follows:

$$-[(St^a + M^p) > (St^a - M^p)] \to -M^p$$

These conditions limit the initial list of interventions that are *prima facie* mandated under Theorem 3 to result in a reduced menu of possible interventions under primary macro-allocation.

VALUES AND PREFERENCES

However, that menu may still be too large to be fundable under the resource limitations that obtain. At this point, public preferences enter. That is to say, the members of society not only access the health care services, but they also fund them. The principle of autonomy therefore entails that society should have a say in how this funding occurs. This, in turn, means that societal values and preferences should be taken into account when deciding between competing and otherwise equal rights/obligations respecting those services.

The temptation is to say that society should choose more or less directly the menu of appropriate services that will be offered. Oregon has gone some way in this direction. However, preferences do not determine the structure of ethical obligations. They can function in that manner if and only if the matter is morally neutral in the relevant respects. Consequently, the use of values when deciding how competing obligations should be met is appropriate if and only if the obligations concerning which the preferences are expressed have the same ethical status. This means that in the context of exclusionary health care resource allocation, it would be inappropriate to allow preferences about medically necessary modalities to be trumped by preferences for those that are merely quality-enhancing.

These considerations suggest the following theorems:

THEOREM 5: *Public preference determinant*

First,

a. *determination of effectiveness range*
Public values/preferences for primary macro-allocation are ethically appropriate to determine the range of act/effectiveness coefficients within which

primary macro-allocation service should be funded from the menu as previously identified;

and second,

b. *choice within a domain*
Public values/preferences for ranking primary macro-allocation modalities are ethically determining (under conditions of exclusionary limitation) if the modalities ranked are within same domain.

To illustrate, this means that public preferences may determine whether modalities that have a 30–40 percent act/effectiveness coefficient should be funded as opposed to, say, modalities that have a 10–25 or a 30–35 percent coefficient. Likewise, it means that public preferences may determine whether heart as opposed to liver transplant should be provided as long as both have the same act/effectiveness coefficients. On the other hand, it rules out as inappropriate public preference-based decisions favoring such things as wheelchairs as opposed to bypass surgery. Wheelchairs are a quality-enhancing modality and therefore have to be decided upon under the rubric of primary quality-enhancing macro-allocation.

SECONDARY MACRO-ALLOCATION

However, the preceding theorems do not guarantee equitable treatment and therefore are seriously incomplete. That is to say, Theorems 1 and 2 require that the health services that are offered by society must also take into account the health care *needs* of those persons who have needs beyond those served by Theorem 3. However, if differing needs are not met—and by assumption 1 and Theorem 5 it is possible that this may be the case—then those whose needs are not met under public preference–determined primary macro-allocation may lose out. As a result, they may be unable to take advantage of the opportunities otherwise available in society. This would violate equality and justice and hence constitute discrimination

Theorems 1 and 2 and the initial assumptions on which they are based therefore license the inference of a *prima facie* duty to provide appropriate resources to those groups whose needs are not covered under primary macro-allocation.[8]

THEOREM 6. *General theorem of equitable treatment*
Since all person are equal as persons yet have different health care needs, equity requires that due allowances be made for these differences when differential treatment is necessary to retain or restore their ability to take equal advantage of the opportunities that are available in society.

This follows from Theorems 1 and 2, and Assumptions 1–4 above. Formally, Theorem 6 capitalizes on the fact that equity is a topological, not an arithmetic relation.

Following the schema as set out under primary macro-allocation, this general obligation of secondary macro-allocation can be translated into a specific macro-level duty as follows:

THEOREM 7: Prima facie *duty of secondary macro-allocation*

If the health status of an identifiable group of persons within society is measurably[9] lower than that of the statistical norm for society and the health care needs of that group are not met by primary macro-allocation, then a secondary macro-allocation directed at alleviating those needs is *prima facie* mandated, and *vice versa*.

If *St* is health status, *u* is an identifiable group of persons, *a* is average person in society, *t* is time, *pf* is *prima facie*, and *Ms* is secondary macro-allocation, then the theorem may be expressed symbolically as follows:

$$(St^u_{tn} < St^a_{tn}) \equiv M^s_{pf}$$

The theorem is stated as a bi-conditional because it is ethically inappropriate that the health status of an initially disadvantaged group be raised above that of the statistical norm as a result of secondary macro-allocation. That would constitute reverse discrimination. The implications of this will be explored more fully a little later.

LIMITATIONS

Since secondary macro-allocation falls within the general mandate to provide publicly funded health services, it is important to emphasize that it is governed by the same ethical considerations as primary macro-allocation. This means that outcome and effectiveness measures apply in equal degree. Specifically, it means that secondary macro-allocation is ethically mandated if and only if there is an identifiable intervention that has a positive act/effectiveness coefficient. Further, this coefficient must fall within the range that is considered acceptable for actions funded under primary macro-allocation.

THEOREM 8: *Theorem of equitable effectiveness distribution*
A *prima facie* obligation of secondary macro-allocation becomes an actual obligation if and only if the act/effectiveness coefficients of the measures targeted by the secondary macro-allocation fall within the range of act/effectiveness coefficients considered acceptable for measures provided under primary macro-allocation

If *r* stands for a real obligation and *A* the act/effectiveness coefficient, then this can be represented symbolically as follows:

$$(M^s_{pf} \to M^s_r) \equiv (A^s_{tn} \geq A^{tn}_p)$$

This theorem captures the fact that to go outside of the range provided by society for other persons would constitute reverse discrimination. It will be noted that there is no parallel theorem dealing with the determination of act/effectiveness coefficients. The reason lies in the fact that separate determination would identify outlier needs as ethically distinct from mainstream needs. This would violate equality and justice. The act/effectiveness range, once identified by society, must remain the same for all.

Still, the preceding conditions impose limits on secondary macro-allocation in terms of act-directed outcome measures. The interventions are need-focused, and therefor specific to a type of health care problem and a type of intervention.

However, as in the case of primary macro-allocation,[10] a particular intervention may produce an outcome that falls within the ranges indicated, while its effect on the overall health status of the individuals is negligible or even non-existent. For instance, this would be the case when treating (successfully) the kidney failure of someone dying in the last stages of AIDS. In situations like these, the otherwise mandated intervention reduces to palliative measures in an extended sense of the term. That goal may be achieved more appropriately by using other measures. Consequently, we have a further theorem of limitation:

THEOREM 9: *Limitation of secondary macro-allocation*
If the health status of the initially disadvantaged group after secondary macro-allocation is not equal to or better than that prior to the secondary macro-allocation, where the retention of or improvement in health status can be traced to the secondary macro-allocation, then the obligation to provide targeted secondary macro-allocation ceases.

$$-[(St^u + M^s) > (St^u - M^s)] \rightarrow -M^s_r$$

This parallels a similar condition under primary macro-allocation by ruling out as ethically inappropriate resources expenditures on useless interventions.[11]

Further, equity requires that the health status of groups that legitimately receive secondary macro-allocation must not become greater than that of the statistical average health status of other members of society, since that would constitute the reverse discrimination that was mentioned before. Therefore if one combines Theorems 6, 7, 8, and 9 one gets the following:

THEOREM 10: *Excessive improvement:*
The health status of groups that receive secondary macro-allocation must not become greater than the statistically average health status of other members of society.[12]

$$-(S(t^u_{tn} > St^a_{tn})) \rightarrow -M^s_{pf}$$

PALLIATION

Many persons do not die catastrophically but fall terminally ill. Likewise, some persons may encounter health conditions that cannot be treated by currently available health care modalities. The principle of impossibility entails that curative efforts need not be extended on their behalf. Nevertheless, the principles of equality and justice, and of autonomy and respect for persons, entail that care should not be abandoned in their case. Consequently,

THEOREM 11: *Duty of Palliation*
All persons have the right to appropriate palliative efforts.

This follows from Theorems 2–4 and 7 and 8, where it should be kept in mind that what constitutes appropriateness for a given intervention is defined relative to that intervention. This means that the appropriateness of palliative efforts must be measured in terms of comfort and absence of pain.

CONCLUSION

The preceding provides a way for using statistically derived health care need indicators, public preferences ,and outcome considerations to provide an ethically appropriate model of macro-allocation. It does not deal with the need for research to advance the state of health care; nor does it deal specifically with the question of how the size of a health care budget should be determined. However, the latter can be derived by combining primary and secondary macro-allocation indicators and taking the nature of the act/effectiveness ranges into account.

ACKNOWLEDGMENTS

The research for this paper was supported by the Canadian Government under its Strategic Studies Programme, Network Centre of Excellence for Health Information Science, HEALnet (Health Evidence Application and Linkage Network), Medical Informatics Section. The paper represents part of an ongoing project in this section.

NOTES AND REFERENCES

1. That is, the impossibility-making condition not being under control of the person who otherwise would have the relevant duty.
2. President's Commission for the Study of Ethical Problems in Medicine and Biomedical and Behavioral Research, *Securing Access to Medical Care*, 3 vols. (Washington D.C.: U.S. Government Printing Office, 1983), Vol. 1, "The Ethical Implications of Differences in the Availability of Health Services," at 1–4.
3. Norman Daniels, "Equity of Access to Health Care: Some Conceptual and Ethical Issues," *Milbank Memorial Fund Quarterly*, Vol. 60, No. 1 (1982), reprinted in *Securing Access to Medical Care*, Vol. 2: "The Ethical Implications of Differences in the Availability of Health Services," pp. 41–47.
4. Allen Buchanan, "The Right to a Decent Minimum of Health Care," in *Securing Access to Health Care*, esp. at 210 ff. and 222 ff.
5. The Oregon approach is a partial example of a socially determined preference approach that fails in this regard.
6. This follows from Assumptions 4 and 6.
7. One can distinguish further between modalities that are life-saving and/or preserving, and modalities that are quality-enhancing. Since there is a fundamental duty to preserve life, life-saving/preserving modalities *prima facie* take priority over those that are quality-enhancing. This relationship becomes important when public preferences are factored into the preceding equations. However, the general presumption should be that the overall size of the health care budget should be functionally determined relative to the needs established under appropriate primary and secondary macro-allocation. The recursive functional nature of this in terms of the resources that are available will not be dealt with in this paper.
8. David Gauthier, "Unequal Need: A Problem of Equity in Access to Health Care," in *Securing Access to Health Care*, Vol. 2, at 179–205.

9. That is, if the difference in the ability to take advantage of opportunities open to other members of society can be linked to difference in health status.
10. Cf. Theorem 4b, *supra*.
11. This does not mean that no intervention would be appropriate; merely that the type of intervention has to be reconsidered. Palliative efforts alone may be mandated. *Vide infra*.
12. As with primary macro-allocation, public preferences play an appropriate role in determining which ones should be offered. Since some of the modalities that are mandated under secondary macro-allocation are life-saving, whereas others are merely quality-enhancing, parity of reasoning demands that the same general conditions apply here as in the case of primary macro-allocation. This can be expressed as a derivative theorem of public preference under Theorem 5b regarding secondary macro-allocation.

The Ethical Professor of Medicine
Challenges for the Twenty-first Century

FREDERICK H. LOWY

Rector and Vice Chancellor, Concordia University, 1455 de Maisonneuve Boulevard, W., Montreal, Quebec, Canada H3G 1M8

INTRODUCTION

The behavior of physicians in their daily relations with patients and health care colleagues, as well as when faced with ethical dilemmas, is shaped to a large extent by the basic assumptions that contribute to their moral frame of reference. While some of these assumptions owe their origins to social, religious, and other influences in physicians' personal lives, others can be traced to the important orienting influence of their medical school professors. It is they who serve as their early medical role models. Given the importance of role modelling in shaping human behavior, it is likely that the messages they transmit to their students, both the overt and those that are inadvertently sent, are as important in determining these future physicians' attitudes and actions as are formal codes of ethics, institutional ethics committees, and even formal ethics courses in medical school curricula. Empirical evidence for this is provided by, among others, Hebert, Meslin, and Dunn,[1] who found that the ethical sensitivity of medical students increases after formal medical ethics courses in the preclinical years and then actually declines during the later years of clinical education. Sulmasy *et al.*[2] similarly found that interns' and residents' knowledge of ethics declined during postgraduate training. One possible explanation for these findings is the influence of the behavior and mentorship of clinical educators.

It is valuable, therefore, to consider the ethical stance of medical educators with particular attention to the challenges that confront the ethical professor of medicine at the turn of the millennium.

SOME HISTORICAL NOTES

Important among the features that distinguish the professions from other occupations is the willing acceptance by the professional of a fiduciary relationship with a client (or patient or student). To establish and maintain this, the professional undertakes to employ skills, experience, and knowledge on behalf of the client, rather than use them to advance his/her interests at the client's expense. The responsibility attendant on such a relationship of trust is a thread that runs through all writings on medical ethics from the Code of Hammurabi, through Hippocrates and Maimonides and Percival to the modern bioethics literature. The role modelling by medical teachers to their junior colleagues and students is the chief method whereby this and related values were transmitted. But for most of the 3,000 years of recorded medical history, the task was simple in comparison with the moral complexities of today and those we can foresee in the twenty-first century. Until relatively recently, physicians practiced in homogeneous communities of which they were part and they shared the community's moral values, values that were largely not in dispute. That is, it was clear to all what was right and acceptable and what was wrong and unacceptable. Further, medical treatment was largely based on a personal doctor–patient relationship in which the personality and caring attitude of the physician were often the most important curative factors since diagnostic and therapeutic options were limited. Physicians therefore valued, cultivated, and developed interpersonal skills that made them successful healers and, in their socializing roles as teachers, transmitted these values and skills to those who entered the medical profession. I refer here to attitudes and behaviors toward patients characterized by what are usually considered virtues rather than duties, viz., compassion, empathy, respect, loyalty, commitment, fidelity, availability, and so on. Medical practice involved the alleviation of pain and discomfort and the amelioration of other symptoms by treatments that became only gradually more sophisticated and effective, together with a doctor–patient relationship that bolstered hope and confidence and provided much comfort.

Throughout most of the history of medicine, as Jay Katz[3] has so eloquently pointed out, it was a "silent world of doctor and patient" with respect to seeking or even permitting patient participation in decisions. Informed consent and patient autonomy were not issues and physicians were rarely troubled by the ethical dilemmas that occupy today's burgeoning medical ethics literature. They knew what was good for their patients, ans they assumed that their own values and those of their patients were synonymous and communally shared. The principal ethical challenge, as Jonsen[4] has pointed out, was resolving ethically the conflict between duty to patients and self-interest. Indeed, it was to this challenge that classical and medieval codes of conduct were directed. Examples are the Hippocratic Code and the prayer of Maimonides. The latter, a clear exhortation to self-effacement and virtue, concludes "May neither avarice nor miserliness, nor the thirst for glory or for a great reputation engage my mind; for the enemies of truth and philanthropy may easily deceive me and make me forgetful of my lofty aim of doing good to Thy children." (Quoted by Pellegrino and Thomasma).[5]

The ethical physician's activities were both inspired and circumscribed by models combining duties, virtues, and medical etiquette that provided reliable, if often unattainable, standards of conduct. They were summarized and held up as guidelines, at least for physicians in the English-speaking world, by Thomas Percival at the turn of the 18th century.[6]

How different is the situation today! We live in a pluralist world. Almost every major city in the world contains health care providers and patients from a variety of ethnic, cultural, linguistic, and religious backgrounds and, most important, various and sometimes conflicting values and expectations.

It is not possible to assume that a particular physician and a particular patient share objectives, wish to attain the same benefits from treatment, or avoid the same harms from the illness. Nor, for example, can it be assumed either that the patient desires to put himself/herself in the doctor's hands (according to the traditional paternalistic model) or that the patient wishes to be the ultimate decision-maker when important choices must be made (according to the autonomy model currently popular, especially in North America).

Further, the pattern of medical practice has shifted dramatically during the century that is now terminating and especially the last 50 years. With the availability of powerful, precise technical diagnostic and therapeutic tools the scientifically inspired and technology-driven medical specialist has become the major clinical role model for young physicians and medical students in most modern faculties of medicine and, especially, in tertiary-care teaching hospitals. This model, and its implications for socializing medical students, interns, and residents into the profession, is in many respects in conflict with the traditional model of the physician. (In reaction to this shift, university departments of family medicine and psychiatry and community hospitals are attempting to return to a modified version of the traditional model and so-called "alternative medicine" is moving from the suspect fringes toward mainstream acceptance.)

In this paper, an attempt is made to examine the effects of these changes on the responsibilities of the ethical professor of medicine at the turn of the millennium.

THE ETHICAL PROFESSOR

Before undertaking this examination, it is important to stress that I will not be focussing on those few medical educators who have special training in bioethics and who function as experts in this field. Rather, I propose to examine the role of the many professors of medicine[7] who, by their teaching and by example, inculcate generations of students into a way of thinking and practicing their profession. They are mostly clinicians whom medical students encounter after their preclinical years and under whose guidance interns and residents treat patients in teaching hospitals and community settings. They are the role models who, in my view, have the greatest influence on how physicians treat patients and how they evaluate themselves. (Occasionally, a preclinical teacher or basic scientist is also influential in this way but in the main it is the clinician-professors who serve as the major role models for future physicians.)

In referring here to "the ethical professor" and in the next section "the ethical professor of medicine," it is not my intention to delineate an elite subgroup nor to suggest that those who do not adhere in all respects to the points made are unethical. The intention is to propose standards that approach the ideals of the medical profession and the legitimate expectations of patients, students and, indeed, society at large.

It goes without saying that the ethical professor of medicine, like all ethical university professors, fulfills basic professorial responsibilities. Implicitly or explicitly, the ethical teacher is guided by some basic principles relevant to these responsibilities. Although, of course, very few university teachers stop to articulate these, rather applying them intuitively, it is nevertheless worthwhile to look at some of these principles. A good framework for this is a series of nine principles developed by the Canadian Society for Teaching and Learning in Higher Education:

1. Content competence. This is especially important in fields in which new information is generated at a rapid pace. The ethical professor exposes students to accurate, up-to-date, and representative knowledge, not only in areas of personal interest to the teacher, but also in all areas relevant to the objectives of the course. Students who are taught by an active researcher have the great advantage of exposure to the cutting edge of the field, often being given access to material that is still unpublished or that has recently appeared in journals but is not yet in their textbooks. However, they risk being given a course that is skewed by the research interests of the professor. If the latter is working in an area that is theoretically controversial—and this applies to many emerging areas of research—there is the risk that such a clinical investigator will proselytize on behalf of the favored theory by dint of enthusiasm and selective presentation of research findings. The ethical professor, of course, does not do this.

2. Pedagogical competence. This is obviously a primary responsibility of the ethical teacher. Different material is often most effectively taught by different methods and the sensitive teacher recognizes that different learning styles and varying student capacities require flexibility in presenting material. Throughout most of the history of medical education, the classical apprenticeship model was the mainstay and it is still important. This model has many advantages, especially for the professor and also for the student and junior physician, but pedagogical advances have led to more sophisticated models of medical education. These provide fewer advantages for the clinical professor (in terms of assistance in the conduct of personal practice and research), but provide a more flexible, better-balanced experience for undergraduate and graduate students. The ethical professor will give priority to the educational needs of students.

3. Dealing with sensitive topics. Given the social, cultural, and religious diversity of students, it is inevitable that some topics will be uncomfortable and even distasteful for some students. This will be discussed more fully in the next section when the impact of the current technological explosion upon medical practice is considered.

4. Student development. "The overriding responsibility of the teacher is to contribute to the intellectual development of the student...and to avoid actions...that detract from student development." In addition to the obvious responsibility to facilitate learning and independent thinking, there are other obligations that ethical professors must meet and actions that must be avoided. As role models, and frequently idealized by students seeking heroes to admire, professors have the capacity to elevate students' self-confidence and self-esteem, but also to shatter these by insensitivity, disrespect, or frank discrimination and exploitation. The ethical professor recognizes this, respects students' vulnerability, and capitalizes on students' potential for growth.

5. Dual relationship with students. A close association with students raises the possibility that non-educational relationships can develop that conflict with the optimal attainment of pedagogical goals. Relationships with graduate students (including medical interns and residents) are especially susceptible to deleterious conflicts of interest. These are the students with whom professors work most closely as research collaborators, teaching assistants, and professional junior colleagues. The dual relationships that are most to be feared (in that they are likely to impair professors' objectivity and detract from students' autonomous development) are those that involve sexual or other close personal links. There is an inherent power differential between professors and students. Any power differential carries with it the risk that the more powerful party will exploit the less powerful to the latter's detriment. In recent years, considerable attention has been given to sexual exploitation of students by their academic superiors, and no more needs to be added here. Many universities have developed formal codes of conduct to protect students from such exploitation.

Another form of exploitation that is at least as common is the appropriation by the professor of intellectual property that rightfully belongs to the student or, at the very least, is rightfully shared. The ethical professor will see to it that authorship, ownership, or acknowledgement as appropriate are awarded to students for their intellectual and practical contributions to publications, patents, and grant applications. Nor will the ethical professor assign research work that advances his/her interests, but is unrelated to the student's needs. Again, many universities have found it useful to produce guidelines or regulations to govern the sharing of intellectual property and the conduct of research by students. Yet another possible abuse of power occurs when the professor is strongly committed to an ideological or political or religious position and subtly coerces or indoctrinates students to become followers.

Conflicts of interest or commitment are inherent in many relationships and are not *ipso facto* improper. Ideally, they are to be avoided since they increase vulnerability to impropriety and they are usually perceived to be improper even when they are not. Students who have dual relationships with professors are not only vulnerable to exploitation; the other side of the coin is that they are often perceived by their fellow students to be the objects of professorial favoritism.

6. Confidentiality. Students who confide in professors are clearly entitled to confidentiality. The same applies to their grades and the professor's evaluation of their work and potential. Without student consent, academic records and confided personal material should not be released. A conflict that arises between loyalty to students and the duty to veracity to others relates to letters of reference that professors are so often asked to write. Clearly, the ethical professor is honest in providing assessments, at students' requests, to other universities, prospective employers, etc. However, it is only fair to warn the student if the professor feels obliged to give a negative assessment.

7. Respect for colleagues. Professors have a duty to respect the competence and dignity of their colleagues even when there is profound ideological or pedagogical disagreement. This is especially important when fellow professors are also fellow health professionals. Failure to observe this principle occurs when derogatory remarks or gestures are made that indicate contempt for a colleague. This can be destructive to the colleague's reputation with students or patients. A problem occurs when there is reason to suspect the colleague is incompetent, unethical, or impaired. Here, responsibilities to the institution, the academic discipline, and the students require that action be taken. Understandably, one is usually reluctant to take up this challenge, but the ethical professor will do so. The action to be taken will vary with the situation and the regulations of the academic and professional institutions involved.

8. Valid assessment of students. This principle speaks for itself and does not require elaboration. An important point is that students should not be assessed on knowledge and skills that were not part of the educational objectives and not relevant to the ends of the studies.

9. Respect for institution. The university and the academic discipline deserve respect and loyalty. Professors who disagree with policies and practices should attempt to have these changed via internal mechanisms that, increasingly, are available in most countries. Where this is impossible and the issue involves fundamental values the ethical professor should seek employment elsewhere. I recognize that this may be a counsel of perfection that in some circumstances cannot be followed without self-destructive consequences to career and family. However, the alternative of covert sabotage of the institution from which one accepts remuneration is hardly to be endorsed.

A more common problem *vis-à-vis* the institution is a conflict of commitment. Many professors, especially in professional programs, act as paid consultants to external agencies or practice their professions part time. Such activities often benefit the institutions as well as the professors themselves. However, the potential for abuse of such opportunities is well known, with the result that students and the institution are deprived of the professor's time, attention, and energy, which are instead devoted to more lucrative external activities. The ethical professor respects and follows the guidelines or regulations governing such activities that many institutions have put in place.

NEW CHALLENGES AT THE END OF THE TWENTIETH CENTURY

Today's physician is caught between two models. In the traditional beneficence model, physicians took responsibility for the welfare of their patients, made decisions on their behalf and acted as emotional and spiritual mentors. As noted earlier, this is giving way, at least in North America, to a rights-driven model in which (in its extreme form) the physician is merely the technical expert who presents advantages and disadvantages of the various treatment options from which the patient must choose; the technologist physician specialist then executes the choice. In the traditional model the physician's own values have decisive influence even if lip service is paid to respecting patients' views. In the physician-as-value-neutral-technologist model, the responsibility for even life and death decisions is that of the patient, whose values are determinative.

In this admittedly oversimplistic portrayal, patients choose between the comfort of being cared for by a benevolent but intrusive caregiver at the expense of autonomy, and the satisfaction of freely applying their own values to a difficult decision-making calculus, but at the expense of emotional isolation from an expert they would have liked to rely upon. At the close of the 20th century, several developments intersect to complicate the picture. These include the technological breakthroughs that, qualitatively as well as quantitatively, expand the range of the possible; the increasingly pluralistic nature of most societies with respect to culture, ethnicity, religion, and social structures; instant communications with new (at times untested) treatments described on the Internet and recommended to patients before their physicians have heard of them; funding policies that provide disincentives to optimal care for individual patients; and, in some countries, a litigious public ready to bring suit against health professionals who take too much or too little responsibility in particular cases.

How does the physician who strives to be ethical (and, more importantly, the professor of medicine who serves as the role model) cope with all this? Beneficence and autonomy are both valuable principles as are, indeed, many others such as justice in the allocation of resources and time; respect not only for humans, but all animals;

gender and minority group equality; and so on. The challenge is how to practice so as to uphold ethical principles and, when principles are in conflict, to achieve a satisfactory balance.

Medical practice is also complicated by the very progress that permits today's physicians to offer so much more to patients suffering from formerly crippling or rapidly fatal diseases. The technology that makes this possible also multiplies the therapeutic choices, including the weighing of adverse effects and possible iatrogenic harms versus expected benefits. What is more, as is so well known, scientific advances have provided therapeutic options that raise fundamental moral questions for everyone—health care professionals and their patients, legislators, philosopher,s and theologians. These questions need not be sought in specialized bioethics journals. They are also now to be found throughout the academic literature and the popular press. Examples abound: Is any form of doctor-assisted termination of life acceptable? Are there limitations on the application of new reproductive technologies? Are legal or administrative controls needed to regulate genetic engineering, including the cloning of mammals? Is the harvesting of organs from the dying for transplantation to others ethical? What about the use of fetal tissues? Xenografts? The issues are complex and vexing.

The specialized, technologically focused, positivist utilitarian physician has an easy way out of such dilemmas. Welcoming the current trend toward patient autonomy and decision-making, this physician claims the technical ground and abandons the moral ground. Trained by super-specialist medical professors in tertiary-care institutions, this physician recognizes only a responsibility to diagnose the disease process (as opposed to being concerned with the broader problem of patients' subjective experience of illness) and to provide the patient with the various therapeutic options. What the patient decides to do is not the physician's problem. Within this narrow view of ethical responsibility, this physician undertakes only to avoid exploiting the patient by not advocating a treatment that will advance the physician's financial or career interests. Otherwise, this physician attempts to be value-neutral.

This philosophical stance, presented here in extreme form for expository purposes, is a reasonable projection into the near future of trends that are all too evident today in North America. While these trends are fuelled by several factors, an important one is the role-modelling provided by many of today's medical professors.

What, then, is the appropriate stance of the medical professor at the birth of the twenty-first century who wishes to teach and practice ethically? My prescription is as follows. In addition to the responsibilities of all ethical university professors discussed in the previous section, the ethical professor of medicine must avoid being such a value-neutral medical scientist. (Space does not permit a justification of the assertion, which I believe true, that this is not possible even if it were desirable.) Today, more than ever—in the face of ethical pluralism and our huge technological potential—patients and their families need a caring, beneficent, emotionally involved guide who does not shrink from moral complexity. The remarkable scientific progress during the twentieth century has not eliminated the need for such a guide. The contrary is true.

The ethical professor of medicine teaches and practices in recognition that someone who is ill has a disorder to which biological, psychological, cultural, and spiritual factors contribute, in proportions that vary with the person. The ethical professor of medicine intervenes, or assists others to intervene, with respect to those factors, pathogenic in a particular case, that are amenable to the intervention, consistent with the patient's wishes and values.

The person who is ill and who seeks help needs neither an authoritarian doctor who imposes decisions that disregard his/her values nor an emotionally or morally disengaged technologist. What the patient does need is a professional partner who will guide decisions to the extent the patient—appropriately informed—wishes. This physician partner will not shrink from revealing his/her own relevant values, but will be guided by the uncoerced choices that the patient makes. (Only in very rare occasions, in my view, will it be necessary for a conscientious physician to withdraw from the care of a patient whose treatment choices are so at variance with the physician's moral values as to be unacceptable. On such occasions, the ethical physician has no choice but to transfer responsibility to another suitable and available colleague.)

What I am prescribing is a reversal of the pendulum swing that gained momentum during the past half-century in order to restore the priority of the physician healer for whom interpersonal sensitivity and traditional virtues are again important means to the therapeutic end. This is not to denigrate the benefits of the scientific advances that can be expected to accelerate as the clinical implications of molecular biology and genetics are further exploited. But they too, like the doctor–patient relationship, are means to a desirable end and not ends in themselves.

Finally, what about ethical medical practice and medical teaching in a pluralistic society in the face of new practice options that challenge the values of some students and patients? Here I would distinguish these two groups. A patient's values, as expressed in informed voluntary choice, must be respected whether or not these values are shared by a majority of the community. But a physician must be prepared to help people with a variety of values, including some at variance with those of the physician. Therefore, I believe the ethical medical professor has a duty to prepare students for practice in the twenty-first century by presenting, fairly, the range of views on the morally vexing questions of the day, including those examples given above without, however, failing to disclose his/her own ethical position. What the ethical medical professor will not do is to model technologically advanced medicine as an end to itself or as a purportedly value-neutral enterprise.

NOTES AND REFERENCES

1. Philip C. Hebert, Eric M. Meslin, and Earl V. Dunn, "Measuring the Ethical Sensitivity of Medical Students: A Study at the University of Toronto," *Journal of Medical Ethics*, Vol. 18 (1992), pp. 142–147.
2. D. Sulmasy, G. Geller, D. Levine, and R. Faden, "Medical House Officers' Knowledge, Attitudes and Confidence Regarding Medical Ethics," *Archives of Internal Medicine*, Vol. 150 (1990), pp. 2509–2513.
3. Jay Katz, *The Silent World of Doctor and Patient* (New York: The Free Press, 1984).
4. Albert Jonsen, "Watching the Doctor," *New England Journal of Medicine*, Vol. 308 (1983), pp. 1531–1535.
5. Edmund D. Pellegrino and David C. Thomasma, *For the Patient's Good: The Restoration of Beneficence in Health Care* (New York: Oxford University Press, 1988), p. 121.
6. C.D. Leake (Ed.), *Percival's Medical Ethics* (Baltimore, MD: Williams & Wilkins, 1927).
7. In this paper the terms "medicine" and "physician" are used broadly to include surgery, psychiatry, and all other medical specialties.

8. Harry Murray, Eileen Gillese, Madeline Lennon, Paul Mercer, and Marilyn Robinson, *Ethical Principles in University Teaching*, Society for Teaching and Learning in Higher Education (Toronto: York University, 1996).
9. Harry Murray *et al.*, *op cit*, p. 6.
10. See, for example, Melanie L. Carr, Gail E. Robinson, Donna E. Stewart, and Dennis Kussin, "A Survey of Canadian Psychiatric Residents Regarding Resident-Educators Sexual Contact," *American Journal of Psychiatry*, Vol. 148 (1991), pp. 216–220; D.C. Baldwin Jr. *et al.*, "Student Perception of Mistreatment and Harassment during Medical School," *Western Journal of Medicine*, Vol. 155 (1991), pp. 140–145.

Open Heart [*Shiva M'Hodu*]

JOHN LANTOS
*Robert Wood Johnson Clinical Scholars Program, University of Chicago Hospitals,
5841 S. Maryland Avenue, Chicago, Illinois 60637-1470, USA*

INTRODUCTION

Nobody knows what medicine will be like in the next century, but two opposing visions can be summoned up: The first is a vision of dreams and ideals, and the second one of limits and frustrated intentions. The optimistic vision is that we are only at the beginning of a biologic revolution that will augment and transform medicine's powers exponentially. New drugs, devices, diagnostic tests, and new abilities to manipulate the human genome will allow the elimination or cure of most of the ills from which we now suffer. These interventions will not only be medically effective, but cost-effective as well, just as polio vaccine was both better and cheaper than the iron lung. It will be a century of cheap health.

The pessimistic view is that medicine will exacerbate both our physiologic and our political suffering. New discoveries will lead to new problems, particularly new "half-way" technologies that cannot cure diseases, but can only prolong the end stage of life into a long, drawn-out, expensive technological ritual of suffering. Medical care will consume more and more resources but we will get less and less value for our expenditures. We will create a culture of illness. Medicine will be our nemesis.[1]

There is little debate about these competing visions within medicine or health policy. Within medicine, the first, optimistic view is virtually taken for granted, while many health policy analysts and bioethicists seem to subscribe to some variant of the second view. To a certain extent, religious thinking supports the first view. But by either view, medicine and health care are conceptualized as fundamental political rights. Individuals are thought of as having a nearly universal moral obligation to preserve and protect life at any cost. This profoundly Judeo-Christian view informs the public policies of most Western countries, even those, such as the United States, that have not gone so far as to create a universal political entitlement to health care or those like the Netherlands, which allow physician-assisted suicide or euthanasia.

One place where there is discussion of these issues is in recent fictional and autobiographical literature about doctors and medicine. In this genre, the open-endedness of the format and the relative intellectual marginality of the discipline allow questions to be raised about doctors and medicine, healing and illness, suffering and dying, that cannot be raised in any other discourse. Literature is thus *avant garde* in raising these issues and beginning to question the patently messianic vision of medicine as a sort of secular salvation.

In this paper, I will discuss some recent works of literature about doctors and medicine. My particular focus will be on A.B. Yehoshua's recent novel, *Shiva M'Hodu* or *Open Heart* as it has been translated from Hebrew into English.

OPEN HEART

I want to begin my examination of the themes in the book by focusing on a scene in which Rubin, the young physician, finds himself unexpectedly sexually attracted to a patient. Rubin, an ambitious young surgical resident has traveled to India with the CEO of his hospital, a powerful man named Lazar. They are accompanied by Lazar's pudgy and pushy wife, Dorit. They have gone to rescue the Lazars' 24-year old-daughter, Einat, who developed severe hepatitis while she was backpacking around India. As the novel opens, Einat is languishing in a primitive Indian hospital in the town of Gaya, "a remote but holy town surrounded by temples." (p. 9)

Worried, Lazar wants a physician to accompany him to India and to help bring her safely back to Israel. When first asked, Rubin cannot decide whether or not to go. He has been struggling in his surgical career, and doesn't want to take time off lest this disappoint his Department Chairman and lead to his ouster from the program. On the other hand, he suspects that impressing the hospital's CEO might open up career opportunities that he cannot quite define but that seem tempting. A modern Israeli, Rubin thinks of himself as a deeply moral person, but he is not very introspective. He wants to do good, but can't figure out a metric to evaluate various forms of the good. He finds the messiness of his intrapsychic struggles disturbing so he puts them out of his mind. He seems to represent scientific Western medicine at it most raw—powerfully ambitious and phenomenally unaware of its own motivations, goals, or inner structural life. In the end, under some pressure, and for reasons he doesn't fully understand himself, he decides to go to India.

India presents a deep and powerful challenge to Rubin's sense of himself as someone who is competent, who knows what's going on. Early in their trip, Rubin, Lazar and Dorit spend a night in a train compartment with an elderly Indian man, a minor government official, who had recently retired and is now traveling to the town of Varanasi to immerse himself in the holy waters of the Ganges before he dies. Yehoshua writes,

> Every time he pronounced the words "before I die," Mrs. Lazar's eyes lost their smile and her face clouded, as if she refused to countenance his thoughts of death even by listening to them. But she was wrong. The thought of death only gave the old Indian pleasure. Since nothing in the universe was ever lost, all that was left for him to do was ensure his rebirth in more advantageous conditions, which he was now about to do by bathing in the holy river.

"Unbelievable," Lazar exclaimed in Hebrew, "this man is actually convinced that someone is going to bring him back to life again after he dies!" (p. 55) At that point, Yehoshua notes, Lazar's breathing sounded heavy and Rubin, an astute diagnostician, was afraid that Lazar's heart wasn't functioning normally.

These contrasting attitudes toward life and health, illness and death, recovery and rebirth form the central tension of the book. Western doctors are allowed the pursuit of a certain kind of scientific truth. They ask questions about what *works* so that they don't have to ask questions about what is *right*. The pursuit of knowledge becomes a moral quest, and knowledge itself thus becomes goodness. Within this moral framework, it seems that the more we understand about what is true, the more knowledge we accrue, the more our understanding reaches to the genetic level, the molecular level, and ultimately the atomic level, the more we will be able to be really good doctors. Beyond scientific knowledge, there is no other universe, no counterweight, no other concerns.

The vulnerable and impressionable young Dr. Rubin is drawn to the exotic and chaotic Indian rituals, especially those involving the burning of the dead on funeral pyres by the rivers. These rituals move him deeply, mysteriously, and in ways that he describes but cannot fully articulate:

> We saw women in saris descending the steps slowly and gracefully, cupping their hair in their hands and dipping it in the water, and half-naked men diving deep into the river and disappearing for a long time before they reemerged, purified. In the distance, all along the riverbank, we saw many more ghats [Hindu burial pyres] teeming with pilgrims, all performing their religious duties in a tumultuous silence. And then, in the gathering dusk, loudspeakers began hoarsely changing long prayers, and many of the bathers came out of the water and stood on the riverbank or the steps to pray and perform complicated yoga exercises. The boatman abandoned his oars and kneeled down to pray while the boat was swept toward the next ghat, where spirals of white smoke rose from a big red funeral pyre.... When the chanting finally stopped, the boatman rose from his knees and picked up the oars with a dreamy look in his eyes. I said to him in a friendly tone, "Shiva," because I had read in Lazar's guidebook that Varanasi was the city of the god Shiva, the Destroyer. His dark face immediately filled with interest, and he nodded his head but corrected me: "Vishvanath," and, dropping the oars, he spread out his arms to embrace the whole of the universe. (p. 67)

Throughout the trip, Lazar and his chubby, clinging, and spoiled wife Dorit alternately praise Rubin for his medical knowledge and then oppose every medical recommendation that he makes. They are both reverential and skeptical of the authority of medicine. They respond to Rubin's "orders" as if they were bargaining points, the opening gambits in a business deal to be negotiated. When they cannot prevail, they run off on errands which seem to Rubin to be frivolous and inappropriate responses to the seriousness of the situation—they shop for shoes, change hotel rooms, fiddle with travel arrangements to try to save a couple of hours on the return trip.

While the Lazars are off on these inexplicable errands, Rubin is left with Einat, alone and worried. He is not sure exactly how sick she is. He knows that if she returns from India alive, his trip will be a success and Lazar will be in his debt. But the opposite will be true if he fails. He feels enormous pressure, but in an entirely self-centered way. He doesn't seem to care much for Einat herself.

At one point, however, Lazar and Dorit leave Rubin and an Indian nurse to look after Einat. The nurse is a young, pretty, gentle Indian girl in a blue sari. While the nurse watches, Rubin anxiously examines Einat. Yehoshua writes,

> I helped her to take off her shift and asked her to lie on her back, so that I could feel not only her shrunken liver but also her kidneys, which were a little enlarged. The Indian girl watched me curiously as I avoided touching her exposed breasts, which in comparison to her skinny body were actually rather full... In this cool bare room, the strong presence of the attractive Indian girl standing behind me merged with the enjoyable sensation passing through my hands kneading Einat's bare stomach, and I felt a faint flare-up of lust. I reminded myself to masturbate tonight when I went to bed.... (p. 107)

This small scene in a complex novel is simultaneously a perfect illustration and a devastating critique of the uncomprehending way in which Rubin, the doctor of the future, conceptualizes both medical ethics and lust. Both seem to be merely physiologic problems. He imagines that the simple and rational hygienic precaution of masturbating before sleep will protect him from the powerful longings stirred up by his naked patient, the gentle Indian girl, his trip to India, his annoying but attractive substitute parents, his career disappointments, and the emptiness of his lonely life in medicine.

The novel meanders over vast psychological, medical, and religious territories. At its center is a realistic depiction of the medicine practiced in a modern teaching hospital. In preparation for writing it, Yehoshua spent time observing the world of the modern hospital, talking to doctors, watching open-heart operations. He comes away troubled by his visit to the land of medicine. Medicine is powerful, perhaps even miraculous, in its ability to see inside the body in phenomenal new ways, providing a new understanding of health and disease, sickness and suffering—things that were terrible mysteries throughout the history of humankind. But the people working within medicine seem uncomprehending, blinkered, more concerned with their careers than with their patients, with attaining technical skill than with healing, with building empires than with building trust.

OPEN HEART AND FURTHER LITERATURE

Yehoshua is not the only novelist so concerned. Over the past decade, numerous novels have taken the medical enterprise as their topic, and their authors have found the most troubling moral issue not in the areas where bioethics has traditionally focused its concerns—such as informed consent, the right to die, abortion or cloning—but rather the spiritual state of doctors and the implications that holds for the spiritual aspirations of medicine. To be more precise, the almost haughty and prideful spiritual emptiness of some doctors suggests not just that medicine seems to have lost its soul, but also that the doctors themselves seem unable to recognize that loss as something to be concerned about. For novelists, this tension might be highlighted by comparing and contrasting American medicine and doctors with those who take a different approach.

Richard Powers, an American novelist, wrote a book called *Operation Wandering Soul*, which is set in a children's hospital in Los Angeles. In that book, a surgical resident named Kraft is taking care of an incurably ill 12-year-old from Southeast Asia named Joy. Her father, Wisat, a traditional Laotian healer, is baffled by the strange combinations in American medicine. He notes the seemingly phenomenal magic and technical skill of American medicine, but also senses a strange and profound emptiness. "The trouble with Americans," he tells Dr. Kraft, "is they think everything begins and ends here, this time. No return, no earth. Imagine. No ancestors! How can one live? It must be terrible. Even their smallest action dies right after the deed is done!" Wisat believes that "no one who thinks deeds are their own consequences should be allowed to saw into the spirit house of another's marrow."(p. 250) Such a practitioner should be outlawed from healing, he says, not so much for the sake of the patient's karma as for the surgeon's. Kraft's attention drifts from the argument. The surgeon's *karma*? His medicine is about bodily healing, about measurable physiologic outcomes. Questions about his own soul, about who and what the healer is working for, are not just unanswerable, but unintelligible. Questions about the relationship between disease in this patient and the diseases of the ancestors may make sense if framed as questions of molecular genetics or environmental toxins, but as spiritual questions they make no sense.

It is hard to convey the depth of this sort of culture clash. On the one hand, we all acknowledge it. We have all read modern anthropology; we are all postmodern. We pay lip service to the notion that our way is just one way—we say we believe in multiculturalism, tolerance, pluralism. On the other hand, our beliefs in these matters are extraordinarily thin. We **talk** as if we are postmodern, pluralistic, and tolerant, but we **live** as if we know that our culture is right, and our tolerance of other ways of living has limits that we only discover when a controversy forces us to see them.

A recent book by Ann Fadiman, *The Spirit Catches You and You Fall Down*, describes this culture clash perfectly. Fadiman tells the true story of a Hmong family, the Lees, living in California, whose daughter Lia is not well. According to the doctors, Lia has a seizure disorder and needs to take medication. According to the family, Lia's soul has wandered off, and she should be treated by a Hmong healer who specializes in recapturing errant souls. Throughout the book, Fadiman humorously contrasts different approaches to every life event, from birth to death:

> If Lia Lee had been born in the highlands of northwest Laos, he mother would have squatted on the floor of the house that her father had built. She would have caught the baby with her own hands, reaching between her legs to ease out the head and then letting the rest of the body slip out onto her bent forearms. No birth attendant would have been present. Her husband cut the umbilical cord. They washed the baby with water carried from the stream. Soon after the birth, while the mother and baby were still lying together next to the fire pit, the father dug a hole at least two feet deep in the floor and buried the placenta. In the Hmong language, the word for placenta means jacket. It is considered one's first and finest garment. When a Hmong dies, his or her soul must travel back from place to place, retracing the path of its life geography, until it reaches the burial place of its placental jacket, and puts it on. If the soul cannot find its jacket, it is condemned to an eternity of wandering, naked and alone. (pp. 3–5)

> But Lia was not born in Laos but in the Merced Community Medical Center in California's Central Valley, at 7:09 PM on July 19, 1982. Her mother was lying on a steel table, her body covered with sterile drapes, her genital area painted with a brown Betadine solution. The doctor artificially ruptured her amniotic sack by poking it with a foot-long plastic "amni-hook." After birth, her mother received a dose of Pitocin to constrict her uterus. Lia weighed 8 lbs, 7 oz, noted to be "appropriate for gestational age." Her Apgar scores were 7 and 9. She was placed in a steel and Plexiglas warmer, where a nurse fastened a plastic identification band around her wrist and recorded her footprints by inking the soles of her feet with a stamp pad and pressing them against a newborn identification form. She received an injection of vitamin K in one of her thighs, two drops of silver nitrate in each eye, and was bathed with Safeguard soap....

> Lia's mother found Lia's birth a peculiar experience, but she has few criticisms of the way the hospital handled it. She thought the doctor was gentle and kind, she was impressed that so many people were there to help her, but she felt that the nurse who bathed Lia with Safeguard soap did not get her quite as clean as she had gotten her newborns with Laotian stream water. (pp. 6–7)

This passage works on a number of levels. It expertly conveys the equally strange nature of both sets of birth rituals, describing them in terms that lead us to question the beliefs that inform them. Why, in the American hospital, is the mother "draped?" Why Betadine? Why do they take her footprint? Why the silver nitrate? To each question, an answer can be framed in narrow medical terms—to keep the field sterile, to prevent infection—but the net result is a culture of microbiologic paranoia. The rituals create the world for us as a hostile and threatening place, full of invisible demons that must be placated and appeased. By contrast, everything in the Hmong birth ritual is designed with a different set of appeasements and harmonies in mind. Interestingly, both sets of rituals work and, by pragmatic implication, both types of explanation may be correct. Lia's mother had 13 children the Hmong way in Laos. She had no perinatal mortality.

The passage comes early in Fadiman's book and presages a controversy about the treatment of epilepsy. Lia's seizures are difficult to control: her parents don't give her the prescribed medicine, they don't understand or approve of many aspects of Western medicine, and they see their own rich and well-developed alternative traditions as preferable to those of the American pediatricians. The story is tragic. As Lia's seizures get worse and worse, the doctors charge the parents with medical neglect, and the state child protection agency concurs. Lia is removed from the family and placed in foster care. Her seizures continue. The family is "counseled," and they agree to treat Lia the Western way. She is returned to the family, where, in spite of treatment, she eventually has a major seizure associated with an episode of septic shock and is left in a persistent vegetative state.

It is not clear, as the story is told, whether better treatment might have prevented this and, if so, whether the better treatment might have been Hmong or Western. The doctors think the parents were noncompliant. The Lees think that the medicines were harming her and that being removed from the home was emotionally devastating. A pediatric neurologist suggests that her seizure medicine, Tegretol, may have in fact weakened her immune system and made her more susceptible to sepsis. The author carefully explains all the theories about Lia's illness, avoiding taking sides and allowing the participants to tell their own versions of the story.

"I am very sad," her mother says, "and I think a lot that if we were still in Laos and not in the United States maybe Lia would never be like this. The doctors are very very knowledgeable, your high doctors, your best doctors, but maybe they made a mistake by giving her the wrong medicine and made her hurt like this." (p. 258)

Maybe they made a mistake! Yehoshua's novel focuses on the issue of mistakes, of accountability, and becomes an inquiry into the ways that doctors understand whether or not they've done the right thing. By implication, it offers guidance for nonphysicians who try to interpret the rightness or the wrongness of controversial or ambiguous medical interventions.

Two ambiguous medical events frame the action of *Open Heart*. One is a blood transfusion that Rubin decides to give to Einat while they are traveling home from India. On the trip home, Einat is very weak. She has recurrent nosebleeds. In order to diagnose her condition, Rubin has made an exhausting trip to Calcutta with some blood samples, and finds that her liver enzymes are elevated, her clotting factors depleted, and that she is hypoglycemic. He decides that she needs a pint of blood, but does not trust the Indian hospital blood banks. Instead, he decides to give her a direct transfusion from her mother Dorit using techniques learned in the military for emergency battlefield transfusions.

The transfusion, done in a hotel room in New Delhi, goes smoothly and seems to help. Rubin feels confident and heroic, even though Lazar appears skeptical:

> I knew that everything I did here was being registered down to the last detail, and that when we got home he would waste no time in asking Hishin and the rest of "his" professors if it had really been necessary to perform the blood transfusion so urgently. But I was calm and sure of myself, ready not only to justify the urgent transfusion to all the professors in the hospital but also to demand the respect due to me for my diagnosis and ingenuity in a medical emergency. (pp. 115–116)

The transfusion is "successful." Einat feels better, her nose stops bleeding, she is stronger, and she makes the trip back to Israel in stable condition. Rubin is proud of what he has done. But when he gets home, people begin to question the appropriateness of this intervention. Levine, the Chief of Medicine, and an expert in hepatitis, sharply criticizes Rubin's decision to have performed the transfusion as "not only completely unnecessary but also irresponsible and perhaps even dangerous." (p. 201) Rubin defends himself, "If the transaminases [liver enzymes] rose to levels of a hundred and eighty and a hundred and fifty eight, it's clear that the clotting factors were also impaired.... so why not strengthen the poor girl with some fresh, safe plasma, from someone as close as her mother, to help her overcome the bleeding? And the fact is, after my transfusion, the bleeding stopped." (p. 202) "It stopped on its own, not because of you. The clotting factors, which you thought you were giving her in your transfusion, are enzymes, not blood cells, and they behave completely differently in a transfusion. They're absorbed and disappear—they're ineffective unless they're diluted in a special serum to bind them and prevent them from dissolving." (p. 202)

The argument is heated, arcane, and impossible for even a medically informed reader to deconstruct. Who's right? Who's wrong? Dr. Hishin, the Professor of Surgery, is not so sure. He says to Rubin, "I'm behind your idea, especially from the psychological point of view, and as I've often told you, psychology is no less important than the knife in your hand." Lazar was skeptical at the time, but becomes convinced that the transfusion saved his daughter's life. One of Rubin's friends thinks it was a crazy and dangerous intervention, one that could help only a little for Einat but that inexcusably put the mother at risk for getting hepatitis herself. As readers, we can't figure it out. Was the transfusion a mistake or a life-saving intervention? Was Rubin heroic, crazy, or lucky? Perhaps he was crazily heroic, or heroically lucky. Did he save a life, or merely endanger one? Who really knows what works and what doesn't? Who has the authority to judge?

In a sense, Yehoshua is saying, you had to be there. You had to see how Einat looked. You had to feel India around you. The transfusion may have made no sense, objectively speaking. But in the context, it worked, in some strange way, perhaps by cementing a relationship between mother and daughter at a crucial point. And, who knows, perhaps the weakening of that bond may have been as important a cause of Einat's weakness as her liver infection, low glucose, or inadequate clotting factors. Earlier in the book, Rubin speaks to family members of a patient who has just been operated upon and tells them that she has "been reborn." Einat's transfusion was, in a sense, a ritual of rebirth, taking life blood from her mother as she did in the womb.

The second ambiguous event occurs toward the end of the book. Lazar develops symptoms of the heart problems that Rubin perceptively intuited while they were on the train to Varanasi. He requires open-heart surgery. Because he is the hospital CEO, there is some scrappy in-fighting to determine who well "get" the case, whether he should be under the care of the Chief of Medicine or the Chief of Surgery. In the end, an outside surgeon from Jerusalem is called to Tel Aviv to perform the operation. Surgery goes well, but postoperatively, Lazar develops irregular heartbeats. Rubin notices them, and points them out to Levine. Levine still dislikes Rubin as a result of Rubin's "reckless and unjustifiable" decision to transfuse blood to Einat in India, so he disdainfully ignores Rubin's concerns about Lazar's cardiac arrhythmias. Perhaps he is right to do so. After all, he seems to know more cardiology than Rubin, just as he seemed to know more about hepatitis. And when Rubin goes to the library to read about postoperative arrhythmias, he notes that "no clear conclusions emerged from my reading. It appeared that there were atrial beats that could look like ventricular beats." Uneasy, he decides to be quiet.

But Rubin's concerns were prescient. Lazar dies as a result of the arrhythmias, a death that may have been preventable. Or may not have. "Perhaps the immediate cause of death had been the arrhythmia," one doctor notes in reviewing the case, "...but the deterioration in Lazar's condition stemmed from an infarct caused by an occlusion in one of the bypasses."(p. 368) The department chiefs cover up for each other, and, try as he might, Rubin is unable to find anybody who will support his contention that an avoidable mistake was made. As readers, we cannot tell whether Rubin just has a vendetta against Levine, whether the physicians at a leading Tel Aviv teaching hospital are incompetent or corrupt, or whether medicine itself is far less certain or scientific than it pretends to be.

And we are not reassured by Rubin. Prior to Lazar's death, he has been floundering in professional and moral amorphousness. Unable to make it in surgery, blackballed from medicine by the vindictive and depressed Levine, he moonlights as an anesthesiologist, takes a fellowship in England, drifts. In love with Dorit, he cynically marries the mystical Michaela, Einat's friend and traveling companion, whose trip to India left her believing a strange melange of ideas about the transmigration of souls. These ideas, for Rubin, become a playful excuse for an amoral permissiveness. Nothing matters because our souls our eternal, flit in and out of our bodies, inhabit other bodies, have wills of their own. There is no self, really, and so, no moral accountability. He becomes a sort of New Age demon, justifying any action, no matter how despicable, by explaining it in terms of a shallow pseudo-Indian jargon. He is the sort of moral thinker that Alasdair McIntyre,[5] in *After Virtue*, perhaps imagined us all to be: McIntyre describes us as equipped only with the shards of destroyed moral systems which we use as makeshift tools or cobble together in bizarre and irrational ways, quite different from the function for which these ideas were intended when they were part of a comprehensive moral system.

After Lazar's death, Rubin goes to visit Dorit, and finds her distraught, consumed with loneliness and despair. She also has a fever, and has sent for him. In an eerie and disgusting scene, Rubin offers his services as a physician in order to console her and earn her confidence. Then, in the process of examining her, he seduces her. She takes off her sweater so he can auscultate her lungs. He diagnoses a viral infection, and prescribes a couple of sleeping pills. Then, the doctor notes,

> Dori obediently swallowed the two pills I gave her to bring her temperature down and went to take off her clothes and put on a fresh, flimsier nightgown. Then she got straight into bed, asking me only to...put the light on in the hallway before I left. But I didn't want to leave yet.... Waves of love and desire began to stir in my double soul, and a thrilling new pleasure kept me rooted to the spot.
>
> ...I lifted the blankets to join myself to the warm source of the mystery. I began passionately embracing and kissing Dori once again. She was startled and began to struggle, but even in the depths of my fatigue, I was stronger then she was. I...felt her ripe, mature body relaxing between my hands. (p. 415).

He is not troubled. He has been imbibing half-baked Indian ideas about the transmigration of souls and imagines that Lazar's soul is in his body, so that he is not fucking the wife of a man who had just died, not using his medical authority to get into the bed of his patient, but only somehow carrying Lazar's soul back to Dorit for one last visit. Here, certainly, is the most ironic of Yehoshua's meanings of *Shiva M'Hodu*, a bereavement ritual brought from India to Israel.

This critique of medicine ends on an entirely ambiguous note. Unlike the moral denoument in classical Greek tragedies, the breaking of taboo in Yehoshuas's tale is not followed by terrifying self-revelation and penitence. No bad things happen. Nobody is punished. Nobody is even sure whether what they did is right or wrong. Rubin meets with Einat one last time, and says to her,

> "Tell me, Einat, did I make a mistake when I fell in love with your mother instead of falling in love with you?" ... She shook her head quickly, as if trying to repulse me, and mumbled, "No, you didn't make a mistake."
>
> "Your mother and father took me to India to fall in love with you, and I behaved like a doctor," I went on. "Was I wrong? Tell me, was I wrong?" She went on shaking her head with a tormented expression on her face and said, "No, you weren't wrong." (p. 489–490)

Recall the earlier scene where Rubin felt the flare up of lust. His therapeutic masturbation did not do the job it was supposed to do. His lust did not entirely dissipate. He managed to "behave like a doctor" towards Einat, but then, in a mysterious and ambiguous medical ritual, created a rivulet of blood connecting Einat to her mother and his lust flowed mysteriously down that narrow stream.

Through these mysterious events, Yehoshua asks what we find at the heart of medicine when we peel away layer after layer. Is it still subject to the ancient moral rules, the laws written into the tragedies? Can doctors now sleep with their patients? Is there punishment for sin, for transgression? Are we on the right path?

No matter how piercing his gaze, the mystery remains elusive. Things happen. People trust or do not trust one another. Doctors are by turns narcissistic, ambitious, irrational, well-meaning, brilliant or compassionate. They have powerful tools and amorphous goals. For the author in *Open Heart*, medicine and the doctors seem to be strangely impersonal and amoral. They judge each other but their judgments seem strangely arbitrary. We are left thinking that the quest for truth will never reach its goal, that the things we discover do not so much add to the total of our knowledge but instead drop out of the equations, leaving us no closer to solutions.

We are better at curing disease and keeping people alive longer than we have ever been before. But we can't keep people alive forever. Because there are more people alive on earth today than at any time in the past, there are also more people dying, on any given day, than at any given time in the past. Medicine's successes highlight medicine's limitations. This inevitable phenomenon raises the question of whether doctors have a role or responsibility in caring for those who are dying, oor whether their work should be limited to those who can be cured. If the latter, then who will care for the dying? Somehow, the answer to the question of whether we need doctors or we need medicine seems tied to the question of whether we know what makes a good doctor. Yehoshua highlights how difficult it is to know whether there is good medicine, and how, in the end, all we can try to decide is what we have always tried to decide, namely, whether someone is or is not a good doctor. And that question, as Yehoshua elucidates it, is profoundly mysterious, qualitative rather than quantitative, mystical rather than scientific.

When Levine dresses down Rubin for the blood transfusion, we cannot decide whether or not he is right about the instability of clotting factors. But we know that he is not treating Rubin fairly, he is not a good teacher, and so, we are not surprised when it turns out (or does it?) that he is not such a good doctor, either. Similarly, we feel that Rubin has transgressed, but there seems to be no context for considering these sorts of moral judgments within a discourse of medicine in which quality is defined by outcomes, or by discoveries, or by nonjudgmental respect for anchorless autonomy.

At Lazar's funeral, Hishin, the chief surgeon, delivers a eulogy. He recalls, as if he were there, the train ride to Varanasi and the profound effect that it had on Lazar. He seems to pay tribute to the wisdom of the East, noting that "perhaps ... the people of the world whom we call 'backward' and 'undeveloped' ... can give us a truer sense of the universe through which we pass so quickly ...." But his appreciation is tempered by his surgeon's realism. He goes on to say that, in his view, there is no such thing as a soul and never has been. "He himself, he announced, had spent his whole life prying into the most secret corners of the human body and had not yet come across any traces of a soul. Further, he assures the audience, "his brain surgeon friends argued that everything they found and touched was pure matter." (p. 381)

This eulogy reads like a manifesto. The surgeon, the highest star in the medical hierarchy, is also the most thoroughgoing materialist. Illness and health are irreducibly physiologic problems, not spiritual ones. In the hospital that Yehoshua describes, as in most modern hospitals, the non-mechanistic aspects of medicine are moving to the periphery. These hierarchies are set up by people who, like Rubin, imagine that all human desires, needs, ideals, aspirations and even loves are, like lust, physiologic balances that must be judiciously controlled rational hygienic exercises.

CONCLUSION

The central tension of these novels is the implicit tension between medicine and bioethics—how do we construct an argument or a belief system that will allow us to decide when knowledge or technical power will cause more harm then good? How do we direct our quest? How do we know whether we're on the right track? Rubin, the "ideal man," is idealistically open-minded. He wants to be like all the father figures—the chief of surgery, and of medicine, and anesthesia, the CEO, the fatalistic Hindu, and even Stephen Hawking. He tries to cobble together a personal moral system from these building blocks, but they do not fit together.

Nothing fits together, at least not straightforwardly. William Carlos Williams, a pediatrician and poet, knew better than most that, in the end, the doctor's task must be assessed by something other than mortality statistics or other conventional measures of success. Williams has an almost stoical acceptance of suffering when he writes,

> We know the plane will crash, the train will be derailed. And we know why. No one cares, no one can care. We get the news and discount it, and we are quite right in doing so. It is trivial. But the hunted news I get from some obscure patient's eyes is not trivial. It is profound: whole academies of learning, whole ecclesiastical hierarchies are founded upon it ....

For Williams, the mysteries of science are dwarfed by the mysterious process by which he, as a physician, becomes drawn in by his patients. He is not interested in impossible systems which promise the relief of human suffering. Instead, he is interested in the human capacity to go out in the middle of the night to make a house call, to struggle with the curious mixture of disdain and respect that we feel when invited to observe the unrelievable suffering of strangers. The tough business of medicine has little to do with the successes. It will always focus on the failures. In another novel of medicine, *The Cunning Man*, by the Canadian Robertson Davies, the young hero wants an old Native American shaman to teach him to be a healer like she is. Impossible, she snorts! Laughingly, she tells him that he has the wrong kind of eyes, the wrong kind of brain, and the wrong idea of what it means to learn to be a healer. It's not about mixing the right potions. In order to become a healer, she says, "you have to go crazy, starve, sweat nearly to death." (p. 41) It's not something you do with your mind.

Yehoshua's novel piles up layer upon layer of elusive meanings. Even the title resonates with ambiguity. *Open Heart* refers both to real and metaphorical hearts, to confessions of truth or of love (as in "opening your heart" to someone) as well as to a particularly invasive surgical procedure. During open-heart surgery, the heart is stopped and the patient may be considered temporarily "dead." In the book, one of the doctors describes a post-operative patient as having been "reborn." In Hebrew, the book is entitled *Shiva M'Hodu*, which, like *Open Heart*, is a bit of a pun. The word "shiva" can mean "return" and "Hodu" means India, so the title might mean "return from India." "Shiva" can also refer to the dangerous Hindu deity who is thought to be the Destroyer of the World. In the book, a baby is named "Shiva." The baby is born to an Israeli couple living in London, but both the man and the woman have been to India—their romance blossomed there, so their "Shiva" is sort of from India.

For Yehoshua, the future of medicine will depend not only upon the quality of scientific discoveries, but even more on the quality of doctors who understand and are allowed to respect ambiguity and mystery. These doctors, in spite of the latest scientific evidence, must also have the vision and the courage to size up a situation and to take personal risks, as Rubin did in ordering an irrationally dangerous but potentially salvational blood transfusion between a mother and daughter in a foreign country while outside the dying immerse themselves in holy waters and emerge to watch their dead loved ones being burned upon pyres. The future of humane medicine will depend upon doctors who know not only know science, but also the more mysterious byways of the human heart—doctors who understand the deepest nature of things and who are willing to acknowledge the importance of the symbols, resonances and nuances of life in addition to physiologic and biological knowledge.

NOTES AND REFERENCES

1. Ivan Illich, *Medical Nemesis. The Expropriation of Health* (New York: Pantheon, 1976).
2. A.B. Yehoshua, *Open Heart* [translated by Dalya Bilu] (New York: Doubleday, 1996).
3. R. Powers, *Operation Wandering Soul* (New York: Harper Perennial, 1994).
4. A. Fadiman, *The Spirit Catches You and You Fall Down* (New York: Farrar, Straus & Giroux, 1997).
5. Alasdair McIntyre, *After Virtue* (Notre Dame: University of Notre Dame Press, 1984).
6. W.C. Williams, *The Doctor Stories* (New York: New Directions, 1984), p.124.
7. Robertson Davies, *The Cunning Man* (New York: Norton, 1992).

Truth Telling

ANTONELLA SURBONE[a]

Memorial Sloan-Kettering Cancer Center, New York, New York 10021, USA

INTRODUCTION

Truth telling is an essential step in medicine and in the patient-doctor relationship. I shall try to examine the epistemic, pragmatic and ethical dimension of truth telling in medicine. It must first be said that neither "truth" nor "telling" are abstract words, nor are they value-neutral. The act of truth telling in medicine is indeed an exchange involving moral agents (the patient, the doctor, and society) with their sets of values and norms, which in turn are derived from culture, personal and religious beliefs, and traditions. Through their variance, complex and differentiated patterns of truth telling emerge in different contexts: hence the different practices and degrees of truth telling throughout the world.[1] In the present work I wish to go beyond those differences (which one might see as belonging to the "sphere of the expressive") to explore the underlying philosophical assumptions and questions which are inextricably intertwined with the ethical and pragmatic dimension of truth telling in medicine.

THE EPISTEMIC DIMENSION OF TRUTH TELLING

Epistemology, as the theory of knowledge, is concerned with truth. Whether it is Plato, Nietzsche, or Foucault speaking, whether we equate it with the highest good or we deny such intrinsic value, in the pursuit of knowledge we are interested in knowing the truth.[2]

According to the *Oxford Dictionary of Philosophy*, the central questions of epistemology include the origin of knowledge; the place of experience and of reason in generating knowledge; the relationship between knowledge and certainty; the relationship between knowledge and error; and the changing forms of knowledge that arise from new conceptualizations of the world.[3]

All these questions are directly related to the issue of truth telling in medicine, and I shall first analyze the relationship between truth and science insofar as it has an impact on truth telling. Western epistemology can be said to be born with Plato, whose initial epistemologic works were deeply connected with ontology.[4] Indeed, the early and middle Plato defines knowledge in terms of its object. In *The Republic*,[5] Plato describes different degrees of knowledge according to what the objects of knowledge are. Knowledge requires *logos*,[6] and real knowledge (which he calls "science") is only that of ideas, which are eternal and immutable, and are characterized by "being." Of these we have noetic knowledge, an immediate intuition. On the contrary, knowledge of the things of the world is of a lesser degree (it is *doxa*, opinion), for these things are temporal and subject to change and are characterized by "becom-

---

[a]Current address: 1045 31st Street, N.W., Washington, D.C. 20007, USA.

ing." Of these, we can only speak in terms of *dianoetic* knowledge, or discourse. Plato never excludes that the things of the world exist and can be known, but he establishes the primacy of the knowledge of absolutes and calls it *science*.[7]

Plato's last dialogue on epistemology is *Thaetetus*,[8] a very modern work, which-frees epistemology from ontology and is concerned with the distinction of three types of knowledge: knowledge through sense perception, propositional knowledge, and pragmatic knowledge. Despite *Thaetetus* and despite most of modern epistemology, in medicine we seem to hold the ontological view (whether we realize it or not, whether we admit it or not). What we have done is a reshuffling of Plato's early thinking, leading to a worrisome conclusion: modern science, seen as eternal and perfect, combines intuition and discourse; it no longer reflects Platonic ideas, but rather the real state of the world. Truth only belongs to science, the scientific method is the only true method of inquiry, and science is equal to objectivity.

The term "objectivity" implies the existence of an object, and the underlying assumption of such epistemic view is that truth corresponds to an external object and describes it accurately.[9] Aristotle defined truth as "to say of what is that it is, and of what is not that it is not."[10] The dominant Western epistemology, relying heavily on the Enlightenment and on the principles of positivism and empiricism, further attached to truth the ideas/ideals of pure objectivity and of value-neutrality.[11] The basic assumptions of such dominant epistemology[12] are that knowers are detached neutral spectators who acquire knowledge by observation, and present it in propositions: truth then is a kind of sameness, and falsity a kind of diversity from the given.[13] Propositions can be verified by others, again through observation. The purpose of knowledge is to foster our capacity to control the external world.[14] This view of knowledge rests on the fact/value distinction as an effective way to maintain the equation knowledge = science.

Other theories of truth have been proposed which deny the primacy of the object and of correspondence to it, and rather privilege more holistic and more pragmatic views, where subjectivity is often taken into account, and knowledge is seen as "situated."[15] Disease is unfortunately one of the most solid proofs that there is an external reality, which occurs independent of our wish and escapes our control.[16] Hence, a narrow-correspondence view of truth in medicine is flawed not insofar as it rests on the recognition of the undeniable reality of disease, but rather because it ignores the role of the knower in generating truth: it lacks a sufficient account of the subjective and contextual dimension of knowledge. Recognizing that knowledge has subjective and contextual dimensions does not mean that we abandon epistemology to enter the psychology of subjectivity, nor that we end with the pessimism of cognitive and cultural relativism.[17] On the contrary, it implies questioning the pure objectivity and the value-neutrality of knowledge (and for us, of medical knowledge), by recognizing that there is a living subject, the knower, who has both reason and emotions, and who holds a certain power position in a certain context. (The knower in medicine is both the doctor and the patient, and they know differently.)

TRUTH TELLING VERSUS TRUTH MAKING

If we remain within the dominant "context-independent" model, the conclusion is generated that "knowledge worthy of the name must transcend the particularities of experience to achieve objective purity and value neutrality."[18] Then, in medicine and in the patient-doctor relationship we privilege the objective dimension of disease, and tend to ignore that disease is first a subjective event, a unique and disrupting—when not devastating—event in a person's life. As the subjective dimension of disease can hardly be measured with scientific methodology, we prefer to discard it as non real. We all do so because we have equated "real" with "scientifically measurable": this is the idolatry of scientific truth which we all share, whether doctors or patients. Truth is perceived as only the opposite or absence of lie; truth is seen as a static object, merely waiting to be described and verbalized; and medical truth is assumed to reside only in the objectivity of quantifiable data.[19] Hence, the emphasis on the diagnostic aspects of disease, where the more objective data are located. Hence, the obligation we feel to overwhelm our patients with obscure quotes from the scientific literature and with statistics about morbidity, mortality, and survival. (And too often we do so even when not requested, even on the first encounter with a new person-patient, without taking into account the patient's cultural and personal context). Truth telling literally becomes the act of someone (the doctor, being the only knower) who knows the truth and tells it to someone else (the patient, being only the listener).

In this perspective, disease becomes reified. Reification of disease[20] serves the purpose of maintaining the supremacy of some over others—the most powerful over the more vulnerable. The power in the patient-doctor relationship is on the doctor's side, for the relationship itself is an asymmetrical one, due to the unique state of dependency created in the patient by disease itself.[21]

There is, however, a quite different way to frame the issues of truth and truth telling in medicine. Truth is not a static object external to us and awaiting our neutral discovery: truth is rather a relational state, which develops in time and space because of interactions. Truth is not only something to be *told*: truth is rather something that we *make*. Both the patient and the doctor contribute to this process of truth making, where the "methodological solipsism" of those who hold that we can think effectively apart from considerations of social practice, is surpassed.

Interactions in medicine take place between the patient, the disease, the doctor, the medications, with their efficacy or lack of efficacy, and finally with the context. The patient-doctor relationship always has a third party, society.[22] Society includes both the micro-environment and the macro-environment, where each one of us acquires and develops his/her own set of beliefs. Personal beliefs, religion, and tradition all play an active part in the development of the medical truth, a development that occurs within a relationship, requiring the active intervention of all partners. In such perspective, truth telling acquires two different meanings: on one hand, it is the duty and act of honesty of the more informed partner (the doctor, who is consulted because of his/her scientific knowledge); on the other hand, information is just a first step towards something that goes beyond it: communication. Information is never exhaustive of truth, which, on the contrary, is created only in communication, a bi-directional process by definition.

In this perspective, the subjective dimension of disease is as important as the objective one, and sensitivity—both cultural[23] and personal[24]—is required to gain access into subjectivity. Sensitivity implies respect for language as a form of life.[25] For instance, where autonomy is synonymous for "isolation," truth telling in the American way is unlikely to be beneficial to the patient or to foster his/her dignity.[26] Even in the American context, objective medical information needs not to be imposed onto, say, an unprepared patient, with a different cultural background or with different beliefs,[27] only out of fear of litigation, nor out of the abstract affirmation of the supremacy of our Western beliefs (a worrisome and widespread form of cultural hegemony[28]). Different practices of truth telling should be accepted and respected: they should be seen as stemming from differences in the modulation and expression of the same basic principles of human dignity, embedded in different contexts. Cultural differences in truth telling seldom give rise to differences in the effectiveness of truth making.[30]

THE EPISTEMIC RESPONSIBILITY OF THE DOCTOR

Disease, as previously said, undeniably carries an objective dimension, and the doctor[31] has an epistemic responsibility towards it, towards his/her patients, and to society in its entirety. The previous discussion of truth and truth telling in medicine, and of the cultural variability with respect to degrees of truth telling, might appear to lead to the easy conclusion that subjectivity and relativism should triumph, and that we should thus feel relieved of our professional responsibilities. On the contrary, I maintain that the doctor first has a professional accountability, which is primarily based on his/her respect for the scientific truth, as well as for the existential truth of the particular patient. This accountability is at the same time towards evidence and towards the individual and the community.[32]

The dichotic view of the "great yet uncaring doctor" (too busy knowing to have any time left for personal or cultural sensitivity) contrasted with the "kind, yet not so expert doctor" (too involved in the emotional turmoil of the patient to have any time left to read scientific journals) is nonsensical insofar as neither of them would be able to establish a therapeutic relationship with his or her patients. The knowledge of the former is kept at such a distance from the patient that it becomes incommunicable: truth telling remains a matter of information only, and fails to reach the level of communication. The warmth and compassion of the latter are at best temporarily comforting, but are again non-therapeutic, as such a doctor betrays his/her epistemic responsibility. There is no such thing as "unethical science" or "non-scientific ethics": the epistemic dimension of truth belongs to science as well as to ethics.

THE PRAGMATIC DIMENSION OF TRUTH

A dynamic relational account of truth within the context of a relationship maintains that the patient-doctor relationship is based on mutual obligations[33] and oriented towards a specific goal: that such relationship be therapeutic.[34] In this perspective, truth in medicine can be understood as instrumental. Instrumental does not mean that truth should be defined in terms of its utility (as James put it), but rather that pragmatic aspects do contribute to make meaning possible, as Wittgenstein suggested in saying that "meaning is use."

Indeed, truth telling has a pragmatic dimension, first because it is by definition an act. Action belongs to the sphere of the practical and is oriented towards a goal. The goal of truth telling in medicine is to achieve therapeutic efficacy.[35] Truth telling finds its justification in the context of (and in view of) a therapeutic project. We have recognized the existence of a medical truth, which precedes (and in part is independent of) the therapeutic success: truth telling in medicine, however, is not merely descriptive. Truth telling in medicine is *praxis*: its goal is therapy (cure and care).

The patient-doctor relationship, as praxis, is at the same time a contractual relationship based on obligations, and an asymmetrical relationship based on the particular needs of one partner. In both instances, the patient-doctor relationship is based on trust.[36] And the patient primarily trusts the doctor's ability and expertise to understand his/her disease, and to treat it properly. The patient's trust is based on the assumption that his/her particular disease has an objective dimension, which can be known through scientific methodology, and can be taught and learned. Notably, the doctor learns through generalization what the patient knows through his/her direct singular experience. The assumption, however common to both the patient and the doctor, is that there is indeed a medical truth (whether spoken or unspoken), and that the doctor recognizes it and acts upon it.

In this sense, medical truth is—in part at least—a matter of correspondence, and the doctor is accountable for adhering to such truth in order to achieve therapeutic success. But medical knowledge is primarily *techne*, it is praxis.

Finally, truth exists in ambiguity[37]: there is a certain vagueness in truth, even in scientific medical truth. The dichotomy *truth/falsity* is often replaced by a more complex reality of vagueness, both epistemic[38] and existential. It is via this ambiguity that we access the ethical dimension of truth telling.

THE ETHICAL DIMENSION OF TRUTH TELLING

The first ethical responsibility of the doctor is his/her professional responsibility, which is not alleviated by recognizing the ambiguity of truth in medicine. On the contrary, respecting such ambiguity calls for an expansion of the doctor's responsibility to include the understanding of the patient's personal and cultural context.[39]

The epistemic relationship between knowledge and certainty, and between knowledge and error, finds a correlate in the two main areas of truth telling in medicine: diagnosis and prognosis. As previously said, the diagnostic aspect of disease is where the more objective data lie, and where the epistemic responsibility of the doctor is first founded. Prognosis, as the ability to predict the likely course of a patient's disease, is far less objective; however, it is often said to be what is distinctive of the medical profession. Rather than recognizing the element of uncertainty in prognostication, modern medicine aims at increasing its accuracy and precision. While this is an important task, all of us who have practiced long enough are very familiar with the uncertainties of prognostication, and we are left with the unsettling feeling that stressing certainty over uncertainty in prognostication betrays the complexity of life. It seems that we are again trying to reify disease, and to distance all subjective elements from the patient-doctor relationship. By reciting survival statistics in front of our patients, rather than contributing to their self-determination, we most often acquire a tremendous power. The power that modern medicine seems to have lost in terms of how the figure of the physician is perceived (no longer a god), we re-establish through our easily pronouncing life and death sentences. Diagnosis and prognosis are formidable tools indeed, and the magic can continue.

The play between certainty and uncertainty (both at the epistemic and at the ethical level) is particularly evident in the rapidly developing field of human genetics, where the intertwinement of scientific knowledge and normativity is strikingly evident. By knowing our genome, we accomplish two major tasks: we find out about genetic diversity and we are in the position of making predictions about the future. *First,* genetics proves us that knowledge is subject to change (in its forms at least) under the influence of new developments and new concepts of the world.[40] This suggests that truth is also subject to change, both in the scientific and in the normative realms. *Second,* whether or not genetic diversity will be felt to be compatible with human equality[41] depends not on the scientific meaning of genetic diversity,[42] but on the meaning and value that society attributes to "diversity," to "sickness," and to "predisposition to a sickness." *Third,* we all agree that the predictive power of genetics is quite limited, since genes do not exist alone, and the interactions between genes and the environment are far from being known and even further from being controllable. Yet, we already have some experts (and to a certain extent all physicians will have to quickly become experts in this field), who can make predictions about future diseases based on the genome of their patients. Where is the truth here? Is it true that genetics expands the control we have on our lives, or is it true that it can paralyze us? Is it true that we can predict the future, or is it true that too many other unknowns are at stake? More pragmatically, is it true that knowing herself to be BRCA1-positive will enable a woman to exercise more effective prevention; or is it true that a BRCA1-positive woman can be denied health care or a job or the adoption of a child? Indeed, these are *all* truths: the truth for each person (whether us or our patients) is likely to be a unique whole, where some elements will figure more and others less. As a consequence, the act of truth telling about genetic risks, for instance, is clearly not a neutral one, and the power held by those who make the predictions is tremendously high.

The second ethical obligation of the doctor is the correct use that he/she makes of all these formidable tools, which allow him/her to convert the symptom experienced into "a disease" (diagnosis always brings about an ontological change in the patient[44]) and to predict the future (whether through prognostication or through risk assessment). If used in the context of a relationship where reciprocity exists asymmetrically, these tools contribute to enable our patients to make informed choices about their lives. If, on the contrary, diagnosis, prognosis, and risk assessment are used to reify disease and to stigmatize our patients, then they only reinforce the already existing power imbalance between the doctor and the patient: truth then becomes another of the asymmetries of life.[45]

When we use truth telling to subjugate the person in front of us, to label her, to make her silent, to quickly move on to the next patient, then we are serving power, not knowledge. Then Nietzsche's question: "This unconditional will to truth—what is it?" is hardly answered in terms of truth. For truth is never the result of an imposition. Truth is something emerging, being discovered and being created, in the patient-doctor relationship, as in any other instance of our lives. And truth is about freedom.

"AND YOU SHALL KNOW THE TRUTH, AND THE TRUTH SHALL MAKE YOU FREE" (JOHN 8:32)

If truth is something dynamic that we make in a historical context, and not only something static that we describe, then truth indeed contributes to freedom. Medicine also is about freedom: freedom from symptoms and from disease, but also freedom to make informed choices. In the medical vocabulary we often hide the importance of the word "freedom": suffice to think of some common abbreviations in medicine, such as DFI (disease-free interval) and DFS (disease-free survival)—they are indeed potent reminders of what medicine is about. Truth telling in medicine is a precious instrument of this freedom, and as such shall be used.

So medicine is about freedom. Truth is about freedom. Freedom is about wholeness. Truth as formulated in language is always partial, as Bradley strongly suggested, and not everything can be verbalized.

The aim of truth telling is "truth" and not "telling." If "telling" becomes an impediment to truth,[46] then we should find truth in its wholeness beyond the spoken word. If not everything can and should be expressed in words,[47] then we shall not be afraid to venture beyond words.

This is only possible when the patient-doctor encounter is not an isolated technical event, but a relationship: there the unspoken finds its proper place, and truth can unravel in its integrity and dignity. There we cease to categorize about the universal human nature, and we dare facing that particular person in front of us, emerging in her wholeness and uniqueness. Such person, our patient, likely loves truth as much as we also do—as physicians and as human beings first.

Because this is what we are in the patient-doctor relationship: human beings. If Wittgenstein was right in one of his letters to Russell in 1914, saying: "How can I be a logician before I'm a human being? Far the most important thing is to settle accounts with myself...," maybe what we really need to do is settle our own account with truth first. Maybe we will realize that at the existential level what we say "isn't necessarily true, but it explains, just by the fact of saying it, our existence,"[48] and that this we also share with our patients. Then, we can take the responsibility of truth telling beyond the narrowness of information and the abusiveness of power. Only then, we can enter the challenging, yet so rewarding, world of the patient-doctor relationship, and tell the truth and make the truth.

This is possibly a new concept of truth in medicine. But "concepts are like multiple waves, which go up and down; but the plane of immanence is the unique wave, which both surrounds them and unfolds them."[49]

NOTES AND REFERENCES

1. A. Surbone, "Information, Truth and Communication: For An Interpretation of Truth-telling Practices Throughout the World," in Antonella Surbone and Matjaz Zwitter (Eds.), *Communication with the Cancer Patient. Information and Truth* [Volume 809 of the *Annals of the New York Academy of Sciences*] (New York: The New York Academy of Sciences, 1997).
2. Truth here can be the truth we wish to know about falsehood, or about the power relationships that undermine it.
3. *The Oxford Dictionary of Philosophy* (Oxford: Oxford University Press, 1987).

4. The best known and most quoted source of Plato's epistemology is ironically one of his latest works, *Thaetetus,* where indeed Plato surpasses its previous views. In the conclusion of *Thaetetus,* Plato questions his own suggestion that "knowledge is true beliefs plus *logos.*" *Thaetetus.* Trans. by R.A.H. Waterfield (London: Penguin Books, 1987).
5. Plato, *The Republic* (New York: Viking Press, 1977).
6. The view that knowledge requires *logos* recurs in Plato's epistemology. What is meant by *logos* probably varies according to different stages of Plato's thinking, but the fundamental view is that there is something which, added to true belief, converts it into knowledge, and this appears to be primarily the ability to analyze, to work out the reason. The best known example is found in *Meno,* where Socrates elicits a correct answer to a mathematical problem from an uneducated slave. That is not yet knowledge: it is only when the slave understands why the proposition is correct, that he can be said to have knowledge. (*Meno,* 85c) (*Meno* (97e-98a), *Gorgias* (465a), *Phaedo* (76b), *Symposium* (202a), *Republic* (533b-c), *Thaetetus* (201c-210d), in Platone, *Opere complete* (Bari, Italy: Biblioteca Universale Laterza, 1996).
7. One might notice that the necessity of defining knowledge with a single term or sentence that can be substituted for the word "knowledge" every time we use it is also platonic. This was the Socratic method of definition. The reality of knowledge, as modern philosophy and epistemology shows, is likely more complex and admits of more than one definition. This is particularly relevant to our discourse on truth telling in medicine.
8. Plato, *op cit.*
9. The correspondence theory of knowledge, also known as adequacy or adherence theory, is the view that truth consists in correspondence with the facts. Such theory assumes that at the basis of knowledge there is "a given," and hence a foundation of knowledge upon which knowledge is built through confirmation and inference. Any correspondence theory of knowledge privileges the role of experience as a mean of discovering the given truth, while undermining the role of beliefs in accessing the facts.
10. Aristotle, *Metaphysics* (1011b), in *The Basic Works of Aristotle* (New York: Random House, 1941).
11. Lorraine Code, "Taking Subjectivity Into Account," in L. Alcoff and E. Potter (Eds.), *Feminist Epistemologies* (New York: Routledge, 1993).
12. Alfred J. Ayer, *Logical Positivism* (New York: The Free Press, 1959).
13. This is the classical philosophical theory of the priority of nature, and of truth as correspondence.
14. One might add: "to our benefit."
15. Opposite to the correspondence theory, the coherence theory of truth affirms that the truth of a proposition consists in its being coherent among a body of other propositions not defined in terms of truth. According to coherence theories there are no given foundations, and the stability of the whole is maintained through the coherence of its parts. Beliefs are privileged, as we can only see and speak of truth within a pre-existing set of beliefs. One of the major criticisms of coherence theories of truth is that they underestimate the role played by experience not only in acquiring knowledge, but also in controlling our sets of beliefs. Other theories of truth include the identity theory, where wholeness is stressed, and the existence of any partial truth denied; the redundancy or semantic theory, offering a minimalist view of truth; and pragmatic theories of truth, affirming the instrumental role of truth with respect to its use.
16. Lorraine Code writes: "The fact of the world's intractability to intervention and wishful thinking is the strongest evidence of its independence from human knowers." *Op. cit.,* p.20.
17. Francesco Bellino, *I Fondamenti della Bioetica* (Roma: Citta' Nuova, 1993).
18. Lorraine Code, *op. cit.,* p. 19.
19. Antonella Surbone, "Informed Consent and Truth in Medicine," *European Journal of Cancer,* No. 14 (1994), p. 2189.
20. The concept of reification is the basis of *History and Class Consciousness,* written by George Lukacs in 1923, and subsequently withdrawn upon the Third International

accusation of "subjectivism." According to Jurgen Habermas (writing on Lukacs in his 1987 *Theory of Communicative Action*) "reification is a peculiar assimilation of social relationships and subjective experiences to things, which we can perceive and manipulate." The reified thing is given, not made. Through the process of reification, objective intrinsic power is attributed to things, whereas those same things are the result of actions and of interactions. Positivistic reified science, according to Lukacs, transforms social products into natural immutable facts, which in turn appear foreign and deprived of any possibility of control by human beings. By "reification of disease" I intend to suggest a similar process of estrangement, leading us to privilege the objective elements of disease to the detriment of its subjective interpersonal dimension. See George Lukacs, *History and Class Consciousness* (Cambridge, Mass.: MIT Press, 1971), trans. R. Livingston.
21. Edmund D. Pellegrino, "Altruism, Self Interest, and Medical Ethics," *JAMA*, No. 258 (1987), pp. 1939–1940.
22. Antonella Surbone, "The Patient-Doctor-Family Relationship: At the Core of Medical Ethics," in L. Baider, C.L. Cooper, and A. Kaplan De-Nour (Eds.), *Cancer and the Family* (West Sussex, England: John Wiley & Sons Ltd., 1996).
23. Lawrence O. Gostin, "Informed Consent, Cultural Sensitivity and Respect for Persons," *JAMA*, No. 274 (1995), pp. 844–845.
24. For a moving and convincing account of the importance of sensitivity and respect in medicine, see the recent book by Dr. Jerome Lowenstein, describing his experiences as Director of the Humanistic Medicine Program at New York University. Cf. J. Lowenstein, *The Midnight Meal and Other Essays About Doctors, Patients, and Medicine* (New Haven: Yale University Press, 1996).
25. Language is the vehicle for truth telling, and a precious instrument for communication. But there is often a major gap between the spoken word and the word that is heard, as we all know from our experience with patients. Then language can even become an obstacle of communication.
26. A. Surbone, "Truth Telling to the Patient," *JAMA*, No. 268 (1992), pp. 1661–1662.
27. Jerome Lowenstein, *The Midnight Meal, op. cit.*, p. 76.
28. The initial work on cultural differences in medicine originated as a reaction to Western cultural imperialism. See Ian E Thompson, "Fundamental Ethical Principles in Health Care," *British Medical Journal*, No. 295 (1987), pp. 1461–1465.
29. Edmund D. Pellegrino, "Is Truth Telling to Patients A Cultural Artifact?," *JAMA*, No. 268 (1992), pp. 1734–1735.
30. Dr. Levy from Zimbawe, writes that in her country "it is not uncommon for a specific disease to be attributed to an expression of displeasure by an ancestral spirit, and the remedy will be seen to lie in acts of appeasement. Another cause of illness is believed to be the casting of spells by grudge-bearing individuals. Faith in traditional healers is deeply ingrained in Shona culture. It is believed that the traditional healer will determine the cause of illness and decide what must be done to propitiate the offending spirit.... Occasionally a healer may recommend that the patient consult a doctor; others advise against any approach to the formal health centers....There is no word in the Shona vocabulary for cancer.... No Shona patient has ever asked me how long he or she has to live." Dr. Levy's success in communicating with her cancer patients and in providing cure and care is undeniable evidence that it is making the truth that counts, not reciting information. (Lorraine M. Levy, "The Cancer Patient in Zimbawe," in A. Surbone and M. Zwitter (Eds.), *Communication with the Cancer Patient: Information and Truth, op. cit.*
31. Throughout this essay, the word "doctor" is used as a short form for "health care worker." It is clear that truth telling is also the responsibility of nurses and of anyone else engaged in a therapeutic relationship with a person/patient.
32. Lorraine Code, *Epistemic Responsibility* (Hanover, NH: University Press of New England, 1987).
33. That obligations in the patient-doctor relationship are mutual is well exemplified by the case of truth telling. In fact, it behooves both partners to tell the truth, and reciprocity certainly must exist with respect to truth telling (the doctor not only has a duty to be truthful, but he/she also expects the patient's narrative to be truthful to

what the patient experiences, for correct diagnosis, prognosis, and treatment to be possible).
34. That the patient-doctor relationship aims at being therapeutic is the presupposition of the relationship itself. The sick person consults a professional for his/her expertise in the medical field and asks him/her for care and cure.
35. Doctors are rarely consulted for information only: even when this occurs, such as, for instance, in the case of genetic counseling, the information sought by the patient is strictly instrumental to his/her decisions about prevention or about family planning, and a therapeutic dimension, albeit indirect, is present. Throughout this essay, the sentence: "truth telling in medicine," refers to truth telling to patients. Truth telling is also to the scientific community, and in this perspective its goal, at times, can be mere information or speculation, not necessarily directed at therapy.
36. For a thorough discussion of the role of trust in ethics, see Annette C Baier, *Moral Prejudices: Essays on Ethics* (Cambridge, MA.: Harvard University Press, 1994).
37. For an extensive and illuminating discussion of ambiguity, see Merleau Ponty's work on perception and our knowledge of the body. Maurice Merleau-Ponty, *Phenomenologie de la Perception* (London: Routledge & Kegan Paul, 1962).
38. The concept of epistemic vagueness is far more challenging and less intuitive than that of existential vagueness, with which we are all very well acquainted in our personal lives. Epistemic vagueness can be found even in the most basic observations, which often admit of borderline cases. Moreover, the emergence of new realities and of new discoveries often makes the classification of new cases hard enough that they become vague. The impact of technology on modern medicine well illustrates the point: suffice to consider the definition of death in the context of organ transplants.
39. The discussion of cultural variability and of cross-cultural stability is now particularly lively because of the multi-ethnicity of most of our societies and of the increasing value that democratic societies attribute to pluralism.
40. This inevitably prompts a reconsideration of the classical philosophic tenet that knowledge and becoming exclude one another. Science is not only about being, as Plato thought.
41. Paul Reilly, "ASHG Statement on Genetics and Privacy: Testimony to United States Congress," *American Journal of Human Genetics*, No. 50 (1992), pp. 640–642.
42. Indeed when we will know all the secrets of our genome, we will all be subject to genetic diversity. That should be enough to discourage any discrimination based on genetic information. Yet, there is something in our collective unconscious which makes genes seem to all of us as carrying some deeper, more drastic, more inevitable sense of diversity and of sharing in the risks associated with such diversity.
43. Antonella Surbone, "The Moral Challenge of Genetic Testing for Breast Cancer," *Medicina e Morale* (1999).
44. Aristotle wrote that "it is not because I think that you are pale, that you are pale. Rather, it is because you are pale, that he who says this has the truth." However, consider what happens when the doctor makes a diagnosis (i.e., gives a name to a symptom). When the feeling of palpitations becomes a mitral valve prolapse, a new ontological state is created in the patient.
45. "Differences between true and false do not exist apart from the practice in which these values are produced and evaluated and statements made to circulate as true, as known or probable.... The practical conditions situate truth amid the major asymmetries of social power, undermining its status as common good." Allen Barry, *Truth in Philosophy* (Cambridge, MA: Harvard University Press, 1995).
46. As seen previously in Dr. Levy's account, in some culture the word for *cancer* does not exist. What would the Western use of such a word do to the truthfulness of such patient-doctor relationships? Western language would be very likely an impediment to establishing a truthful relationship in that context. Similar considerations need to be made when speaking to a Western patient who does not want to know about his/her disease (mastering silence can be very important too).
47. One of the most quoted propositions of contemporary philosophy is Wittgenstein's "Whereof we cannot speak, thereof we must be silent." It also is one of the most often ignored, in our cult of verbalization.

48. Cesare Pavese, as cited in Stein Husebo, "Communication, Autonomy and Hope. How Can We Treat Seriously Ill Patients with Respect?," in Antonella Surbone and Matjaz Zwitter (Eds.), *Communication with the Cancer Patient: Information and Truth, op. cit.*
49. Gilles Deleuze, *Quest'est Que C'est Que la Philosophie?* (Paris: Minuit, 1991).

The Evolution of a Hospital Ethics Committee

G.H. GROWE

Medical Director, Blood Transfusion Services, Vancouver Hospital,
855 West 12th Avenue, Vancouver, British Columbia, Canada V5Z 1M9

INTRODUCTION

The introduction of an ethics program as an integral and important part of hospital practice has not been an entirely smooth one in our institution. There has been concern about the commitment both from the administration and from the practising physicians. Although the members of the committee have been loyal and hard working and most have participated for at least five years, during the first few years their efforts seemed to have little impact. The issuance of our first policy regarding resuscitation in 1989 piqued the interest of some doctors and satisfied certain basic administrative needs. This event appears to have been a turning point, and, since then, more meaningful dialogue has developed within the hospital community, although some highly contentious issues have even led to resignations from the committee. Advances have been made through the guidance of a few expert individuals, but the successes and "personality" of the committee are due, in the main, to our collaborative style and broad-based representation.

EARLY DEVELOPMENT

In 1986 an interest group consisting of several physicians and an ethicist, wrote to the medical advisory committee of the Vancouver General Hospital (VGH) suggesting the establishment of an ethics committee. Clinical activities such as the palliative care program had already presented certain ethical questions regarding pain medication protocols and heroic treatment for dying patients, and the matter of informed consent became of considerable interest because of legal cases that had arisen. By this time, certain social attitudes had also begun to have an impact on health care such as an increased appreciation of patient autonomy; a general distancing of the population from traditional religious ties, and a response to the women's movement. Societal attitudes toward physicians and modern medicine were also changing: there was a notable decline in respect for the position of the physician in society; and many significant technologic developments strained at the boundaries of human moral comprehension (e.g., the support of immature and malformed newborns, the life-sustaining ability of intensive care programs, and the diversity of tissue transplantation possibilities). At this time, the only health care institution in Vancouver to have a functioning ethics committee was the British Columbia Children's Hospital (BCCH). However, there had been a ten-year history of academic interest at the medical school, and a program had been introduced to the undergraduate medical students with the assistance of Dr. E.H. Kluge of Victoria.

Questions were raised as to (1) why an ethics committee was necessary; (2) how it would interfere with the practice of physicians and surgeons; (3) who would constitute the members of such a committee; and (4) what issues were suitable to be brought to it. Certain health care workers and academics in our community were well versed with some of the relevant philosophical concerns and practices through their participation in the above-mentioned undergraduate medical program. But many practicing physicians were concerned about the threat to their primary role in patient care by such a committee, and to some degree this attitude continues today. Another major contention then, and now, was the resistance of many physicians and surgeons to the concept of a "health care team" and to the value of interdisciplinary activity. Current attitudes reflected by training programs in the medical school will likely socialize physicians into practicing in a more collaborative way. However, major obstacles to this integration are the provincial statutes and the responsibilities designated by hospital bylaws, which place the legal onus for decision-making completely on the shoulders of the physician.

THE HEALTH CARE ENVIRONMENT IN VANCOUVER

With a population of more than two million, the Vancouver region has a number of suburban as well as city-core, university-affiliated hospitals. There are two large general hospitals, plus the BC Cancer Institute, the BC Children's Hospital (BCCH), and one obstetrical/women's complex associated with the University of British Columbia (UBC). As well, there are six small hospitals, a number of which were founded by Roman Catholic orders and which have an affiliation with one of the large general Catholic hospitals. The Canadian Catholic Hospital Association has taken an active role in preparing background material for its affiliated institutions covering a wide range of situations with ethical content. The hospital in which I practice, the Vancouver General Hospital (VGH) complex, consists of approximately 1,200 total beds, of which more than 400 service chronic-care patients. No pediatric or obstetric patients are seen in this institution. The restricted nature of our hospitalized population has resulted in the focus of the ethics committee to be directed mainly toward matters of consent and end-of-life issues.

There has been no organized plan for the community. The hospital programs first developed with little interaction, and the university filled the major gaps for professional education and research review. In the year 2000 there are now ethics consultation groups at all of these various hospitals. These are mandated by the B.C. Hospital Act for purposes of hospital accreditation. Dr. Sidney Segal at BCCH was a pioneer not only in neonatal health care, but also in developing ethics programs in the community. At the pediatric facility, he and his group concentrated on problems that arise at the outset of life, such as those related to abnormal birth, fetal-alcohol syndrome, and the competency of impaired parents and of minors. The UBC Faculty of Medicine developed its own committee to provide both undergraduate and postgraduate education to the medical community. A separate ethics committee was also developed in the Faculty to deal specifically with research and clinical trials. The Faculty of Applied Research Ethics under the directorship of Dr. Michael McDonald was established at UBC in 1993, and close ties through cross appointments have developed between the various university groups and the hospitals. The BC Transplant Society, through its own committee, has dealt separately with the issues related to organ retrieval and provision. The hospitals are now dealing more actively with clinical problems related to transplantation and tissue harvesting within their own institutions. With regionalization of health care, several facilities have joined together and their ethics committees have also merged.

EARLY DAYS OF THE COMMITTEE

The attention of our VGH group has been drawn specifically to patient-related matters within our institution. In 1986, informed consent and the lack of guidelines for resuscitation were cited as the primary concerns to require our attention. At the outset, the ethics committee was commissioned to report formally to the medical advisory committee (MAC), and copies of our minutes were distributed to hospital administration and the Board of Trustees. The initial committee consisted of four physicians, three nurses, one administrative representative, one social worker, one chaplain, one lawyer, and one philosopher from a local university, who had a special interest and expertise in medical ethics. During the first two years the members met every month, shared among themselves information and articles related to ethics, and began to arrange educational rounds in the hospital for staff and trainees. The members either volunteered or were recruited by the chairman, who was appointed by the MAC. The following were the terms of reference: (1) to make recommendations on policies related to ethical matters; (2) to promote activities and education related to ethical issues; (3) to promote and develop research related to current ethical matters; and (4) to support a clinical consultative service related to ethical issues. In the first five years we were able to make reasonable inroads on the first two matters, but felt quite limited in our ability to comply with the latter two.

EVOLUTION OF THE COMMITTEE AND ITS ACTIVITIES

Committee Structure and Function

From an initial composition of twelve, the official size of the committee grew to sixteen. Additional members represent long-term care, the human rights and diversity office, the UBC ethics program, and the community at large. There is little ongoing legal input, but advice is solicited when needed. Usually, there are more than twenty persons at our monthly one-and a half-hour meetings, as guest observers and students frequently attend. Most of the detailed work is done by subgroups outside of the meetings, so the large group acts mainly to provide broadly based input and develop policy initiatives. The usual monthly agenda includes working group reports on policies under development; highlights from recent meetings of interest; the circulation of reprints, and discussion by the ethicists about their current clinical consults. A formal primer has not yet been completed for new members, but the chair introduces them individually to the program. Very few of the participants have opted to resign, so the chair has had to orchestrate the gradual turnover of personnel.

Policy Development

This section is the lengthiest of the paper, and it deals primarily with our most complex evolving policy, related to resuscitation procedures in the hospital setting. I use it as an example of our operational style and our ability to respond to change. I have taken care to outline in some detail the underlying thoughts and efforts of the first attempt. At six years, and then at nine years, this policy required review, and this narrative explains how we proceeded with the venture.

The initial policy guideline was presented to and passed by the hospital board and distributed in August of 1989. (Although it took a year to draft it carefully, we were naive in our expectation of its acceptance. The program for its introduction was inadequate.) It outlined conditions of ill health where an attending physician's decision that a patient should not be resuscitated would be clinically appropriate and ethically acceptable.

The physician was to assess the patient and write a clear statement of prognosis in the progress notes of the chart specifically when resuscitation would not be medically indicated. It was also agreed that this process was to be repeated should the prognosis of the patient change. The not-to-resuscitate order was also to be written on the doctor's order sheet. It was stressed "that all necessary measures be taken to assure the physical, mental and spiritual comfort of the patient." Patients were categorized into four groups: the majority who were expect to be successfully treated and leave the hospital; those where an expected outcome was not known, but a presumption must be made in favor of life support; those with a hopeless short-term prognosis, not expected to leave the hospital alive; and a large number of cases that did not clearly fall into the above categories, (especially those patients with chronic and debilitating mental or physical illnesses). It was also pointed out that if a mentally competent patient had indicated instructions in a "living will" that he/she did not wish to be resuscitated, these instructions should be considered. However, at that time, there was little experience in Canada regarding living wills, and therefore an uncertainty as to how to proceed. It was explained that patients falling into the first two categories above should have resuscitative measures instituted immediately, but it was also clearly stated that there was no legal or moral imperative to provide treatment to those not expected to live (the third category). If a concern arose about the prognosis, physicians were encouraged to obtain an independent second opinion, and patients and their families were always to be advised of any decision regarding resuscitation. For mentally incompetent patients, a process was established so that surrogate decision-making was available, and there now has been enacted an Adult Guardianship Law in the Province. Physicians were encouraged to take the time to discuss the reasons for the decision about resuscitation with the other hospital health care staff.

Over the succeeding years, although the categorization of patients and indications for resuscitation appeared reasonably clear, it was found that very limited discussion was taking place at the bedside, and very few specific orders were being written. There were reports by nurses that unwarranted resuscitative procedures were being undertaken frequently. Because of these concerns, a task force to readdress the issue was formed in 1995, and over the following year it reviewed local outcomes and the relevant medical and ethical literature and eventually revised the policy.

The review was chaired by the Vice-President of Medicine who was a long-standing member of the ethics committee. The working group consisted of several members of the ethics committee, including our senior ethicist, representatives from the hospital wards, and the office of the Ombudsman of the Province of British Columbia. In order to try to understand the lack of compliance by physicians, decisions were made to review our institutional success with resuscitation, to review recent evidence-based articles on the subject, and to widely canvass hospital staff. A number of focus groups were held throughout the hospital so that unique issues could be addressed from the various constituencies. Universally, it was clear that there was an obligation felt by the nursing staff to commence cardiopulmonary resuscitation (CPR) when a patient apparently died, unless there was a "Do Not Attempt Resuscitation" (DNAR) written order. Physicians had frequently expressed their discomfort and reluctance to write such orders, and the nursing staff felt that the natural outcome was that CPR attempts were being made in inappropriate circumstances.

The literature reviews regarding CPR showed that since the procedure had primarily been developed to deal with acute cardiac events, not surprisingly this was the major area in which there was a reasonable although modest chance of success.[1] Both the reports in the literature and our own internal review showed that the success rate of CPR in patients who sustained cardiac arrest due to a primary cardiac event was about 20%. When the cardiac arrest occurred in a patient with cancer, the overall success rate was 5.8%, and in the context of metastatic cancer not one of our patients survived of the more-than 100 treated. Similar studies done on patients with severe infection showed only a 5% positive response. The literature also indicated that certain risk factors were directly related to the eventual chances of success or failure of CPR at the time of "death."[2] Those conveying independent, but negative impact on the success included: age, malignancy, pneumonia, kidney failure, high blood pressure, angina, infection, heart failure, coma, liver disease, stroke, and severe lung disease. It was an extreme rarity for any patient to survive CPR if his/her death was not witnessed. The other important differentiating cardiac factor was whether there was asystole (the heart stops beating completely), or whether there was ineffective action (fibrillation). When there was no heart action, survival was a rarity. Also, resuscitative attempts with arrhythmias lasting longer than 20 minutes were associated with an extremely poor outcome. Complications of CPR itself were also noted, and these included fracture of the breastbone and ribs. There was also evidence of potential lasting brain damage following attempts at resuscitation, even if the cardiac status was restored.

Among the negative emotional and ethical issues reported were the discomfort of family and friends, especially in matters related to the patient's dignity, privacy, and spirituality. There was also palpable unease of the staff when they were trapped into applying a therapy that they felt best withheld. In this context, the question often arose as to whether the resources of the hospital could be better spent on palliative and other support care.

The revised report stated at the outset that there were conditions of ill health where an attending physician's decision not to attempt to resuscitate was both clinically appropriate and ethically acceptable. There is reference to the negative factors cited above. A decision not to attempt resuscitation meant the acceptance of death without intervention, if and when it might occur, but did not imply a restriction on any other useful form of treatment.

During the course of the review, other related issues surfaced, which caused further revisions. There were continuing tensions related to matters of patient autonomy and physician responsibility. It appeared necessary to reaffirm the view that no physician was obligated to provide a course of therapy such as resuscitation that he or she considered contraindicated. On the contrary, a physician's first obligation was to do no harm unless in the pursuit of a clearly desirable outcome. This position was supported legally by the Manitoba Court of Appeal (December 1997).[3] Popular television had contributed to this dispute with its overly optimistic portrayal of heroic-treatment outcomes.[4] There were also problems related to the incompetent patient in terms of what was considered a "best interest" versus a "substituted judgement." The task force's opinion was that for the incompetent patient the "best interest judgement" was most appropriate. And finally, many physicians continued to express difficulty not responding actively to iatrogenic events, even when the patient had already indicated a preference for no CPR. There was a recent heated and unresolved debate on this topic in *The New England Journal of Medicine*.[5]

As our committee was preparing its report, the Canadian Medical Association (CMA) published in 1996 its most current position on CPR, and in it recognized many of these same difficulties. The CMA encouraged health care facilities to make use of interdisciplinary committees with access to legal and ethical consultation to develop such policies and programs for their implementation. The CMA guideline writer, John Williams, noted that historically "it has been interpreted to mean that unless there is a written DNAR order, resuscitation has to be attempted, no matter how futile it appears to be."[6] He went on to say that the main feature distinguishing the revised CMA statement (October 1994) compared with the original one of 1984 was "that it changes the prevailing view of resuscitation as an intervention which will be undertaken unless there is a DNAR order. Resuscitation interventions are now considered to be like all other medical treatments—they will be undertaken in some situations but not in others." He went on to say "a second distinguishing feature of the revised policy is that it is not restricted to terminally ill patients."[7] The new statement did away in a sense with DNAR orders and replaced them with notations on the patients' charts that resuscitation is or is not indicated. The CMA was working toward a principle where an order to resuscitate needed to be written, rather than the lack of a DNAR order's resulting in automatic resuscitation.

In the introduction of the newly formulated guidelines it was stated that "many physicians and nurses experience, at present, a large gap between what they feel they should do and what they feel they are obliged to do for patients at the end of life. These policy guidelines are intended to help physicians and other care providers make appropriate decisions and to have them feel strongly supported by the hospital community in making the appropriate decisions. It is emphasized that a decision not to attempt resuscitation means the acceptance, without intervention, of death if and when it occurs, and does not imply a restriction of any other potential form of treatment unless specified." The term DNAR was changed to DNACPR—do not attempt cardiopulmonary resuscitation—in order to avoid confusion between CPR and other forms of supportive therapy. It was recommended that a DNACPR order should be included in the management of a patient having compassionate terminal care and that this order must not affect the provision of any other form of treatment or care that was appropriate. Direction was given to encourage discussion of these matters with competent patients and their families and to deal with incompetent patients appropriately. It was also noted "that there was no legal or ethical obligation for a physician to offer CPR to a patient if this would result in a course of action deemed to be contrary to the patient's best interest."

A number of other points were clarified. Orders were to be written by a licensed physician, and a resident or other trainee could not do so unless there was full knowledge and agreement by the attending physician. In reference to the use of advanced directives, it was now agreed that these should be obeyed by the health care providers. This reflected a change in common practice over the six-year period. Another suggestion was that if disagreement arose between members of the health care team on any major aspects of care, an ethics consultation should be considered. The ethics committee discussed at length the question about whether the current "reverse onus policy" was appropriate. It was recognized that CPR was the only form of treatment in the entire field of medical care in which a written order is required in order for treatment not to be provided. The prevailing view of our committee in 1996 was that it was not desirable in our hospital setting to write the order "resuscitate if required," as was suggested by the CMA. The guideline placed clear responsibility on the physician to actually write the DNACPR order, and stated that it was unethical for a physician not to do so when appropriate. It was recognized that honest and open communication between the physician, patient, family, and the rest of the health care team would be critical in ensuring that these difficult orders would be appropriately written, interpreted and carried out.

In order to implement these guidelines throughout the hospital an active strategy was established to circulate the information to all attending members of the medical staff and to the medical and administrative heads of all functioning areas. Each department and division was asked to meet and discuss the new guidelines. Members of the task force and the ethics committee were available as resource persons, and offered to assist practitioners who expressed difficulty understanding or complying with the guidelines. The public affairs office in the hospital produced a pamphlet in order to inform patients and the public about these new guidelines, and it was translated into several languages. The resuscitation team of the hospital had participated in the guideline development and agreed to provide the clinical data for an outcome evaluation. The second review of the matter was concluded in 1999. It was disappointing in that it revealed much the same number of unwarranted resuscitation attempts and little progress in convincing physicians to write clear orders. However, many more of the hospital staff and patients were aware of the situation and more discussions were taking place. These findings have been circulated again to the staff with emphasis on the poor procedure outcome results.

Although the DNACPR policy was the most prominent, other reviews and guideline development were undertaken at the request of committee members, hospital units, or administration. In the early years, matters related to informed consent were of major concern. One particular issue that arose was related to the need for consent for HIV testing purposes, since there never had been a requirement for a consent for any laboratory test. It was felt that this particular issue was so sensitive that formal consent should be written. This policy was instituted in 1990 and initial evaluation showed good compliance.

As our institution incorporated more chronic-care beds, the number of cases requiring evaluation for cessation of therapy increased, especially for severely neurologically damaged patients. As there had never been a formal policy or procedure in place, a proposal was made to incorporate surrogate input into the decision-making process with the care team. After a guarded neurologic prognosis was rendered for stroke or head-injured patients, the approach was to map out a treatment plan with staged temporal evaluations. If no objective improvement was noted, then a decision to withdraw tube feeding and other support could then be better understood and accepted.[8] Other unique problems might arise in chronically ill person. Recently, an opinion was rendered by the ethics committee to deny the request of a high-level quadriplegic to drink by straw, because of the potential for aspiration.

As the ethics committee became more accepted within the hospital, new and controversial topics were presented to it. The group has been asked to render suggestions regarding the implementation of stereotactic brain surgery to manage otherwise uncontrollable severe mental illness. Our forum was able to provide the milieu for discussion of this rather sensitive area, as brain surgery for psychological problems had been abandoned in Canada for thirty years. Another concern for hospital administration was the problem of caring for foreign patients temporarily residing in Canada, as our universal health care system basically addresses the needs of Canadian residents only, and itself is in financial turmoil. The ethics committee underscored the concept that emergency care must be offered to all, but that our limited resources should be reserved primarily for residents, and only in very unusual circumstances should health care facilities be made available electively to others. Another very contentious issue raised for discussion has been the matter of managing patients with severe brain injury who have not as yet been declared "brain dead."[9] Under Canadian law should these patients progress to true brain death, they then would become potential organ donors. Within our institution there was considerable disagreement among the trauma surgeons, neurosurgeons, and ICU and emergency physicians as to the appropriate management of these people. The ICU staff frequently found themselves in the difficult situation of maintaining persons with no future, and found at times that their supportive measures resulted in rendering them in a persistent comatose state. The committee's opinion recommended against this type of "elective ventilation" because of the potential long-term harm to these injured patients and the ramifications that might be visited on their families. This debate now continues outside the confines of our committee, and is receiving broader attention through the BC Transplant Society and public forums.

EVOLUTION IN THE EDUCATIONAL MISSION

The committee members began with a modest ambition of self-education and the presentation of relevant cases at departmental rounds in the hospital. Because of our long-term connection with the Medical School, many of our members had already gained considerable experience teaching in undergraduate seminars. The Faculty of Medicine ethics office designed a problem-based case text for undergraduates, which was widely used by our members.[10] Subsequently, as university ties were established further through the Centre for Applied Ethics, we were able to share other scholarly activities such as graduate seminars and visiting academics. At least once yearly, a notable scholar in the field of ethics visits for a week at the Medical School and participates with the ethics committees of the major hospitals.

A senior nurse participated as a member of the ethics committee while she earned her doctoral degree in ethics. She was able to incorporate her experience into her dissertation and has subsequently become one of the two members of our consultative staff, as well as a lecturer at the University of Victoria.

As postgraduate specialty committees of the Royal College of Physicians and Surgeons of Canada have incorporated biomedical ethics as part of the core curriculum for all graduate programs, the demands on our members for teaching medical specialists have also increased considerably.

In response to the significant challenges presented by the reorganization of our regional health care system, our group felt that there was a need for a major focus on interdisciplinary and inter-institutional collaboration. Ethics programs are offered to students in the community in social work, pharmacy, nursing, audiology, speech language pathology, medicine, rehabilitation science, and nutrition science. To prepare a welcoming environment for these students, who are eager to work in interdisciplinary groups, our committee plans to continue the education of the workers currently in our health care institutions.[11] Meetings have brought together participants from acute and long-term care agencies in the region to review common goals and problems. The variety of interdisciplinary projects so far undertaken include protocols related to paraplegic and quadriplegic patients with pressure ulcers; special interventions with those living at risk during rehabilitation; and the ethical management of non-cooperative patients.

EVOLUTION OF CONSULTATIVE ACTIVITIES

For more than eight years the committee felt uneasy about its inability to provide adequate clinical consultation. Although able to find elective time for the development of guidelines and policies, most of the members found it extremely difficult to be available, on an urgent basis, to deal with patient problems on the wards. As well, many of the members felt somewhat inadequate to this responsibility and a great deal of the onus therefore fell on the shoulders of a willing, but overworked, voluntary member of our committee, our external ethics consultant, Dr. Alister Browne. After a consult was requested, he would organize an *ad hoc* team of one or two other members, usually with a clinical background, to review the case and assist him in the discussion with the staff, patient, and family. Comments and opinions were provided verbally or noted in the patient's record, but no formal consult was written. In 1994, the committee members issued a formal report to the hospital board and administration stating that they felt that this was not an appropriate way to continue because of the increasing complexity and numbers of consultations. It was recommended that an ethicist with special qualifications, including professional experience and special personal characteristics[12] be hired, at least on a part-time basis, to address the hospital's needs. In 1996 two such persons were hired: Dr. Browne, who had already provided much of the expertise, and Dr. Rosalie Starzomski, the nurse on our committee who had completed her Ph.D. thesis and was now teaching. These two remain as members of the ethics committee, and make two or three consults per week. This liaison has proved to be quite productive, as they are able to draw on members of the committee for clinical assistance and also alert the committee regarding the types of cases prevalent in the hospital. The consultants produced a pamphlet entitled *Ethics Resources Available at Vancouver General Hospital.* In it is a description of who provides the help, what type of help by consultation is available, as well as instructions on how to reach the consultants. Also included are references to previous guidelines developed and the type of educational programs available within the hospital. Their appointment and role was featured in publications addressed to all staff and the public. In each case, when consulted, they meet with an interdisciplinary group on the ward and the family as often as necessary, and ultimately generate a timely letter of opinion addressed to the attending physician.

An important observation made years ago during the consultations on the wards was that many problems arise primarily from miscommunication between staff members or between hospital staff, patients and their families. Often they were not problems of a truly ethical nature. Several examples should serve to illustrate this problem. In one case, a decision was made by the attending physician to treat a young stroke victim with a profound neurologic defect, and little chance of recovery, with hyperbaric oxygen. The family had read about this application and the physician agreed to a trial of therapy. The nurses on the unit felt that this was unproven therapy, that it might well deprive worthy cases of access to hyperbaric therapy, and really was research. The ethics committee representative acted as a catalyst, and in the course of the discussion the physician explained that he had considered this program as "desperate therapy," not as research, and that he had advised the family that this treatment would be stopped if, and when, needy cases arose. He had also arranged for an objective evaluation of the patient's condition on a stepwise basis over a period of time. The unfortunate part was that he had not explained this in any detail to the nursing staff; but once informed, they were satisfied with this approach. Another such event occurred when the family of a patient on a neurosurgical ward accused the staff of withdrawing supportive care. During the discussion it was revealed that the normal plan of staged changes of therapy during the prolonged recovery phase had not been clearly explained to the family or the patient. Once they realized that this was the standard method of caring for such patients, the family was satisfied.

THE CURRENT SITUATION

As stated in the introduction to this paper, the incorporation of our ethics committee and its program into the hospital environment has not been without obstacles. However, it is clear that some important advances have been made, especially in relationship to the policies crafted, and the adoption of the recommendation to employ formal ethics consultants. The committee views the current situation with professional staff readily available as the appropriate approach to the provision of consultation within our institution. The lack of more general acceptance of the DNACPR has been a disappointment. We have not relied on charismatic leadership, but our members individually have continued to hone their skills in ethical analysis and teaching, and our enthusiasm has spread to other institutions. We continue to promote the concept of the need to recognize an ethical component to the restructuring of our health care organizations in the community. On reviewing a recent commentary by Dr. Francoise Baylis regarding the principal issues that a modern hospital ethics committee should address,[13] I found with satisfaction that we have clearly made substantial inroads. In order to best capitalize on the resources of ethics talent in Vancouver, it now might be appropriate to develop a more regional ethics centre incorporating all or most of the hospital and university activities

ACKNOWLEDGMENTS

I wishes to acknowledge the assistance of Nomi Kaplan and Margaret Wilson in the preparation of this manuscript; and the support of my colleagues on the Ethics Committee as the inspiration for this paper.

NOTES AND REFERENCES

1. M.H. Ebell, "Prearrest Predictors of Survival Following In-Hospital Cardiopulmonary Resuscitation: A Meta-Analysis," *Journal of Family Practice*, Vol. 34 (1992), pp. 551–558
2. E.B. Cohn, M.D. Lefevre, P.R. Yarnold, M.J. Arron, and G.H. Martin, "Predicting Survival from In-Hospital CPR; Meta-Analysis and Validation of a Prediction Model," *Journal of General Internal Med.*, Vol. 8 (1993), pp. 347–353.
3. Manitoba Court of Appeal, Nov.14/97 *Child & Family Services of Central Manitoba v. R. Lavallee and S.L. Hay etc.*
4. S.J. Diem, J.D. Lantos and J.A. Tulsky, "Cardiopulmonary Resuscitation on Television: Miracles and Misinformation," *New England Journal of Medicine*, Vol. 338 (1996), pp. 1578–1582.
5. D. Casarett and L.F. Ross, "Overriding a Patient's Refusal of Treatment after an Iatrogenic Complication," *New England Journal of Medicine*, Vol. 338 (1997), pp. 1906–1907.
6. J.R. Williams, "How is the New Statement on Resuscitative Interventions Different from the Original?," *Can.adian Med. Assoc. J.*, Vol. 151 (1994), pp. 1182-1183.
7. H. Brody, M.L. Campbell, K. Faber-Langendoen and K.S. Ogle, "Withdrawing intensive life-sustaining treatment: Recommendations for compassionate clinical management," *New England Journal of Medicine*, Vol. 336 (1997), pp. 652–657.
8. D.P. Price, " Organ Transplant Initiatives: The Twilight Zone," *Journal of Medical Ethics*, Vol. 23 (1997), pp. 170–175.
9. A. Browne and V.P. Sweeney, *Biomedical Ethics, Syllabus*, publication of the Division of Health Care Ethics, University of British Columbia, 1997 (personal communication).
10. A. Browne, M. Burgess, G. Growe *et al.*, "Charting a New Course for Interdisciplinary Collaboration," Abstract and Presentation, Canadian Bioethics Society 9th Annual Conference (October 1997).
11. F. Baylis, *A Profile of the Health Care Ethics Consultant: From the Health Care Ethics Consultant* (Clifton, NJ: Humana Press, 1994).
12. F. Baylis, *Standards for Acute Care Organisations: A Client-Centred Approach* (Canadian Council on Health Services Accreditation, 1995).
13. Manitoba Court of Appeal, Nov.14/97 *Child & Family Services of Central Manitoba v. R. Lavallee and S.L. Hay etc.*

Developments in Abortion Laws
Comparative and International Perspectives

REBECCA J. COOK

Faculty of Law, University of Toronto, Toronto, Ontario, Canada M5S 2C5

INTRODUCTION

The historical Anglo-Saxon Common Law treated abortion as an offence, but considered pregnancy to begin only when it was first evidenced through "quickening." This evidence became available at a time that coincides in general with the end of the first trimester and beginning of the second trimester of pregnancy, that is, at about the twelfth or thirteenth week of gestation. Accordingly, a woman's absence of a single or two consecutive menstrual periods was not legal evidence of pregnancy, notwithstanding any medical practice to measure the length of gestation from the beginning of the last menstrual period.[1]

English law on abortion changed in 1803, when legislation was enacted making abortion before quickening a crime, although not punished as severely as the performance of abortion after quickening. The purpose of the Act was to deter action taken upon women, by administration of "any deadly Poison, or other noxious and destructive Substance or Thing with intent to procure miscarriage," because of injuries and deaths that women suffered through such interventions. The Act probably also applied to women attempting their own abortions. Following statutory amendments in 1828 and 1837, the offence of abortion was incorporated in the Offences Against the Person Act, 1861, section 58 of which became the foundation of the abortion prohibition in many jurisdictions of the Common Law world. The section provides that

> every woman, being with child, who, with intent to procure her own miscarriage, shall unlawfully administer to herself any poison or other noxious thing, or shall unlawfully use any instrument or other means whatsoever with the like intent and whosoever, with intent to procure the miscarriage of any woman whether she be or be not with child, shall unlawfully administer to her or cause to be taken by her any poison or other noxious thing, or shall unlawfully use any instrument or other means whatsoever with the like intent, shall be guilty of felony.

Of the several significant developments in the understanding of this law, three warrant special attention. First, in 1869, the Roman Catholic Church redefined the mortal sin of abortion to apply not simply from quickening, as before, but from conception. This reinforced the secular criminal law with religious support, and made defense of the criminal law a matter of concern to religious interests and institutions. Second, in 1938 in the celebrated *Bourne*[2] case it was judicially determined that the crime of acting "unlawfully" was not committed when pregnancy was terminated in order to preserve the life or enduring health of the woman acted upon. Third, in 1973 the United States Supreme Court, in *Roe v. Wade*,[3] reverted to the law that existed at the time the United States Constitution was drafted at the end of the eighteenth century, and held that later legislation restricting abortion before the second trimester, that is, before the historical time of quickening, violated women's constitutional rights and was subject to judicial scrutiny.

These three developments are of contemporary significance to comparative and international development of abortion law. First, much argument about the role of abortion law is influenced by religious convictions. Many supporters of restrictive criminal legislation are unmoved by evidence of its practical dysfunctions and consequent cost of women's lives and health, because they consider the law essential to the prevalence of a moral order based on religious principles. Second, criminal legislation punishing abortion does not apply to interventions to preserve women's lives or health, but affords physicians a defense when prosecuted. In practice, restrictive laws often operate to the detriment of women, however, because they deter medically indicated procedures of benefit to women's health by exposing physicians to liability to prosecution. Third, the trimester approach to legal control of abortion continues to commend itself to popular support and legal reform, in that democratic voters and legislators often accept that medical termination of early pregnancy requires less regulation and control, in the interests both of developing fetuses and women, than do interventions later in pregnancy.

Legal developments in the last decade reflect the historical concern of early English legislation with health, in that laws addressing the crime and punishment of abortion have been moderated to take account of the need for the health and welfare of pregnant women. Further developments have placed women's entitlements to promotion of their health and welfare in the wider setting of respect for women's human rights to self-determination, in matters of reproduction and other choices in life including, but beyond, motherhood. Nevertheless, legal principles concerning crime, fetal interests, the health of women and existing children and respect for human rights remain interwoven.

Different balances of these components are reflected in legislation, judicial interpretations of prevailing laws and constitutions, and proposals for legislative reform. Legal reform and understanding of existing law are increasingly responsive to empirical findings from epidemiologic and related studies in social and health science, for example, on maternal mortality associated with high-risk pregnancy and unsafe abortion. For instance, a liberal abortion law enacted in Guyana in 1995 emphasizing women's health responded to evidence of high rates of abortion-related mortality under the previous restrictive law. In 1988, the Supreme Court of Canada similarly held a restrictive criminal abortion law unconstitutional for impinging on women's health care by denying them in practice access to legal services the legislation offered only in theory. In contrast, constitutional interpretation in Poland in 1997 has negated a liberal abortion law directed to women's health in favor of fetal interests held to have constitutional protection over women's interests.

CRIME AND PUNISHMENT

In the Anglo-Saxon Common Law tradition, practices are permissible unless a prosecutor or plaintiff shows them to be in violation of a prohibitive provision. Accordingly, therapeutic abortion is legally permissible, and enacted law will express only criminal prohibitions, punishing behavior that is undertaken "unlawfully." Written law will emphasize crime and punishment, but the scope of lawful abortion remains unwritten and interpretable by the courts, the definition of crime being read to punish as little as necessary to achieve the purpose of the written Act. In systems of codified law, where all rights must be contained within the framework of the code, abortion has tended to be addressed through penal or criminal codes rather than through codes that codify rights of access to health services or that define rights of medical practice. Thus, the modern history of abortion law has emphasized the criminal nature of the practice and the punishment of those who perform it and of women who request its performance. It has been seen above that the criminal provisions of secular law are frequently invoked to support religious values inherent in unborn life.

Constitutional laws have been brought into play in contests over the scope of permissible abortion by inclusion of declarations that protected human life begins at conception. Some constitutions include explicit language to this effect, and others have been judicially interpreted to contain a similar finding. Further, both constitutional and regular courts have on some occasions found that the constitutionally protected interests of unborn life prevail over the interests of pregnant women in reproductive self-determination, life-style and social choices, and even health except where ill-health endangers life itself. Courts have accordingly upheld criminal prohibitions of resort to abortion, and struck down as unconstitutional laws that remove criminal sanctions from abortion undertaken for non-therapeutic reasons.

In Poland, for instance, the Constitutional Tribunal ruled in May 1997 (K 26/96) that a liberalizing abortion law of 1996 on family planning, human embryo protection, and legal conditions for pregnancy termination was incompatible with constitutional provisions that the Tribunal found to protect human life in every phase of its development. The Court emphasized that the phase of development of human life commenced at conception, and that, while women's lives could be constitutionally protected against fetal life when endangered by continuation of pregnancy, abortion could not be permitted on such vague grounds as a woman's difficult life conditions or difficult personal situation. The Tribunal found a constitutionally imposed duty of motherhood and family protection, and that the constitutional interests of unborn human life could not be at the disposal of vague criteria of women's conditions or situations, particularly when such conditions or situations were to be determined, as the previous law provided, by women themselves. The Tribunal made no specific reference to religious or spiritual principles, but the assumption of the protection of such values in the Constitution pervades the ruling. No attention was given to competing interests of unborn human life and the lives of born children dependent on the pregnant woman's health and welfare.

The Constitutional Court of Colombia upheld the right of a couple to decide the number of their children, but in a 1994 decision (C-133/94) held that the right was not infringed by the criminalization of abortion because the right can be exercised, for example, by contraceptive means, only until the moment of conception. The decision upheld the constitutionality of the criminalization of abortion under Colombia's 1991 Constitution.

In a decision of January 1997 (C-013/97), the Constitutional Court also upheld the constitutionality of a provision setting a lesser punishment for abortion in cases of pregnancy resulting from rape (and non-consensual artificial insemination), but cited two encyclicals of Popes Paul VI and John Paul II to endorse the constitutional protection of human life, both born and unborn. However, a concurring judge recognized constitutional power to decriminalize abortion entirely, and three dissenting judges considered criminalization of abortion not to be constitutionally protected under the prevailing law, pointing out the constitutional obligation of religious pluralism and that parents' rights to decide the number of their children could not be removed from them constitutionally by the act of a rapist. Nevertheless, the majority of the Court relied on the religiously framed sanctity of unborn human life to support the constitutionality of the criminal abortion law.

A number of jurisdictions have amended criminal legislation to accept rape as a lawful indication for abortion. However, experience in some countries, such as Pakistan, shows that provisions of this nature can operate so harmfully to women's interests as to constitute a powerful deterrent not only to abortion, but to exposing rape itself. Islamic law as interpreted in Pakistan contains demanding evidentiary requirements for proof of rape, such as multiple witnesses to the alleged act of non-consensual intercourse. A woman who complains that the intercourse in which she was involved was involuntary on her part, but who cannot satisfy the evidentiary requirements of rape, is herself convictable of fornication or adultery, since she has admitted that intercourse occurred but cannot show that it was a rape committed against her. Accordingly, when women have complained that they were raped, for instance by prison guards or police officers, they have become liable to criminal conviction and punishment for adultery or fornication.[4]

How far states are willing to go to enforce the prohibition of abortion under criminal law is shown in Nepal. In this country, a woman's attempt to terminate her own pregnancy is punishable with up to life imprisonment, and it has been reported that many women are charged, convicted and often imprisoned for some length of time for this offence.[5] In contrast, most legal systems provide a lesser punishment for women acting on themselves than for those who act upon them, and in practice women are often given immunities from prosecution in exchange for their testimony against illegal practitioners of abortion. Immunity is justified when women are entitled to lawful termination of pregnancy on therapeutic grounds, but cannot avail themselves of lawful services because of their practical unavailability or prohibitive cost.

Willingness to prosecute is clearly influenced by governmental philosophies and policies. For instance, in Chile in the early 1980s, the Pinochet regime made it national policy to suppress any activities and services that reduced population growth and, in collaboration with fundamentalist Roman Catholics, applied the law against even therapeutic procedures. At this time, an estimated 1,000 prosecutions per year were reported against women having abortions, many following reports to police from hospitals to which women had gone for treatment for abortion-related complications. Many of the women were young, poor, unmarried, rural immigrants to larger cities and pregnant following rape. In 1983, 15 out of 230 women sentenced to imprisonment (6%) were convicted on abortion charges. However, the subsequent administration was more hesitant to press abortion charges and seek imprisonment. In 1993, 10 of 423 women sent to prison (2.4%) were convicted on abortion charges. In 1984, the Santiago Court of Appeals heard 197 abortion cases, but by 1991 the number had dropped to 45.[6] Nevertheless, by reference to most other countries, Chilean statistics of prosecutions of women on abortion charges remain unusually high.

The threat of criminal proceedings against women who have abortions and against physicians and others who perform such procedures may be contrasted in several countries with the absence of threat of criminal prosecution against men who violate women and cause pregnancies women want to terminate. Criminal laws against abortion do not invariably permit lawful procedures when pregnancy follows rape. For instance, the majority of judges in the Constitutional Court of Colombia invoked the innocence of the conceived embryo or fetus as the reason why its life should be protected even when created as a consequence of a criminal offence. Where abortion is lawful when resulting from rape, criminal procedure may require the rape victim's immediate complaint and compelling evidence that intercourse was non-consensual. Women who are terrified and ashamed may not complain, and be fearful to complain against men who have authority over their lives or in their communities. Further, police may be slow to follow complaints, particularly against authoritative officers, such as their colleagues.

Patients attending physicians for medical care are entitled to confidentiality in accordance with longstanding ethics of medical practice. Confidentiality is particularly important for patients seeking treatment of an intimate or sensitive nature. Ordinarily, patients' rights of confidentiality prevail even over the public interest in the due administration of justice. Physicians are not obliged to initiate reports to police or other law enforcement authorities of evidence they have gained of crimes committed by their patients. However, physicians may be entitled, in the interests of patients' protection, to initiate reports of crimes committed against their patients, such as sexual assault and domestic violence.

In particular cases, legislation compels physicians to report abuse of their patients, such as abuse of children and of elderly and intellectually disabled patients. However, where legislation does not require reporting, courts may decide not to punish physicians who disclose crimes that their patients have committed, particularly where public order and morality seemed to be involved. For instance, in Argentina in 1998, the Supreme Court of the Province of Sante Fe held that a gynecologist was entitled to breach professional confidentiality and to inform authorities that a patient seeking treatment for complications arising from abortion may have initiated the procedure unlawfully.[7]

Illegal abortion raises difficult issues of public policy and of professional and personal ethics for physicians. Unskilled practitioners risk serious harm and death of women they treat, but since the women themselves request such practitioners' services, they are parties to their crimes. Further, where illegal practitioners are not identifiable, the only prosecuted parties may be patients who sought the medical help of doctors who were willing to inform the police.

Some countries, such as Mexico, provide no facilities through which women entitled to terminate pregnancies resulting from rape can avail themselves of lawful procedures.[8] In other countries, provisions allowing for abortion in the case of rape are rarely used or, worse, are misapplied. Under criminally restrictive laws, minor and complex exceptions are liable to be misunderstood, misapplied, and applicable only under compelling, uncontested evidentiary standards, affording judges factual grounds, which are not appealable, to find that conditions of the exceptions are not satisfied. For instance in Bolivia, an eleven year-old girl, raped by her stepfather, who was subsequently imprisoned, was denied an abortion despite the fact that Article 266 of the Penal Code does not punish abortion performed as a consequence of rape. Judicial approval for abortion was requested not on the ground of rape, but on the ground of pregnancy's being a danger to the young victim's physical and mental health, on which the medical evidence proved inconclusive.[9] Persuasive legal evidence is particularly difficult to show concerning abortion requested on grounds of rape, where determination of intercourse itself and of the complainant's consent are often contested, and on grounds of physical and psychological danger to pregnant women, where medical prognoses of continuation of pregnancy may differ.

In contrast to the lack of application of the law in Mexico and its misapplication in Bolivia, a women's health advocacy group in Brazil has developed collaborative arrangements with the police to investigate rape complaints and provide timely access to abortion services in legally justifiable cases, where the evidence of sexual aggression is persuasive.[10]

In light of the many health, social ,and legal dysfunctions associated with criminal abortion laws, the 187 governments that adopted the Platform for Action resulting from the United Nations Fourth World Conference on Women, held in Beijing in 1995, have committed themselves to consider "reviewing laws containing punitive measures against women who have undergone illegal abortions."[11] This commitment governs not only women acting alone to terminate their pregnancies, but also women who are chargeable in principle for inciting, aiding, or abetting offences for which others may be charged who act unlawfully with intent to terminate the women's pregnancies.

HEALTH AND WELFARE

Modern thinking on abortion law reform directs legislation away from a primary concern with criminalization and punishment towards the protection and promotion of women's health. Although many historical criminal laws accommodated therapeutic abortion, the procedure remains stigmatized, and medical schools give little if any training in performance of procedures except, perhaps, management of incomplete and septic abortion as emergency care. On pragmatic grounds, however, health officials concerned with high rates of emergency hospital admissions for complications of unskilled abortion attempts have come to recognize the need for the safe conduct of therapeutic procedures. However, where laws explicitly provide for medical conduct of therapeutic abortions, meaning procedures indicated by danger to women's lives or permanent health from continuation of pregnancy, they frequently require prior approval by several doctors, including specialists, through cumbersome procedures that in practice make services unavailable or seriously delayed.

In 1988, the Supreme Court of Canada reviewed availability of services that complied with restrictive Criminal Code provisions, which limited hospitals that were eligible to perform procedures and required approval by hospital therapeutic abortion committees. The Court noted that no hospital or health service facility had any duty to establish such a committee, thus confining service availability to eligible hospitals that had such committees. The Court found that abortion services indicated on health grounds were so inequitably restricted and so delayed as to deny women their right to health services and therefore to security of the person guaranteed by the Constitution, and struck down the restrictive Criminal Code provision as unconstitutional.[12]

The Guyana Medical Termination of Pregnancy Act 1995 is expressly based on women's needs for safe health services. The long title of the Act is that it is an Act to reform the law relating to medical terminations of pregnancies, to enhance the dignity and sanctity of life by reducing the incidence of induced abortion, to enhance the attainment of safe motherhood by eliminating deaths and complications due to unsafe abortion, [and] to prescribe those circumstances in which any woman who voluntarily and in good faith wishes to terminate her pregnancy may lawfully do so ...

The Act does not explicitly allow "abortion on request," but permits termination of pregnancy of not more than 8 weeks' duration to be undertaken or supervised by a registered medical practitioner in, for instance, a doctor's office. Pregnancies of 8–12 weeks duration may be terminated only in institutions approved for the purpose, except in emergency.

Terminations of pregnancies of more than 12 weeks' but not more than 16 weeks' duration require opinions of two medical practitioners that there is risk to the pregnant woman's life or physical or mental health or of substantial risk that a child, if born, would suffer such physical or mental abnormalities as to be seriously handicapped. An alternative ground is that the pregnant woman is of unsound mind and not cable of taking care of an infant. The Act also accommodates lawful abortion on grounds of rape or incest, the pregnant woman's HIV-positive status, or clear evidence of use in good faith of a recognized contraceptive method by the pregnant woman or her partner. The assessment of risk of grave injury to the pregnant woman's health shall take into account "the pregnant woman's entire social and economic environment, whether actual or foreseeable" (sec. 6[2]). For termination of a pregnancy of more than 16 weeks' duration, the opinions of three medical practitioners must be obtained that the procedure is necessary to save the life of the woman or to prevent grave permanent injury to the physical or mental health of the woman or her unborn child.

Despite intensely animated and widespread debate about enactment of Guyana's 1995 law, at its enactment major hospitals in the country were found to be unprepared to implement its provisions, concerning the availability of clinical services and regulations for pre- and postabortion counseling for women and their partners.[13] Nevertheless, the 1995 Act reflects a new attitude towards abortion. Even advocates of liberal abortion legislation recognize that abortion usually indicates a failure of reproductive health education and care and, in common with opponents of liberal abortion laws, their goal is to minimize resort to the procedure. The contrast is that they favor improvement in reproductive health services by means of contraceptive counseling and services and improved sexuality education programs, for example, whereas many opponents of abortion law reform also oppose artificial means of contraception and sexuality education programs that include more than advocacy of sexual abstinence.

The health consequences of liberalized abortion laws, and the health costs to women of repressive abortion laws, are most clearly demonstrated in statistics from Romania. Legislation taking effect in 1990 reversed the severely repressive law of the former administration introduced in 1966. During the quarter century of pro-natalist policies, abortion-related maternal deaths per 100,000 live births rose from under 20 in 1965 to between 120 and 150 in 1982–1989. As a percentage of maternal deaths from all causes, abortion-related deaths rose from about 20% to nearly 90% and the rate of maternal mortality, which in 1966 was comparable to that of most other Eastern European countries, was at least 10 times higher than in any other European country by 1989.[14]

The Guyana 1995 law was the first enactment to advance the reproductive health goals of the Programme of Action adopted at the United Nations 1994 International Conference on Population and Development, held in Cairo. The Programme adopted a concept of reproductive health that was based on the World Health Organization concept of "health," but amplifies the implications of this concept across a full spectrum of reproductive health interests. The Cairo Programme looks to a future of reproductive health in which resort to abortion is minimized in consequence of access to a range of educational and clinical services that will enhance women's and couples' ability to achieve families of the size and timing of their choice. Reproductive health as described in the Cairo Programme is:

> a state of complete physical, mental and social well-being and is not merely the absence of disease or infirmity, in all matters relating to the reproductive system and to its functions and processes. Reproductive health therefore implies that people are able to have a satisfying and safe sex life and that they have the capability to reproduce and the freedom to decide if, when and how often to do so. Implicit in this last condition are the right of men and women to be informed and to have access to safe, effective, affordable and acceptable methods of family planning of their choice, as well as other methods of their choice for regulation of fertility which are not against the law, and the right of access to appropriate health-care services that will enable women to go safely through pregnancy and childbirth and provide couples with the best chance of having a healthy infant.[15]

No participant in the discussions in Cairo approved abortion as a desirable method of family planning, although many recognized that, as a necessary back-up service for contraceptive failure, it should be available in conditions of safety and dignity. The intense political lobbying surrounding adoption of the Cairo Programme precluded from its text specific reference to abortion and to expectations that subscribing countries would be required to change their laws. Accordingly, the expression relating to abortion is "other methods ... for regulation of fertility which are not against the law."

RIGHTS AND JUSTICE

The next stage of development in abortion law has been to take it beyond considerations of health towards transcending considerations of protection and promotion of human rights, particularly the human rights of women who for obvious physiological reasons bear the overwhelming burden of unplanned pregnancy and often confront restrictive abortion laws and policies. Movement to advance women's interests in reproductive health and self-determination was furthered in 1995 at the UN Fourth World Conference on Women, held in Beijing.

The Declaration and Platform for Action adopted by 187 UN member states in Beijing reaffirm the Cairo Programme definition of reproductive health, but place such health within a more comprehensive framework of women's interests. The Beijing Platform for Action declares that:

> [t]he human rights of women include their right to have control over and decide freely and responsibly on matters related to their sexuality, including sexual and reproductive health, free of coercion, discrimination and violence. Equal relationships between women and men in matters of sexual relations and reproduction, including full respect for the integrity of the person, require mutual respect, consent and shared responsibility for sexual behavior and its consequences.[16]

The Platform has wider potential to advance women's reproductive self-determination through the response it made to experiences in parts of the world where women have been raped in situations of armed and tribal conflict and "ethnic cleansing." The Platform condemns "torture ... sexual slavery, rape, sexual abuse and forced pregnancy."[17] The reference to forced pregnancy was to both forced initiation of pregnancy and forced continuation of pregnancy. Condemnation of forced pregnancy exposes women's coercion to continue pregnancies against their will, by criminal laws and other means, as analogous to rape and sexual abuse. This reconceptualization of legal denial of women's choice of abortion shows that restrictive laws and governmental policies can be as disrespectful of women's own wishes, interests, and bodily integrity as are rapists who enforce their will upon women to advance their own purposes.

In contrast, the Supreme Court of Canada found restrictive abortion laws unconstitutional because they denied women's fundamental rights. The then Chief Justice of Canada, Chief Justice Dickson, observed that:

> Forcing a woman, by threat of criminal sanction, to carry a foetus to term unless she meets certain criteria unrelated to her own priorities and aspirations, is a profound interference with a woman's body and thus a violation of security of the person.[18]

Respect for women's human rights compromised by restrictive abortion laws was shown in the response of the UN Human Rights Committee to the Report of the Government of Peru, submitted pursuant to its obligations under the International Covenant on Civil and Political Rights. The Committee monitors states' compliance with their obligations under the Covenant. In considering the Peruvian Report, the Committee addressed the human rights of women, including the rights denied them by the criminal abortion law of Peru.

In its Concluding Observations, the Committee expressed its concern "that abortion gives rise to a criminal penalty even if a woman is pregnant as a result of rape and that clandestine abortions are the main cause of maternal mortality."[19] The Committee found that the criminal law subjected women to inhumane treatment contrary to Article 7 of the Covenant. Moreover, the Committee explained that this aspect of the criminal law was possibly incompatible with Article 3, on equal entitlement of men and women to the enjoyment of the rights set forth in the Covenant, and Article 6, which protects the right to life.

The Committee recommended "that the necessary legal measures should be taken to ensure compliance with the obligations to respect and guarantee the rights recognized in the Covenant" and that "the provisions of the Civil and Penal Codes [of Peru] should be revised in the light of the obligations laid down in the Covenant," particularly Article 3 requiring that countries ensure respect of women's rights under the Covenant.[20]

As a result, Peru is responsible at least to require the medical profession to facilitate women's access to safe abortion and related health services as the law permits. Moreover, since prevailing law, which strictly penalizes abortion, was shown to result in inhumane treatment of women and undue maternal mortality, Peru is obliged to consider law reform so that the law encourages compliance with human rights standards for women's health and dignity. A new national policy would have to be established in new law that more adequately balances limitations on abortion with women's rights to safe and humane access to services for preservation of life, health, and dignity.

The Committee on the Elimination of Discrimination Against Women (CEDAW) was established to monitor state compliance with the Convention on the Elimination of All Forms of Discrimination Against Women (the Women's Convention). CEDAW members are persistent in their vigilance of country reports with regard to governmental obligations to protect and promote reproductive health and self-determination. CEDAW members question reporting governments and make Concluding Comments on their reports. For example, in making Concluding Comments on the Report of Morocco at its January 1997 meeting, the Committee:

> noted with concern the high rates of maternal mortality in Morocco, the high number of unattended births, the unavailability of safe abortion and the need to develop further reproductive and sexual health services, including family planning.[21]

At the same meeting, the Committee in its Concluding Comments on the Report of Saint Vincent and the Grenadines noted the "very high rate of pre-teen and teen-age pregnancy" and recommended improved reproductive health services and information for this age group. With regard to the Report of Turkey, it considered that the legal requirement that a woman obtain the authorization of her husband in order to have an abortion was a violation of her right, under the Women's Convention, to equality before the law. The Committee, in its Concluding Comments on the Report of Venezuela, noted with concern:

> the reduction of health budgets, the rise in the maternal mortality rate, the lack of and limited access to family-planning programmes (especially for teenagers), the lack of statistics on acquired immunodeficiency syndrome and women's limited access to public health services. In addition, legislation that criminalized abortion, even in cases of incest or rape, remain in force.[24]

Democratic reform in South Africa has been sensitive not only to international concerns with transcending human rights but also to the need for racial nondiscrimination in its new domestic environment. South Africa's approach to abortion law reform reflects experience in other countries, where it has long been recognized that socioeconomic elites and women associated with influential families in their communities have been immune from restrictive abortion laws, but that such laws have prejudiced the choice, health, and very lives of powerless women who are poor, young, and marginal to the societies in which they live.[25]

The Preamble to South Africa's Choice on Termination of Pregnancy Act, 1996, makes clear in its opening paragraph that the legislation was proposed:

> Recognizing the values of human dignity, the achievement of equality, security of the person, non-racialism and non-sexism, and the advancement of human rights and freedoms which underlie a democratic South Africa" (para. 1).

The Preamble similarly recognizes the constitutional right of persons "to make decisions concerning reproduction and to security in and control over their bodies" (para. 2), and that:

> ...the decision to have children is fundamental to women's physical, psychological and social health and that universal access to reproductive health care services includes family planning and contraception, termination of pregnancy, as well as sexuality education and counseling programs and services (para. 4).

The State accepted the responsibility to provide reproductive health to all, and safe conditions under which the right of choice can be exercised without fear or harm, while believing "that termination of pregnancy is not a form of contraception or population control" (para. 6). Accordingly, the new Act repeals:

> the restrictive and inaccessible provisions of the Abortion and Sterilization Act, 1975 ... and promotes reproductive rights and extends freedom of choice by affording every woman the right to choose whether to have an early, safe and legal termination of pregnancy according to her individual beliefs" (para. 7).

The 1996 Act makes termination of pregnancy legal upon a woman's request up to 12 weeks of pregnancy; up to 20 weeks on physical and mental health grounds, on socioeconomic grounds and in cases of rape or incest; and after 20 weeks if the woman's life is endangered, or there is a risk that the fetus is severely deformed. The Act enables registered midwives who have completed the prescribed training course to perform abortions up to 12 weeks (sec. 2[2]). The law does not require third-party authorizations for married women or minors. Medical practitioners or registered midwives shall advise pregnant minors to consult with parents, friends, or guardians, but the Act makes clear that services for termination of pregnancy cannot be denied because a minor chooses not to consult parents, guardians, or friends (sec. 5[3]).

To understand the human rights and social justice dimensions of the 1996 law, it has to be seen in the context of the law it repeals, the Abortion and Sterilization Act, 1975.[26] The 1975 law extended the previous grounds for abortion beyond saving the life of the pregnant woman to permitting abortion if there was a serious risk to the physical health of a woman or a danger of permanent damage to the woman's mental health, or serious risk of irreparable and serious handicap of the child if born, but did not permit abortion on social or economic grounds.

The 1975 Act required that the abortion be performed by a registered medical practitioner in a state-controlled or designated hospital (sec. 3[1] and 5[1]), and that the abortion be approved by three doctors (sec. 3). The performing doctor could not employ the two certifying doctors, and one of the two must have practiced medicine for at least four years (sec. 3[2][a] [1] and 3[3][a]). To qualify under the mental health exception, one of the two certifying doctors had to be a state psychiatrist (sec. 3[3] [b]).

To qualify under the rape or incest exception, approval had to be obtained both from the district surgeon who examined the patient on a report of the offence, and from a magistrate (sec. 3[3][c] and 6 [4] [1]). The magistrate had to certify that:

> (i) a complaint alleging unlawful carnal intercourse had been lodged with the police and, in cases where a complaint had not been lodged, that there was a good and acceptable reason why a complaint had not been so lodged;

and

> (ii) that on the balance of probabilities, the magistrate was satisfied that unlawful intercourse had taken place. (sec. 4[1][a][i]–[iii])

In the case of incest, the magistrate had to certify that the prohibited degree of relationship exists between the sexual partners, and the woman had to certify in an affidavit that unlawful carnal intercourse occurred (sec. 6 [4] [1] [b]).

Professor Charles Ngwena explains that these excessive certification procedures confined access to only socioeconomically advantaged women, citing a study conducted by the Medical Research Council explaining that an average of 800 to 1,200 women per year qualified for abortion under the old law. Of these women, 66% were white and from urban middle-class backgrounds, at a time when whites constituted only 16% of the general population. Professor Ngwena further explains that:

> according to official estimates, annually, upwards of 44,000 mainly black women had recourse to backstreet abortion, with the consequent toll on health and mortality. About 33,000 such women would require surgery to treat the residue of septic abortion,

with abortion-related deaths amounting to more than 400 a year.[27]

A South African anti-choice activist association sued the Minister of Health for a judicial declaration that the 1996 Act is unconstitutional. They argued that the life of a human being starts at conception and therefore is protected by section 11 of the 1996 South African Constitution, which states that "everyone has the right to life." The judge refused the declaration since "everyone" was a legal alternative expression to "every person," and on historic grounds legal personhood commences only at live birth.[28]

The judge did not find it necessary to address the claim regarding the biological beginning of human life, since he found that, even if it was correct, it did not justify the conclusion that the human life that had begun was that of a legal person. He adopted the observation that "the question is not whether the conceptus is human but whether it should be given the same legal protection as you and me."[29] The judge echoed many other courts that have addressed abortion interests in making clear that the judicial task is not to resolve conflicts about biological facts or spiritual values, but to make determinations of law, according to legal traditions and contexts, guided but not governed by social effects.

Evidence of injustice and human rights abuses from restrictive abortion laws can prove influential in judicial and democratic reform of such laws. In 1988, the Supreme Court of Canada was strongly influenced by evidence of a decade of continuing inequity in women's access to abortion when it was legally indicated on grounds of danger to their lives or health. In Ireland, public reaction against unsympathetic judicial obstruction of access to abortion services by abused young girls in highly publicized cases triggered intense political action for legislative liberalization, resulting in a referendum approving constitutional reform.[30] Similarly, public outrage in Bolivia against judicial denial of abortion for an eleven-year-old rape victim resulted in a legislative bill to ease application of enforcement of the restrictive Penal Code.[31]

CONCLUSION

Trends in abortion law reform show a transition away from reliance on criminal laws imposing liability to punishment, with only limited exceptions, where women's lives or enduring health were at risk, through laws prioritizing protection of women's health, to laws aimed at protecting human rights, including construction of families according to individuals' goals and aspirations. Criminal-based laws reflect a vision of male-ordered or patriarchal societies in which women's reproductive potential is molded to serve a public or religious agenda, and women's reproductive autonomy is considered subversive and a threat to public order and morality. Laws directed to health interests tend to be pragmatic or utilitarian, accepting separation of state functions from religion and addressing the damage to the health of women and families associated with resort to unsafe abortion. Laws serving human rights incorporate but transcend concerns with health, and recognize reproductive autonomy as a significant but not singular aspect of individual and family-based self-determination that is a central component of human dignity.

Modern evolution of abortion law associates repressive enforcement of repressive legislation with totalitarian governments, such as recently experienced in Chile and Romania, fearful that women's achievement of their reproductive choices would subvert governmental pronatalist policies, and indifferent to the impact of punitive measures on the lives of women and families. Legal approaches concerned to minimize harms to health from unplanned pregnancies accommodate abortion, but recognize how resourceful programs of sex education and family planning can reduce its incidence. Countries, such as South Africa, that have newly come to democracy based on an enfranchised electorate, where those who employ political power are accountable to the electorate, are taking initiatives to situate their abortion legislation within frameworks that invoke and implement human rights principles recognized at an international level.

There are, of course, established democracies whose abortion laws remain expressed primarily in restrictive, criminally focused terms. Movement towards legal reform is not universal, and remains strongly resisted within some democratic political establishments, particularly when reinforced by religious authorities that have no commitment to democratic reform of abortion laws. However, experience over the last three decades shows an emerging trend of liberalization, and over the most recent decade has shown further reform.[32] This has been at a slower rate, and in some countries is already facing a backlash. Nevertheless, recent evidence indicates more widespread international recognition that democratic advance is essentially incompatible with laws repressive of women's reproductive choice and self-determination.

Legislatures and judiciaries respectful of women's views, including those that hear women's opinions from within their own memberships, have molded legislation and its interpretation sympathetically to women's interests in health, and in observance of human rights. As state institutions, including legislatures and judiciaries, come to treat women as equal members with men in their societies, it may be anticipated that abortion concerns will evolve from placement within criminal or penal codes, to placement within health or public health legislation, and eventually to submergence within laws serving goals of human rights, justice, and dignity.

NOTES AND REFERENCES

1. B.M. Dickens, *Abortion and the Law* (London: Macgibbon and Kee, 1966), pp. 20–28.
2. *R. v. Bourne*, 1938. [1939] 1 King's Bench 687.
3. *Roe v. Wade*, Supreme Court Reporter, Vol. 93 (1973), pp. 703–763.
4. Human Rights Watch, *Double Jeopardy: Police Abuse of Women in Pakistan* (New York: Human Rights Watch, 1992), p. 53.
5. G. Ramaseshan, "Women Imprisoned for Abortion in Nepal: Report of a Forum Asia Fact-finding Mission," *Reproductive Health Matters*, Vol. 10 (1997), pp. 133–138; Nepal Women's Legal Service Project, *Report: Female Inmates of Prisons* (1989), p. 13.
6. L. Casas-Becerra, "Women Prosecuted and Imprisoned for Abortion in Chile," *Reproductive Health Matters*, Vol. 9 (1997), p. 30.
7. Insurralde, Mirta, T.148 PS. 357/428, Corte Suprema de la Provincia de Santa Fe, Argentina, August 2, 1998.

8. M. Acosta, "Overcoming the Discrimination of Women in Mexico: A Task for Sysiphus," in T*he Rule of Law and the Underprivileged in Latin America* (Indiana: Notre Dame University Press, 1998).
9. T.L. Monje and A.M. DeNicola, "Ignoring the Anguish," *Conscience*, XX (3) (1999), pp. 21–24.
10. J. Pitanguay & L.S. Garbayo, *Relatorio do Seminario a Implementacao do Aborto Legal no Servico Publico de Saude (Report of a Seminar on the Implementation of Legal Abortion with the Public Health Service)* (Rio de Janeiro, Brazil: Cicadania, Estudo, Pesquisa, Informacao e Acao, 1995).
11. United Nations, *Report of the Fourth World Conference on Women,* Doc. A/Conf.177/20 (New York: United Nations, 1995), para. 106(k).
12. *Morgentaler, Smoling and Scott v. The Queen*, Dominion Law Reports (1988), 4th. 44, pp. 385-500.
13. F.E. Nunes and Y.M. Delph, "Making Abortion Law Reform Work: Steps and Slips in Guyana," *Reproductive Health Matters*, Vol. 9 (1997), pp. 66–76.
14. P. Stephenson, *et al.*, "Public Health Consequences of Restricted Induced Abortion - Lessons from Roumania," *American Journal of Public Health*, Vol. 82 (1992), pp. 1328–1331.
15. United Nations, *Report of the International Conference on Population and Development*, Doc. A/Conf.171/13 (New York: United Nations, 1994), para. 7.2.
16. United Nations, *Report of the Fourth World Conference on Women,* Doc. A/Conf.177/20 (New York: United Nations, 1995), para. 96.
17. United Nations, *Report of the Fourth World Conference on Women*, Doc. A/Conf.177/20 (New York: United Nations, 1995), para. 135.
18. *Morgentaler, Smoling and Scott v. The Queen,* Dominion Law Reports (1988), 4th. 44, 402.
19. United Nations, *Report of the Human Rights Committee*, Doc. CCPR/C/79/Add.72 (1996), para. 15.
20. United Nations, *Report of the Human Rights Committee*, Doc. CCPR/C/79/Add.72 (1996), para. 22.
21. United Nations, *Report of the Committee on the Elimination of Discrimination Against Women,* Doc. A/52/38 (Part I), para. 68.
22. United Nations, *Report of the Committee on the Elimination of Discrimination Against Women,* Doc. A/52/38 (Part I) (1997), para. 147.
23. United Nations, *Report of the Committee on the Elimination of Discrimination Against Women,* Doc. A/52/38 (Part I), (1997), para. 184.
24. United Nations, *Report of the Committee on the Elimination of Discrimination Against Women,* Doc. A/52/38 (Part I) (1997), para. 236.
25. A. Jenkins, *Law for the Rich* (London: Victor Gollancz Ltd, 1961).
26. A.E. Haroz, "South Africa's 1996 Choice on Termination of Pregnancy Act: Expanding Choice and International Human Rights to Black South African Women," *Vanderbilt Journal of Transnational Law*, Vol. 30 (1997), pp. 879–883.
27. C. Ngwena, "South Africa's New Abortion Law: a Break with the Past," *IAB News: The Newsletter of the International Association of Bioethics,* Vol. 6 (1997), p. 4.
28. *Christian Lawyers Association of South Africa v. The Minister of Health*, Case No 16291/97, Transvaal Provincial Division, Judgment July 10, 1998
29. G. Williams "The Foetus and the Right to Life" (1994) 33 *Cambridge Law Journal* 71 at 78.
30. J. Kingston and A. Whelan, *Abortion and the Law* (Dublin: Round Hall Sweet and Maxwell, 1997), pp. 180–229.
31. T.L. Monje and A.M. DeNicola "Ignoring the Anguish," *Conscience,* XX (3) (1999), pp. 21–24.
32. R. J. Cook and B.M. Dickens, "A Decade of International Change in Abortion Law: 1967–1977," *American Journal of Public Health*, Vol. 68 (1978), pp. 637–644; R.J. Cook, and B.M. Dickens, "International Developments in Abortion Law: 1977–88," *American Journal of Public Health*, Vol. 78 (1988), pp. 1305–1311; R.J. Cook, B.M. Dickens, and L.E. Bliss, "International Developments in Abortion Law from 1988 to 1998," American Journal of Public Health, Vol. 89 (1999), pp. 579–586.

The Continuing Conflict between Sanctity of Life and Quality of Life

From Abortion to Medically Assisted Death

BERNARD M. DICKENS

Faculty of Law, University of Toronto, Toronto, Canada M5S 2C5

INTRODUCTION

As the twentieth century draws to a close, liberal laws on abortion have become settled in leading countries of the English-speaking world, and in many others beyond. The issue remains emotive, but in Britain, the Abortion Act 1967, although slightly amended by the Human Fertilisation and Embryology Act 1992, is substantially unchallenged. In the United States of America, the 1973 U.S. Supreme Court decision in *Roe v. Wade* (1973),[1] which found a constitutional right to abortion, has withstood the most concentrated move for reversal[2] and attempts to limit its scope tend to be indirect, such as through limitations on funding and provision of abortion services, and proposals to afford fetuses legal protection.[3] In Canada, the Supreme Court in 1988 declared the restrictive criminal law on abortion unconstitutional and inoperative[4] and no new criminal prohibition has been introduced there.

In contrast, legislative and judicial initiatives to allow medically assisted death have been few, and strongly opposed, despite a growing popular interest in and body of support for more liberal laws.[5] Legislation enacted in Australia's Northern Territory to permit such death[6] was promptly circumscribed as a prelude to its nullification. In the U.S. the Supreme Court has denied any fundamental right to assisted death[7] and Oregon voters' increasing approval of permissive legislation has been powerfully resisted. In Canada, a Special Senate Committee rejected adoption of permissive legislation in 1995[8] after the Supreme Court upheld criminalization of medically assisted suicide in 1993.[9] Nevertheless, there is growing momentum to review legal prohibitions, associated in part with apprehension of intrusive medical treatment and fears of indignity at life's end. Four Supreme Court of Canada judges favored legal accommodation of medically assisted suicide, and the majority of five were influenced by the absence of necessary safeguards against abuse such as provided in the Netherlands.[10]

Whether the trend towards liberalization of abortion laws will in time be followed by laws on medically assisted or induced death is a matter that engages, and troubles, many communities and interest groups in countries that have experienced abortion law reform. The issues of abortion and medically assisted death are linked,[11] in that many protagonists in the abortion debate confront each other similarly regarding assisted suicide and euthanasia, and legislators, judges, and commentators employ the reasoning and language heard in the conflict over abortion in argument over assisted death. The underlying difference between participants in both conflicts concerns attitudes towards the inherent sanctity of human life, which limits human intervention in the natural or divinely mandated processes of life and death, and towards the entitlement of human beings to exercise decisive control over these vital processes in order to regulate the quality of human and social experience and achieve a world of their own design.

The purpose of this paper is to address how analysts and commentators approach the relationship between abortion law and law governing medically assisted death, discussion of which is here limited to assisted suicide and voluntary active euthanasia. The issue of involuntary euthanasia or "mercy killing" of non-consenting persons is beyond the present discussion. This paper is further limited to English-language literature, and to legal experience and commentary primarily from the United States of America, Britain and Canada, although reactions to developments in the Netherlands are included. Attention will be directed initially to legal and related analysts and commentators who oppose legalization both of abortion and of medically assisted death, and who resist application of the reasoning that supported decriminalization of abortion to medically assisted death. They represent the so-called Pro-Life protagonists in the debate. Language is often employed instrumentally in the conduct of the disagreement, but the practice adopted here is to refer to protagonists by the titles they give themselves.

Second, attention will be given to adherents to the so-called pro-choice position, who favor both liberalized abortion laws and tolerance of medical means by which individuals may end their own lives when they find survival excessively painful, burdensome, or undignified. Consideration is then given to those who oppose liberal abortion laws, perhaps because of fetal vulnerability, but who consider that non-vulnerable, competent persons, such as terminal patients in unrelievable distress, should be legally entitled to assistance in dying. The reverse is then addressed, concerning those who favor women's choice on abortion, but oppose medically assisted death because, for instance, it may be exploitive of disabled patients or violative of ethical duties that health care professionals owe patients. In conclusion, it will be proposed that reconciliation of opposing views may be approached through promotion of choice, both to continue unplanned pregnancy and burdensome life, through availability of options that individuals may be encouraged and supported, but not coerced, to adopt.

OPPOSITION TO ABORTION AND MEDICALLY ASSISTED DEATH

Religious leaders and activists are prominent in movements that oppose both abortion and medically assisted death. Describing life as a divine creation and gift, both to the individuals who possess it and to their communities, they invoke principles of religious and natural law to protect human life before birth and before natural death. They tend to approve medical interventions for the prolongation of life and postponement of death, consistently with their vision of a divinely ordained mission to heal and to serve life, but they oppose legal acceptance of medical means deliberately intended to abbreviate life, even under a justification or excuse of ending unrelievable suffering. Both abortion and suicide are mortal sins in the doctrine of the Roman Catholic faith, and medical assistance for the purpose of either constitutes complicity that is comparably wrong.

A leading modern natural law theorist, Professor John Finnis of Oxford University, opposed legal accommodation of abortion,[12] referring to injustices that this exercise of women's autonomy inflicts on vulnerable, dependent "persons," whom he claims exist from conception,[13] and he opposes suicide and medically assisted death on the same ground. He asserts that:

> If one is really exercising autonomy in choosing to kill oneself, or in inviting or demanding that others assist one to do so, or themselves take steps to terminate one's life, one will be proceeding on one or both of two philosophically and morally erroneous judgments: (i) that human life in certain conditions or circumstances retains no intrinsic value and dignity; and/or (ii) that the world would be a better place if one's life were intentionally terminated. And each of these erroneous judgments has very grave implications for people who are in poor shape and/or whose existence creates serious burdens for others...
>
> The moral errors underlying claims to a right to assistance in suicide or to voluntary euthanasia are errors which do the most vulnerable members of our communities the great injustice of denying, in action, the true judgments on which depend both the acknowledgment of their dignity and their right to life (and so too all their other rights).[14]

The right to life is the human rights claim that inspires the Right to Life movement, which has developed beyond its historical anti-abortion thrust to oppose medically assisted suicide and euthanasia. In the U.S., the National Right to Life Committee has devoted considerable energy and resources to seek reversal of the 1973 U.S. Supreme Court judgment in *Roe v. Wade* that recognized a constitutionally protected right to abortion.[15] Its members were understandably dismayed when that judgment was not only substantially sustained in 1992,[16] but later applied by the Ninth Federal Circuit Court to recognize a right to assisted suicide. When the Supreme Court reaffirmed the *Roe* decision in 1992, General Counsel for the National Right to Life Committee, James Bopp, Jr., wrote that:

> If America does not gain a toehold on the slippery slope before reaching legal approval of assisted suicide, it should not be expected that the slide will stop at assisted suicide. The distance between assisted suicide and voluntary euthanasia (and even nonvoluntary euthanasia for persons who are incompetent) is even shorter than that between abortion and assisted suicide.[17]

In 1997, the U.S. Supreme Court reversed decisions of the Ninth Federal Circuit and Second Federal Circuit Courts of Appeals, respectively, that were sympathetic to medically assisted death.[18] The Court found that, while states may enact legislation that specifically permits such death, individuals who desire assisted death have no constitutionally protected right to demand or to obtain it. Reaction to the two Federal Circuit Courts of Appeals judgments that allowed medically assisted death included a vast outpouring of literature, particularly on suicide, the withdrawal of life-prolonging medical care, and the moral and legal difference between the two. For instance, a Jesuit law professor argued that the distinction between intentionally killing oneself and intentionally letting oneself die is coherent and morally relevant. The intention artificially to end one's life with intervention by a medical person who shares that intention was found distinguishable from the intention to forego life-sustaining medical care that the patient considers would not be personally beneficial, for example, by not relieving the patient's distress. The Supreme Court reversals were found to be consistent with this distinction in finding state laws constitutional that penalized assisted suicide.[19]

John Finnis agrees on the centrality of intention[20] and accepts the doctrine of double effect. By this doctrine, embraced by the Roman Catholic tradition, no culpability arises for foreseen harmful consequences of a deliberate act that is good in itself if it is undertaken only for another legitimate purpose and there is a proportionate reason for the harm,[21] such as administering drugs for relief of severe pain at a dosage that may in time prove toxic.[22] Finnis explains that:

> in common sense and law alike, there is a straightforward, non-artificial, substantive distinction between choosing to kill someone with drugs (administered over, say, three days in order not to arouse suspicion) in order to relieve them of their pain and suffering, and choosing to relieve someone of their pain by giving drugs, in a dosage determined by the drugs' capacity for pain relief, foreseeing that the drugs in that dosage will cause death in say three days. The former choice is legally and morally murder (in mitigating circumstances); the latter is not.[23]

Finnis also applies the description of murder, however, to the judgment of England's highest court, the House of Lords, in the case of Anthony Bland.[24] Bland suffered crushed and punctured lungs, resulting in prolonged loss of oxygen to his brain, which left him in an exceptionally severe persistent vegetative state and beyond any hope of recovery. He could breathe without assistance, but was dependent for survival on hospital care and on liquefied food pumped into his stomach through a nasogastric tube. After he had survived for about three years in this condition, an application was made by the hospital authority, with his family's concurrence, for discontinuation of tube feeding, which would result in his death. A majority of the judges upheld grant of the application. Lord Goff rejected any approval of euthanasia, but observed that:

> The question is not whether the doctor should take a course, which will kill his patient, or even take a course, which has the effect of accelerating his death. The question is whether the doctor should or should not continue to provide his patient with medical treatment or care which, if continued, will prolong his patient's life...the question is not whether it is in the best interests of the patient that he should die. The question is whether it is in the best interests of the patient that his life should be prolonged by the continuance of this form of medical treatment or care.[25]

The majority of judges found that prolongation of Anthony Bland's life by these means served none of his interests.

Lord Browne-Wilkinson addressed respect for the sanctity of human life, and questioned how it could be upheld when the quality of a patient's life is non-existent because he lacks and will never regain awareness of anything that happens to him. He noted that:

> On the moral issues raised by this case, society is not all of one mind. Although it is probably true that the majority would favour the withdrawal of life support in the present case, there is undoubtedly a substantial body of opinion that is strongly opposed. The evidence shows that the Roman Catholic church and orthodox Jews are opposed. Within the medical profession itself, there are those...who draw a distinction between withholding treatment on the one hand and withholding food and care on the other, the latter not being acceptable.[26]

Lord Browne-Wilkinson approved the key question in the case formulated by Lord Goff, and the answer that, since treatment by artificial feeding served no interest of the patient's, there was no legal duty to continue it and no legal liability for its termination. He remained concerned, however, about not only the moral status of his answer, but also its wider implications. He closed his judgment by stating:

Finally, the conclusion I have reached will appear to some to be almost irrational. How can it be lawful to allow a patient to die slowly, though painlessly, over a period of weeks from lack of food but unlawful to produce his immediate death by a lethal injection, thereby saving his family from yet another ordeal to add to the tragedy that has already struck them? I find it difficult to find a moral answer to that question. But it is undoubtedly the law and nothing I have said casts doubt on the proposition that the doing of a positive act with the intention of ending life is and remains murder.[27]

In his concern with the centrality of intention in the law, particularly the criminal law, Professor Finnis addresses not just intention as to the final outcome of conduct, but also intention or deliberation of the immediate conduct itself. He recognizes that judges in the case of Anthony Bland accepted that the applicant care-givers intended the patient to succumb to starvation, dehydration, or perhaps infection. He questions the merit of the judges' conclusion, however, that, by omitting to supply the patient with foods, liquids, or antibiotics on the ground that such care served no interest of the patient's, the doctors were safe from legal liability.[28] He finds that:

> Intentionally terminating life by omission—starving someone to death, or withholding their insulin, etc. etc.—is just as much murder as doing so by "deliberate intervention" ("commission," "active euthanasia"). Without squarely confronting the issue, at least a majority of the Law Lords in *Bland* [i.e., *Airedale*] slid, via a confused analysis of "duty of care," into a position tantamount to denying this implication of the significance of intention.[29]

By this analysis Professor Finnis, a leading natural law scholar of our day, repudiates as unreasonable the consequentialist or utilitarian reasoning that legitimated the death of Anthony Bland, who had expressed no wishes regarding his death. He rejects reasoning that, *a fortiori*, legitimates the deaths of conscious, competent patients who ask that life-sustaining means be withdrawn,[30] and that might legitimate their claim to medical assistance in suicide. The conviction Finnis holds that

> [a]s a general strategy of moral reasoning, utilitarianism or consequentialism is irrational[31]

also furnishes an attack upon and repudiation of much of the reasoning that supports women's moral and legal claims to abortion.

Judges in the House of Lords expressed their sympathy for Anthony Bland and their pity at the state into which he had fallen, but in recognizing the neurological damage that denied him any of the characteristics of present or future personality, they came close to denying his enduring personhood. The personhood of fetuses and embryos is strongly contested in the abortion conflict. A Yale law professor concerned about medical interventions in life, particularly at its termination, has observed that:

> The "personhood" dispute points to a theme in particular that is common to the claims about abortion and the right to die: that passage into or out of the human community involves extraordinary vulnerability; that the threats come not only or even primarily from biological risks but from social abuses; and that the medical profession is directly responsible for the infliction of these abuses. The proposed technique for protecting against abuse is also similar in the two contexts, though it differs in strategic details of application. The basic protective technique is to control the timing of the socially recognized designation of "personhood." To guard against iatric [that is, medical] abuse via abortion, the social status of "personhood" is bestowed at increasingly earlier stages of fetal and even embryonic biological development; to guard against iatric abuse via technological inflictions—mechanical ventilators, nasogastric tube feeding, etc.—during the process of dying, the social status of "personhood" is revoked at increasingly earlier stages of biological decline.[32]

In an instrumental bid to prevent or obstruct lawful abortion, Right to Life activists seek legal and constitutional acceptance that protected human life and personhood begin at conception. Similarly, they resist termination of mechanical ventilation or artificial feeding of patients in persistent vegetative states by asserting their continuing personhood and its protection by law, and they oppose medically assisted suicide by raising fears that this would lead to involuntary euthanasia of mentally incompetent people. It has been seen that General Counsel for the U.S. National Right to Life Committee has envisioned this progression.[33] In raising the more remote specter of harmful consequences in order to protect a conservative preference, this reasoning takes a consequentialist or utilitarian form more familiar among those tolerant of abortion and some forms of medically assisted death.

TOLERANCE OF ABORTION AND MEDICALLY ASSISTED DEATH

A leading modern advocate of legal accommodation of abortion, suicide without and with medical assistance, and euthanasia, has been the late Cambridge University law professor Glanville Williams. His lectures delivered at Columbia University, New York, in 1956[34] invoked the spirit of utilitarian analysis based on empirical enquiry, and profound scepticism about doctrines of the beginning of human life and how such life should end founded on religious faith. He confronted advocates of criminal laws governing the processes of human life based on religious beliefs with the logical and predictable consequences of such laws, and asked them to offer socially convincing justifications of such consequences, and their related contradictions of professed principles.

For instance, assertions of individuals' moral agency and responsibility are contradicted by claims that individuals' autonomous choices in their lives must be legally denied, and assertions of spiritual dignity are contradicted by legal denial of individuals' choices to govern the physical dignity of their lives and deaths.[35] The emphasis that utilitarian or consequentialist analysts and legal policy proponents place on pragmatic considerations may be countered, however, by the claim that legal and moral distinctions concerning end-of-life decisions that are defended as a matter of principle are inherently more valuable than those that are made on purely pragmatic or prudential grounds.[36]

Empirical evidence in Canada, for instance, shows a significant decrease in women's abortion-related deaths following legal recognition of therapeutic abortion by amendments to the Criminal Code that took effect from late August 1969. Earlier death rates were underestimated because doctors and others ascribed deaths to causes that reduced patients' and perhaps their own exposure to criminal investigations and prosecution, and that preserved deceased women's eligibility for burial in consecrated ground. Nevertheless, experience of women's access to skilled abortion in Canada, although such access was inequitably available, showed a reduction in pregnancy-related deaths from 75 in 1970 to 35 in 1974, and over the same period a decline in stillbirths of 24 percent, in infant deaths of over 20 percent, in neonatal deaths of over 25 percent, and in perinatal deaths of over 23 percent.[37] Although a composite of factors may have accounted for each of these statistics, it appears that the liberalized abortion law contributed to improved maternal and child health and saved the lives of many human beings. This reflects experience worldwide. A world review of induced abortion in 1990 found that:

> The provision of abortion under modern medical conditions has reduced abortion mortality to an extremely low level in developed countries that have legalized the procedure... In developed countries where induced abortion is legal, the procedure is now safer than pregnancy and childbirth. During 1981–85 in the United States, the maternal mortality rate excluding deaths from abortion and ectopic pregnancy was 6.6 deaths per 100,000 live births, a rate that is 11 times that associated with legal abortion.[38]

In contrast, the review observed that:

> The possible effects on maternal mortality of the legal restrictions on abortion can be seen in Romania, where most abortions were prohibited in 1966. Between 1965 and 1984, abortion mortality rose from 21 deaths to 128 deaths per 100,000 live births. Over the same period, maternal mortality from other causes fell from 65 deaths to 21 deaths per 100,000 live births. In 1984 alone, the WHO reports that there were 449 abortion deaths in Romania.[39]

Advocates of abortion law liberalization prefer that the need for abortion should be minimized through, for instance, sex education programs and availability of family planning services, but invoke statistics of this nature to show that their Pro-Choice position is also pro-life, and that Pro-Life denial of legalization and supply of services for abortion is associated with avoidable deaths of women and children.

Canadian evidence has also been found of harms individuals suffer when they attempt unskilled suicide. A study in British Columbia of persons with HIV/AIDS and of others who had been involved with acts of euthanasia or assisted suicide of persons with AIDS showed that, of those with AIDS, 53 percent had taken steps to plan assisted death, often with secretive cooperation of friends, family members, and physicians. The overriding concern motivating such plans was loss of independence, rather than fear of invasive medical technology and pain. Attempted suicide was decriminalized in Canada in 1972, but continuing legal prohibition of others' assistance in suicide left many persons with AIDS in fear that they would have to die alone, without the presence of loved ones, lest those in attendance be charged with crimes. Further, many had grave concerns that their deaths would be bungled by their own unskilled acts or unskilled assistance and that, instead of the comfortable, dignified deaths they desired, they would survive in aggravated injury, disfigurement, distress, dependency, and indignity. The study described several horrific real circumstances under which assisted deaths had been attempted, causing these results.[40]

The case of Sue Rodriguez came to the Supreme Court of Canada from British Columbia.[41] Anticipating death in dependency and indignity from her amyotrophic lateral sclerosis (Lou Gehrig's disease), she applied to the courts for a finding that the Criminal Code prohibition of assisted suicide violated her constitutional rights to liberty and security of the person. Further, since normally capacitated people would commit no crime in attempting suicide, but when disabled she would require assistance that it was a crime for another to provide, and for her to request since she would be a party to the other's crime, she claimed violation of her right to nondiscrimination on the ground of disability. A five-to-four majority in the Supreme Court upheld denial of her application, on the ground that, although she had full mental competence, and had earned the deepest sympathy of all the judges in being unable to manage the manner of her death, the prohibitive provision against assisted suicide must be maintained. This is because

[it] has as its purpose the protection of the vulnerable who might be induced in moments of weakness to commit suicide. This purpose is grounded in the state interest in protecting life and reflects the policy of the state that human life should not be depreciated by allowing life to be taken.... This is not only a policy of the state, however, but is part of our fundamental conception of the sanctity of human life.[42]

In the 1988 *Morgentaler* case, the Supreme Court had declared Canada's restrictive Criminal Code provision on abortion, even as partially liberalized in 1969, to be unconstitutional for violation of women's human rights to security of the person. Chief Justice Dickson observed that:

Forcing a woman, by threat of criminal sanction, to carry a foetus to term unless she meets certain criteria unrelated to her own priorities and aspirations, is a profound interference with a woman's body and thus a violation of security of the person.[43]

In the *Rodriguez* case, Justice McLachlin, who in late 1999 was appointed the first woman Chief Justice of Canada, gave a dissenting judgment based on the 1988 abortion decision. She observed that:

In my view, the reasoning of the majority in *R. v. Morgentaler* [references omitted] is dispositive of the issues on this appeal. In the present case, Parliament has put into force a legislative scheme which does not bar suicide but criminalizes the act of assisting suicide. The effect of this is to deny some people the choice of ending their lives solely because they are physically unable to do so. This deprives Sue Rodriguez of her security of the person (the right to make decisions concerning her own body, which affect only her own body).... This is precisely the logic which led the majority of this court to strike down the abortion provisions of the Criminal Code in *Morgentaler*.[44]

In reply to the majority's view that the criminal prohibition of assisted suicide was necessary for protection of disabled persons who may not truly consent to death, Justice McLachlin did not see why

Sue Rodriguez is asked to bear the burden of the chance that other people in other situations may act criminally to kill others or improperly sway them to suicide.[45]

She added that:

it is not clear that such a provision [prohibiting aiding or abetting suicide] is necessary; there is a sufficient remedy in the offences of culpable homicide. Nevertheless, the fear cannot be dismissed cavalierly; there is some evidence from foreign jurisdictions indicating that legal codes which permit assisted suicide may be linked to cases of involuntary deaths of the aging and disabled.[46]

This may have been a reference to the Netherlands, although the language of the Dutch Penal Code, which invalidated consent to the infliction of death and prohibited assisting suicide and, of course, murder, was at that time closely comparable to that of the Criminal Code of Canada. However, sensitized by harrowing revelations of acutely distressing and prolonged deaths of patients, and aware of judicial reluctance to punish doctors who facilitated deaths in sympathetic circumstances, procecutors developed policy guidelines on initiating proceedings. By prosecutorial interpretation of judicial decisions, physicians who complied with guidelines on assisted suicide and voluntary euthanasia in the Netherlands were unlikely to face prosecution.

The Netherlands has one of the lowest national abortion rates in the world.[47] This is due not to a restrictive abortion law, but to widespread sex education programs and accessible family planning services. The national abortion law is, in fact, one of the most liberal in the world, and indeed many nationals of nearby countries with more restrictive laws go there for this procedure. Similarly, the Netherlands has a very tolerant and accommodating approach to medically assisted suicide and voluntary euthanasia. Some uncertainty existed as to which of the prosecutorial guidelines were applicable in particular regions, but in 1989 the person chairing the Dutch Health Council listed them to be that:

(i) Requests for euthanasia must come only from the patient and must be entirely free and voluntary;

(ii) the patient's requests must be well-considered, explicit, enduring and persistent;

(iii) the patient must be experiencing intolerable physical, mental or other suffering, with no prospect of amelioration;

(iv) euthanasia must be a last resort, alternatives to alleviate the patient's condition having been considered and found wanting, such as by the patient's refusal;

(v) euthanasia must be performed by a physician;

(vi) the physician must have consulted with an independent physician who has relevant experience.[48]

The physician who conducts a patient's euthanasia cannot complete the death certificate by reference to "natural causes," but must report actual circumstances of the death either to the local coroner, who will report the death and circumstances to the police, or to the police directly. The police report the facts to the district attorney, who decides whether or not to prosecute on the basis of the applicable guidelines.[49]

Following the *Rodriguez* case in Canada, the Criminal Justice Branch of the British Columbia Ministry of the Attorney General issued comparable prosecution policy guidelines on Active Euthanasia and Assisted Suicide.[50]

Some commentators are highly critical of Dutch practice, both as originally shaped by the prosecutorial guidelines and as the 1991 Remmelink Committee showed the guidelines subsequently to have been implemented,[51] such as by slipping precipitously down a slippery slope to tolerance of involuntary euthanasia.[52] Many critics also condemn liberal abortion laws,[53] which they approach from a natural law orientation. Opponents of medically assisted or induced death have invoked the experience of abortion law reform to show the danger to which they believe legal liberalization leads. For instance John Habgood, now Archbishop of York, noted in 1974 that:

> Legislation to permit euthanasia would in the long run bring about profound changes in social attitudes towards death, illness, old age and the role of the medical profession. The Abortion Act has shown what happens....[t]here is no doubt about two consequences of the 1967 [Abortion] Act:
>
> (a) The safeguards and assurances given when the Bill was passed have to a considerable extent been ignored.
>
> (b) Abortion has now become a live option for **anybody** who is pregnant.... [B]ecause abortion is now on the agenda, the climate of opinion in which such a pregnancy must be faced has radically altered.
>
> One could expect similarly far-reaching and potentially more dangerous consequences from legalized euthanasia.[54]

What opponents consider dangerous about such law reform, namely its perceived compromise of the sanctity of human life, others may see as liberating individuals to preserve the quality of their lives, and the dignity of their deaths. Some consider the distinction between assisting suicide and performing euthanasia on the one hand, which are usually unlawful, and withdrawing treatment and allowing natural death on the other, which is lawful, to be vanishing, and that a case is growing for legal tolerance of assisted suicide and even requested euthanasia.[55] From a Pro-Choice perspective, laws that accommodate the autonomy of competent people, giving them power over and responsibility for their own lives, are to be favored over prohibitive laws. Tolerant laws reduce coercion, increase available options, enrich the human experience and furnish wider potentials for self-realization, self-determination and self-defense. Human dignity, the quality of life, and the quality of death, are perceived to be enhanced by removal of laws that, to paraphrase language of a Chief Justice of Canada, force people, by threat of criminal sanction, to meet criteria unrelated to their own priorities and aspirations.[56]

OPPOSING ABORTION, TOLERATING MEDICALLY ASSISTED DEATH

Some object to liberal abortion laws on purely secular grounds, such as that abortion ends the life *in utero* of a vulnerable, dependent fetus incapable of forming any wishes in the matter, or because they believe that women suffer subsequent psychological harm when they hurry unreflectively, perhaps in panic at unplanned pregnancy, to abortion practitioners who offer no disinterested counselling. They recognize, however, that the logic of their reasoning compels them to tolerate people who are mentally competent, sufficiently autonomous to be capable of self-determination and sufficiently mature to bear the consequences of their own choices, making a decision to end their own lives, and, if they wish, to seek medical assistance to achieve the comfort and dignity they desire. Lest children be deprived of necessary support, it may be necessary to allow this option only for terminal patients and elderly persons as well as younger persons so sick and incapable of performing routine functions that they are unable to give dependent children the personal support and protection they need.

The issues of tolerating choice in terminal care but defending the unborn as a priority have come together. In some of the United States and beyond, enacted and proposed legislation on advance medical directives and active voluntary euthanasia excludes pregnant women from taking advantage of their provisions. More than a decade ago, it was observed in the U.S. that several proposals for legislation on so-called living wills included terms making such documents inoperative or unavailable during pregnancy.[57] Advance medical directives are historically modelled on Do Not Resuscitate orders, and are often seen as applicable only to rejection of terminal care, thereby warranting their common name of "living wills." In fact, however, terminal care directives are only a species or component of advance medical directives. Such directives may be used, for instance, by women proposing childbirth under general anesthetic and wanting to specify in advance how foreseeable contingencies are to be managed if they occur when the women are unable to exercise judgment or express their preferences. Making such directives unavailable to women when they are pregnant is clearly dysfunctional in this case.

Proposals to render women unentitled to active voluntary euthanasia when they are pregnant[58] may appear somewhat more defensible, in that prolongation of a life a woman finds excessively burdensome would not be compelled for more than nine months, and usually for considerably less. A requirement, such as in practice in the Netherlands, that a request be enduring and persistent, may entail a delay of this length. Nevertheless, degrading the value of women's autonomy when they are pregnant is discriminatory, and appears objectionably paternalistic. The tragic death of both mother and child in the Washington D.C. Angela Carder case,[59] following judicial disregard of the legal rights, autonomy, and dignity of a dying pregnant woman in the cause of preserving the life of her unborn child, serves as an enduring lesson in the perils of awarding fetal life priority over a pregnant woman's preferred terminal care.

The patient was 25 weeks pregnant when it became clear that her adolescent cancer had come out of remission and was threatening her life. She agreed to palliative radiation and/or chemotherapy to relieve her pain in a bid to survive 28 weeks' pregnancy, when the chances that her fetus could survive cesarean delivery would be greatly improved. Unfortunately, her health rapidly deteriorated, her pain greatly increased, and her death appeared imminent. Her family and hospital doctors agreed it was best that she be kept comfortable and peaceful while she died. However, legal counsel for the hospital initiated court proceedings to decide what, if any, interventions should be performed on behalf of the fetus *in utero*. The guardian *ad litem* appointed for the fetus argued that the right to abortion under *Roe v. Wade* ceases at fetal viability, which the guardian claimed had been reached, and that the patient could not thereafter refuse treatment to preserve fetal interests. Over her physician's advice and protests, the judge ordered cesarean delivery. A panel of the District of Columbia Court of Appeals denied the patient's appeal, and the cesarean delivery was performed against her will. The baby died about 150 minutes after birth, the patient two days later. Her death certificate listed the court-ordered surgery as a contributing factor in her death.

Almost three years later, the full court of the D.C. Court of Appeals[60] found that the trial judge and appellate panel had been wrong to order intervention, and that the patient's best interests, as she and her medical advisor perceived them, and her right to bodily integrity, should have prevailed. A leading commentator at the time of the original decision had observed, of the brutal and unprincipled judicial violation of the terminal patient's rights, that:

> This is what happens when judges (and hospital lawyers that call them)... combine rescue fantasies with dehumanization of the dying.[61]

Dehumanization of pregnant women, by appearing to treat them as no more than manipulable incubators, is a risk to which the all-male judiciary in the trial and appellate panel case of Angela Carder[62] may have been prone. Boston University's professor George Annas later observed of the event that:

> The ultimate rationale may be purely sexist: this situation will never apply to males like these judges; they are unable to identify with the pregnant woman and thus need not concern themselves about the future application of their decision to themselves.[63]

Approaches to abortion, and particularly institutional opposition, not least by male-dominated religious bodies, raise obvious issues of gender discrimination, but approaches to terminal care and medically assisted death are also often gendered. The catalogue of the names of leading legal cases in North America in which patients' demonstrated preferences that would result in their deaths have been resisted and legally contested, is dominated by those of Karen Quinlan, Nancy Cruzan, Nancy B., Sue Rodriguez, Angela Carder and other women.[64] Gendered acceptance that critical decision-making is a masculine activity, particularly in matters of life and death such as making war, shooting weapons, insemination for procreation, and judicial imposition of death sentences, and the related inability to accept women as autonomous decision-makers in abortion, may parallel the inability to accept as authoritative women's choices to end their lives. Such decisions therefore are perceived to require or compel initiation of judicial proceedings. However, gender may equally contribute at least in part to the reverse disposition, namely to tolerate abortion but oppose medically assisted death.

TOLERATING ABORTION, OPPOSING MEDICALLY ASSISTED DEATH

Pro-choice attitudes that tolerate abortion are paradoxically sometimes reversed in feminist and related attitudes that oppose choice of medically assisted death. Opposition is rooted in fear of the oppression of people who are vulnerable because of their disability, age, or poverty, and the recognition that the most vulnerable of disabled, elderly, and impoverished populations are usually women.[65] An argument opposing medically assisted death may be pitched at the wider, inclusive level of social justice. It has been observed, for instance, that

> A number of experts—doctors, ethicists, and lawyers—contend that the right to assisted suicide should not be recognized because of its social justice implications. These experts maintain that, in the case of terminally ill patients, the economically, racially, ethnically, or physically disadvantaged could be forced to exercise an "assisted suicide option" should one become available because they will be unable to afford adequate palliative care. The more "advantaged" would have more "free will" to determine whether and when to commit assisted suicide because they will be able to afford adequate care, and thus, their "choice" to exercise an "assisted suicide option" will be more meaningful than that of the more disadvantaged members of society.[66]

This argument, based on U.S. experience, carries less weight, however, in countries where principles of social justice have led to publicly funded national health care systems.

Professor Susan Wolf of the University of Minnesota has shown that the health characteristics that may increase vulnerability to seek assisted suicide and euthanasia— such as depression, inadequate pain relief, lack of health insurance, poverty and difficulty in obtaining satisfactory health care, as well as being the inferior party in relationships with physicians and comparable authority figures whom patients want to respect their views and preferences—affect women disadvantageously.[67] She contrasts abortion and assisted suicide on the ground that the former involves women's right to prevent unwanted (embryonic and fetal) invasions into their bodies, which is essential to women's sexual and personal integrity and feeling of security, whereas the latter involves receiving bodily interventions, to which no right exists. She writes that:

> abortion is indeed about a right to be free of unwanted invasion, the invasion of pregnancy. The state cannot compel women to tolerate that invasion...But it is not at all clear that it covers a right to be free to obtain bodily invasion for the purpose of ending your own life. This is not an artificial distinction. Removing an unwanted pregnancy-from the body reinforces the status quo ante (not being pregnant) and allows a woman to continue her life plan before it was interrupted by unwanted pregnancy. Removing unwanted life-sustaining treatment also restores the status quo ante (life with a disability or illness) and allows a person to continue what may be a dying process. But assisted

suicide removes nothing from the body and restores no status quo ante. It intervenes to change the life course radically.[68]

The U.S. Supreme Court has recognized women's constitutional right to abortion within a framework of privacy and liberty, but Professor Wolf observes that:

This is a concept of liberty as the right to live unencumbered by unwanted pregnancy in order to carve out a destiny other than mother of that child-to-be. There is no support here for a concept of liberty as the right to forfeit one's life.[69]

She also notes that women's culturally conditioned role as caregivers to others imports an expectation of women's self-sacrifice.[70] Physicians and others may fatally reinforce a history of gender inequity by presuming women's preference for ending their lives rather than being a burden to others, such as their children or those on whose constant care they would depend.[71] The tendency is aggravated where women's lives are regarded as less valuable than men's, and particularly where older women's lives are devalued.

Feminist analysts of health care continue to be suspicious of medical paternalism,[72] but the distinction they often draw between legal rights to abortion services, which they endorse, and to medically assisted death, which they oppose, is strongly supported by organized medicine. Support has grown for tolerance of lawful abortion, and even though countless practitioners have personal conscientious objections to participation, the profession recognizes on pragmatic grounds that the costs of prohibiting women's access to safe medical services are inhumane and unjustifiable. The British Medical Association, for instance, urges that the British Abortion Act 1967 be extended to Northern Ireland.[73] In contrast, legal recognition of a patient's so-called "right to die" is resisted, not only because it might create physicians' duty to kill their patients, but also because physicians disclaim any power or legitimate intention to end patients' lives.

Opposing both medically assisted suicide and euthanasia, the British Medical Association (BMA) has long-standing policies that:

the BMA considers that doctors should not assist, either directly or indirectly, their patients to commit suicide

and that equally, while doctors

have a duty to try to provide patients with a peaceful and dignified death with minimal suffering...the BMA considers it contrary to the doctor's role deliberately to kill patients, even at their request.[74]

Accordingly, while doctors who may properly invoke reasons of private conscience to deny abortion services may be legally obliged to refer their patients to practitioners who do not share such reasons, those who deny requests for assisted death have no such duty to refer patients to colleagues of a different persuasion, and may indeed have a duty not to.

In Canada, between 1991 and 1993 the Committee on Ethics of the Canadian Medical Association (CMA) reviewed options on medical responses to controversial issues, and noted its earlier observation that:

It can be argued that for physician-assisted death the CMA should adopt the same position that it has on abortion, namely that this involves a medical decision between doctor and patient.[75]

It was speculated that, like abortion, physician-assisted death can be considered a medical act appropriate for medical administration, with comparable safeguards for conscientious objection.[76] The profession rejected this equation between abortion and euthanasia, however, and its current policy is that members should specifically exclude participation in active voluntary euthanasia and physician-assisted suicide.[77]

In the U.S., the Supreme Court litigation on final appeal from the Courts of Appeals for the Second and Ninth Federal Circuits, in which the Supreme Court declined to expand on its earlier decision upholding the right to abortion, and rejected a constitutional right to physician-assisted suicide, focused and to an extent polarized medical professionals' opinions. The American Medical Association embodied its longstanding opposition to medically aided death in the *amicus curiae* brief it filed with the Court in support of the petitioners, whose argument the Supreme Court upheld.[78] The almost uniform medical professional opposition to any equation between abortion and medically assisted suicide and euthanasia reflects the view that, while abortion is a medical act, whether performed by surgical means or recently developed non-surgical means, assisting suicide and performing euthanasia require no special medical skills or knowledge. Neither practice is taught in medical schools, tested as a condition of professional licensure, nor discussed in standard medical texts.

The risks of aggravated distress due to bungled suicide and unskilled attempts at euthanasia present scenarios of preventable harms to patients that doctors may consider it proper that they be professionally and legally entitled to address. The fact that an apparent assisted suicide request may be more a cry for help than a genuine bid to end one's life[79] that doctors should be available to hear and assess, makes a stronger case for medical professional approachability and involvement. Recent evidence indicates a growing sympathy among medical practitioners for reconsideration of professional organizational opposition to medical involvement in assisted suicide and active voluntary euthanasia.[80] The position may indeed reflect that existing for some decades prior to general liberalization of attitudes and eventually law regarding induced abortion, when the practice was known to be not uncommon among medical practitioners, but almost invariably clandestine.

CONCLUSION: TOWARDS RESOLUTION OF CONFLICT

Pro-life and pro-choice approaches to medically induced abortion, suicide, and voluntary euthanasia are in obvious conflict, but choice offers considerable potential to narrow the scope of irreconcilable difference. It is a mistake and injustice to believe that adherents to the pro-choice position are pro-abortion, since they consider this acceptable only as a means of last resort. When choices exist, for instance through education and access to suitable means, to plan pregnancy, and in particular to avoid unplanned pregnancy, resort to abortion can be largely reduced. Pro-life and pro-choice advocates both favor reduction in the incidence of abortion. Similarly, law has been applied dysfunctionally when pro-life activists who have offered women financial support through pregnancy, childbirth, and recuperation, with placement in adoption of children the mothers find they cannot rear, have been warned that they face prosecution, since it is usually an offense to offer money in order to induce adoption. The choice of childbirth and adoption is no less agreeable in principle to pro-choice than to pro-life advocates, although the issue of children's rights to learn their birth mothers' identities remains contentious. Pro-life advocates may also be sympathetic to women's having options in life in addition to motherhood, and be able to accept the modern reality that women in many circumstances need to have paid employment outside the home in order to contribute to the well-being of their families.

At the end of life, advocates of different approaches to medically assisted suicide and euthanasia may similarly agree that those considering their own voluntary induced death should be offered better choices for living in comfort and dignity until the natural cessation of life. Those who sympathize with medical participation in suicide and euthanasia do not oppose options of palliative care. Disagreements about the sources of financial support for improved care for patients whose lives have become excessively burdensome to them, whether for instance through encouragement of private saving or insurance to provide means of future medical care, private philanthropy, or taxation-supported government action, turn on political and moral considerations. In principle, however, even those holding clear preferences may recognize that inflexibly punitive laws against disfavored options may be ineffective or counterproductive. Experience may show that their preferences for judgment based on moral values are more successfully pursued through legal accommodation of moral choices, rather than the prescription of doctrinaire prohibitions backed by fearsome criminal, professional, and other sanctions. Criminal laws may produce at best mere obedience, and at worst evasion, privileged immunity, misrepresentation, and hypocrisy.[81] Tolerant laws and medical professional codes can be responsive to individual moral choices, and accommodate moral objections through inclusion of conscientious objection provisions that balance competing interests in pragmatically sound laws and in respect for moral convictions.

NOTES AND REFERENCES

1. *Roe v. Wade* (1973), *Supreme Court Reporter*, Vol. 93, pp. 703–763.
2. *Planned Parenthood of Southeastern Pennsylvania v. Casey* (1992), *Supreme Court Reporter*, Vol. 505, pp. 833–1002.
3. See, e.g. A. Tsao, "Fetal Homicide Laws: Shield against Domestic Violence or Sword to Pierce Abortion Rights?" *Hastings Constitutional Law Quarterly*, Vol. 25 (1998), pp. 457–481.
4. *Morgentaler, Smoling and Scott v. The Queen* (1988), *Dominion Law Reports*, Vol. 44 (4th series), pp. 385–500.
5. M. Otlowski, *Voluntary Euthanasia and the Common Law* (Oxford: Clarendon Press, 1997)
6. Otlowski, *ibid.*, at 339.
7. *Washington vs. Glucksberg, Supreme Court Reporter* (1997), Vol. 117, pp. 2258–2293, 2302–2312.
8. Senate of Canada, *Of Life and Death: Report of the Special Senate Committee on Euthanasia and Assisted Suicide* (Ottawa: Publications Canada, 1995).
9. *Rodriguez v. British Columbia (Attorney-General), Dominion Law Reports* (1993), Vol. 107 (4th series), pp. 342–424.
10. *Rodriguez, ibid.* at 386.
11. R. Dworkin, *Life's Dominion: An Argument About Abortion, Euthanasia, and Individual Freedom* (New York: Knopf, 1993).
12. J.M. Finnis, "The Rights and Wrongs of Abortion: a Reply to Judith Thomson," *Phil. Pub. Aff.*, Vol. 2 (1973), pp. 117–145.
13. J.M. Finnis, "The Fragile Case for Euthanasia: a Reply to John Harris," *in* J. Keown (Ed.), *Euthanasia Examined* (Cambridge: Cambridge University Press, 1997), p. 48.

14. J.M. Finnis, "A Philosophical Case Against Euthanasia," *in* J. Keown (Ed.), *Euthanasia Examined, ibid.*, pp. 23–35 at 33–34.
15. *Roe v. Wade* (1973), *Supreme Court Reporter,* Vol. 93, pp. 703–763.
16. *Planned Parenthood of Southeastern Pennsylvania v. Casey* (1992), *Supreme Court Reporter,* Vol. 505, pp. 833–1002.
17. J. Bopp Jr., and R.E. Coleson, "Roe v. Wade and the Euthanasia Debate," *Issues in Law & Medicine*, Vol. 12 (1997), pp. 343–354 at 345.
18. *Washington v. Glucksberg* (1997), *Supreme Court Reporter*, Vol 117, pp. 2258–2293, 2302–2312; *Vacco v. Quill* (1997), *Supreme Court Reporter*, Vol. 117, pp. 2293–2302.
19. K.P. Quinn, "Assisted Suicide and Equal Protection: In Defense of the Distinction Between Killing and Letting Die," *Issues in Law & Medicine*, Vol. 13 (1997), pp. 145–171.
20. Finnis, "A Philosophical Case Against Euthanasia," *op. cit.*, at 28.
21. J.M. Finnis, "Intention and Side-Effects," *in* R.G. Frey and C. Morris (Eds.), *Liability and Responsibility* (Cambridge: Cambridge University Press, 1991), pp. 32–46.
22. D. Price, "Euthanasia, Pain Relief and Double Effect," *Legal Studies*, Vol. 17 (1997), pp. 323–342.
23. Finnis, "A Philosophical Case Against Euthanasia," *op. cit.*, at 27.
24. *Airedale N.H.S. Trust v. Bland (*1993), *Appeal Cases,* pp. 789–899.
25. *Airedale 1993*, at 868.
26. *Airedale 1993*, at 879.
27. *Airedale 1993*, at 885.
28. J.M. Finnis, "Bland: Crossing the Rubicon?," *Law Quarterly Review*, Vol. 109 (1993), pp. 329–337.
29. Finnis, "A Philosophical Case Against Euthanasia," *op. cit.*, at 28.
30. B.M. Dickens, "Medically Assisted Death: Nancy B. v. Hotel-Dieu de Quebec," *McGill Law Journal*, Vol. 38 (1993), pp. 1053–1070.
31. J.M. Finnis, *Natural Law and Natural Rights* (Oxford: Clarendon Press, 1982), p. 112.
32. R. Burt, "Rationality and Injustice in Physician-Assisted Suicide," *Western New England Law Review*, Vol. 19 (1997), pp. 353–369, at 366-367.
33. Bopp and Coleson, "Roe v. Wade and the Euthanasia Debate," *op. cit.*, at 345.
34. G. Williams, *The Sanctity of Life and the Criminal Law* (London: Faber and Faber, 1958).
35. R. Cohen-Almagor, "Reflections on the Intriguing Issue of the Right to Die in Dignity," *Israel Law Review*, Vol. 29 (1995), pp. 677–701.
36. S. Kadish, "Letting Patients Die: Legal and Moral Reflections," *California Law Review*, Vol. 80 (1992), pp. 857–888, at 864–868; K.P. Quinn, "Assisted Suicide and Equal Protection: In Defense of the Distinction Between Killing and Letting Die," *Issues in Law & Medicine,* Vol. 13 (1997), pp. 145–171 at 149 n.19.
37. *Report of the Committee on the Operation of the Abortion Law 1977* (Chair: R. Badgley) (Ottawa: Supply and Services Canada, 1977), p. 47.
38. S.K. Henshaw, "Induced Abortion: A World Review," *Family Planning Perspectives*, Vol. 22 (1990), pp. 76–89 at 81.
39. Henshaw, *ibid.*, at 82.
40. R. Ogden, "Palliative Care and Euthanasia: A Continuum of Care?," *Journal of Palliative Care,* Vol. 10 (1994), pp. 82–85.
41. *Rodriguez* (1993)
42. *Rodriguez*, at 396–397.
43. *Morgentaler* (1988), 402.
44. *Rodriguez* (1993), 415.
45. *Rodriguez* (1993), 417–418.
46. *Rodriguez* (1993), 421.
47. Henshaw, "Induced Abortion: A World Review," *op. cit.*, at 78.
48. J. Keown, "The Law and Practice of Euthanasia in The Netherlands," *Law Quarterly Review*, Vol. 108 (1992), pp. 51–57, at 56.
49. M.A.M. de Wachter, "Active Euthanasia in the Netherlands," *JAMA*, Vol. 262 (1989), pp. 3316–3319 at 3317; Otlowski, *Voluntary Euthanasia and the Common Law, op. cit.*, at 396–397.
50. Senate of Canada, *Of Life and Death: Report of the Special Senate Committee on Euthanasia and Assisted Suicide, op. cit.*, A-59–63.

51. Otlowski, *Voluntary Euthanasia and the Common Law, op. cit.*, at 423.
52. J. Keown, "Euthanasia in The Netherlands: Sliding Down the Slippery Slope?" in *Euthanasia Examined, op. cit.*, at 282.
53. J. Keown, Abortion, Doctors and the Law (Cambridge: Cambridge University Press, 1988).
54. J.S. Habgood, "Euthanasia—A Christian View," *Journal of the Royal Society of Health*, Vol. 3 (1974), pp. 124–129 at 126.
55. D. Orentlicher, "The Legalization of Physician-Assisted Suicide: A Very Modest Revolution," *Boston College Law Rev*iew, Vol. 38 (1997), pp. 443–475.
56. *Morgentaler* (1988), at 402.
57. G. Gelfand, "Living Will Statutes: The First Decade," Wisconsin Law Rev. (1987), pp. 737–822 at 778–780.
58. S. Cole and M. Shea, "Voluntary Euthanasia: A Proposed Remedy," *Albany Law Review*, Vol. 39 (1975), pp. 826–856, at 845–847.
59. B. Steinbock, *Life Before Birth: The Moral and Legal Status of Embryos and Fetuses* (New York: Oxford University Press, 1992), at 155–160.
60. *In re A.C.* (1990), *Atlantic Reporter,* 2nd. Vol. 573, pp. 1235–1264
61. G. Annas, "She's Going to Die: The Case of Angela C.," *Hastings Center Report,* Vol. 18, No.1 (1988), pp. 23–25 at 25.
62. *A.C.* (1990).
63. G. Annas, *Standard of Care: The Law of American Bioethics* (New York: Oxford University Press, 1993), p. 40.
64. S. Miles and A. August, "Courts, Gender and 'The Right to Die'," *Law, Medicine and Health Care,* Vol. 18 (1990), pp. 85–95.
65. M. Nussbaum and J. Glover (Eds.), *Women, Culture and Development* (Oxford: Clarendon Press, 1995).
66. M. Spindelman, "Are the Similarities Between a Woman's Right to Choose an Abortion and the Alleged Right to Assisted Suicide Really Compelling?," *University of Michigan Journal of Law Reform*, Vol. 29 (1996), pp. 775–856 at 826–827.
67. S. Wolf, "Gender, Feminism, and Death: Physician-Assisted Suicide and Euthanasia," in S. Wolf (Ed.), *Feminism and Bioethics: Beyond Reproduction* (New York: Oxford University Press, 1996), pp. 282–317.
68. S. Wolf, "Physician-Assisted Suicide, Abortion and Treatment Refusal: Using Gender to Analyze the Difference," in R.F. Weir (Ed.) *Physician-Assisted Suicide* (Bloomington, Indiana: Indiana University Press, 1997), pp. 167–201 at 173.
69. Wolf, *ibid.*, at 175.
70. Wolf, "Gender, Feminism, and Death," *op. cit.*, at 289.
71. Wolf, "Physician-Assisted Suicide, Abortion and Treatment Refusal," *op. cit.*, at 178.
72. S. Sherwin, *No Longer Patient: Feminist Ethics and Health Care* (Philadelphia: Temple University Press, 1992).
73. British Medical Association, *Medical Ethics Today: Its Practice and Philosophy* (London: BMJ Publishing Group, 1993), at 103.
74. British Medical Association, *op. cit.*, p. 175.
75. Canadian Medical Association, "Induced Abortion," *Canadian Medical Association Journal*, Vol. 139 (1988), 1176A.
76. F.H. Lowy, D.M. Sawyer and J.R. Williams, *Canadian Physicians and Euthanasia* (Ottawa: Canadian Medical Association, 1993), p. 52.
77. Canadian Medical Association, "CMA Policy Summary: Physician Assisted Death," *Canadian Medical Association Journal*, Vol. 152 (1995), 248A.
78. *Washington v. Glucksberg* (1997), *Supreme Court Reporter,* Vol 117, 2258-2293, 2302-2312.
79. E. Stengel, *Suicide and Attempted Suicide* (Harmondsworth, U.K.: Penguin Books, 1964); E. Stengel and N.G. Cook, *Attempted Suicide* (Oxford: Oxford University Press, 1958).
80. Otlowski, *Voluntary Euthanasia and the Common Law, op. cit.*
81. B.M. Dickens, "Legal Approaches to Health Care Ethics and the Four Principles," *in* R. Gillon (Ed.), *Principles of Health Care Ethics* (Chichester, New York: John Wiley, 1994), pp. 305–317 at 305–307.

Advance Directives and Dementia

RON BERGHMANS

Institute for Bioethics, P.O. Box 616, 6200 MD Maastricht, the Netherlands

INTRODUCTION

There is a growing interest in advance directives in health care. In a number of jurisdictions the legal status of advance directives is regulated by law, or legal regulation is being discussed. Advance directives have emerged as a vehicle for people to control post-competence medical interventions.[1] In an advance directive, a person can formulate his or her personal preferences and wishes with regard to medical treatment and care in case of future incompetence, and so he or she can try to maintain a measure of autonomy even after having become incompetent. An advance directive may also designate an agent who will ultimately be responsible for implementing the declarant's instructions, or, in the absence of discernible instructions, for making medical decisions on behalf of the incompetent patient.

The dominant view is that by executing an advance directive a person can exhibit so-called prospective autonomy.[2] A refusal of treatment that is formulated in an advance directive is generally considered to operate as an extension of a competent patient's moral and legal right to refuse treatment, based on the principle of respect for autonomy and individual self-determination.[3] The dominant ethical and legal point of view is that a refusal of treatment by a competent patient should be respected, even if we think that this decision is unwise, and even if this refusal may lead to an earlier death of the patient.[4]

Exemplary for the role of advance directives in the context of patient self-determination is the following statement of the American Academy of Neurology Ethics and Humanities Subcommittee (1996): "Completing and following advance directives (in dementia) is desirable ethically because it permits a type of patient self-determination even in states of incompetence." (p.1181)

The potential benefits of advance directives are obvious. Not only can persons prospectively promote personal values and conceptualizations of dignity, but also the ultimate decision-makers on behalf of the incompetent patient can receive crucial guidance.[5]

ADVANCE DIRECTIVES AND DEMENTIA

Given the greying of the population and the growing numbers of people suffering from Alzheimer's disease and other dementias, the interest for advance directives that specifically deal with medical care in case of dementia and other diseases of old age is also growing.

Such a dementia advance directive, however, raises specific ethical questions because of the fact that in dementia one can speak of people who can become incompetent, but who generally will, for a substantial time period during the progression of this disease, remain conscious. Because of the fact that most demented patients, even in case of incompetence, remain conscious and stay able to have subjective experiences, a conflict may arise between their former wishes and preferences as stated in an advance directive, and their present interests as conscious but incompetent subjects.[6]

In this essay I will deal with some of the ethical problems that are raised by dementia advance directives, as far as they apply to the conscious but incompetent demented person. I will particularly pay attention to one prominent objection against giving moral authority to dementia advance directives that flows from a particular view concerning the relationship between dementia and personal identity. I will argue that this view has some serious flaws.

I will conclude that end-of-life decisions in dementia nevertheless cannot rely solely on the wishes that were expressed in an advance directive, but ought to take into account considerations that are connected to the actual situation and interests of the incompetent demented person. My analysis will be restricted to non-treatment decisions.

ADVANCE DIRECTIVES ARE NOT EQUIVALENT TO DECISIONS MADE BY COMPETENT PATIENTS

As stated, the moral status of advance directives is considered to be an extension of the competent patient's moral and legal right to refuse treatment. However, upon a closer look this extension is not at all self-evident.

Comparing choices made in an advance directive (prospective autonomy) with contemporaneous decisions of competent patients (actual autonomy), several differences can be distinguished.[7]

First, even if, at the time an advance directive was issued, an individual was well-informed about the options available should he or she develop a particular disease, therapeutic options and hence prognosis can change between the time the advance directive is issued and the time it is to be implemented.

Second, advance directives are often framed with certain implicit assumptions in mind about the expected condition of the patient when the treatment decision must be made. The individual's actual condition, however, may be substantially different.

Third, the assumption that a competent person is the best judge of his or her own interests is weaker in the case of a choice about future contingencies under conditions in which those interests may have changed in radical and unforeseen ways than it is in the case of a competent individual's contemporaneous choice. Inasfar as the mental states of persons deviate more from what we are used to, the possibility for "transpersonal introspection" becomes more problematic.[8] Our imagination is constrained by our own experiences, and these "color in" the conscious experiences we attribute to other people or creatures.[9]

A fourth asymmetry is that in the case of an advance directive, important informal safeguards that tend to restrain imprudent or unreasonable contemporaneous choices by a competent individual are not likely to be present. If a competent patient refuses life-sustaining care, those around the person who are responsible for care can and often do urge the patient to reconsider his or her choice. In connection with this asymmetry, we can point at the fact that an advance directive brings with it the inability to reconsider the choices made at the time of application.[10] Persons with Alzheimer's disease lose their ability to change their minds once they lose the ability to make decisions.[11] The problem, then, with advance directives is that at the time you would most likely "change your mind," you don't have enough mind left to change.[12] In this respect we may say that in case of dementia the former self irrevocably binds the later self of the person.

Feinberg[13] asks in this context whether we can be sufficiently convinced that the former self "acting on the basis only of a partial anticipation of the eventual situation, would not himself have chosen to revoke [the advance directive] had he been able to foresee precisely these circumstances in every relevant detail?"

These four morally relevant differences between choices in advance directives (prospective autonomy) and contemporaneous choices of competent patients support the view that more confidence should be accorded to the assumption that an individual is the best judge of his or her own interests in the latter case than in the former.[14] In a number of respects the choices as formulated in a dementia advance directive may fall short of autonomy and are less than fully autonomous decisions. In light of this, in my view dementia advance directives cannot be given absolute moral authority in case of non-treatment decisions involving incompetent demented patients.

PERSONAL IDENTITY

A more principled objection against the moral authority of dementia advance directives is connected to the issue of personal identity. When people become demented, their self and personal identity are subject to more or less deep psychological changes. During the process of becoming demented, these changes may become so profound that the former person is not recognized anymore by significant others.[15] The patient often has little memory of her previous life, her personality has changed, her intellect has deteriorated, and she may have considerably different needs, concerns, beliefs and desires than before. Much of the psychological continuity which is often thought to be necessary for personal identity can be lost.[16]

Rebecca Dresser, following the work of Derek Parfit,[17] argues that the radical personality changes that accompany the process of dementia lead to a loss of the personal identity of the person involved.[18]

Upon this view only facts about psychological connectedness and psychological continuity (Parfit calls them "Relation R") have relevance for personal identity. As Relation R becomes weaker, commitments in time become weaker, and the binding force of the expressed wishes of the former self of a person, as formulated in an advance directive, may become weaker in case of the radical psychological changes accompanying dementia. Phases in a person's life, as a result of deep psychological changes, may be considered as divisions between lives, and the expression that somebody has become "a different person" may not only be metaphorically correct, but also litterally.

Upon the Parfitian theory of personal identity it may be claimed that dementia advance directives in fact are not documents promoting prospective personal autonomy, but in reality are sinister instruments advancing the subjection of other persons.[19] The argument from personal identity thus would severely undermine the moral authority of dementia advance directives. In fact, dementia advance directives ought not to be given any moral authority at all. In the light of this fundamental implication of the personal identity claim, it is necessary to look at some arguments against the view upon personal identity and dementia as defended by Dresser.

OBJECTIONS TO THE PERSONAL IDENTITY VIEW

A first problem with the personal identity view is that the criteria of psychological connectedness and continuity are inherently vague.[20] Connectedness and continuity are not a matter of all-or-nothing, but of more-or-less. The crucial question remains how much connectedness between different mental states (i.e., memories, affects, dispositions) is necessary in order to attribute psychological continuity. In other words: how radical must the psychological changes in time be in order to say that psychological discontinuity exists?[21]

A further question is whether the only facts that matter for personal identity are psychological connectedness and continuity. From a number of different viewpoints it can be argued that other things also matter.

Firstly it can be argued that facts about connectedness and continuity are not sufficient conditions for personal identity, but that the degree of connectedness and continuity among the stages of the life of a person (the strength of Relation R) may themselves depend on facts about how persons think about themselves over time and on facts about how other persons think about us over time.[22] The moral importance of a particular degree of connectedness and continuity is not exclusively determined by facts about connectedness and continuity. To some degree a person can, him- or herself, affect and control Relation R, for instance by trying to preserve particular memories or to erase others.

Another objection against the exclusive importance attached to psychological connectedness and continuity with regard to personal identity relates to the fact that for societal purposes people are treated as the same persons over time. We will want to hold people accountable, both legally and morally, to commitments and responsibilities over time.[23] If the demented person is really a different person metaphysically, morally and legally, then the former competent person has ceased to exist and the demented person has no property, no insurance, and no relatives.[24] The social fabric requires us to attach importance to personal identity that does not derive from the facts of connectedness and continuity themselves.[25]

A last objection against the connectedness-and-continuity view of personal identity stems from a social constructionist perspective on personal identity as developed by Sabat and Harré,[26] who argue that the self of personal identity persists far into the end stage of Alzheimer's disease. The self that is projected in the public domain, which depends for its existence on the cooperation of others, can get lost, but only indirectly as a result of the disease. At least as important is the way in which others perceive and communicate with the patient.

These different objections against the Parfitian/Dresserian view on personal identity deny the exclusive importance attached to facts about psychological connectedness and continuity. It cannot be denied that these facts have importance for personal identity (and for its survival over time), but they do not seem to be the only things that matter in a theory of personal identity. The theory as it stands is insufficient to undermine, independently from other considerations, the moral authority of dementia advance directives.

CONCLUSION

In non-treatment decisions in dementia, an exclusive reliance on expressed wishes and preferences in dementia advance directives, based on the negative moral right of respect for autonomy, involves an unjustified reduction of reality to a single moral principle. This means that dementia advance directives, although they are relevant from a moral point of view, ought not to be considered decisive and having absolute moral authority. Other considerations in specific individual situations, concerning the particular interests of the person who has become demented and incompetent, also have moral weight and deserve to be taken into account in non-treatment decisions.

This view is not dependent on a particular theory about the relationship between dementia and personal identity, but results from the recognition of the fact that a dementia advance directive in a number of different respects can fail to be the expression of a fully autonomous choice of the person involved.

In this paper attention has been paid to the moral significance of dementia advance directives in non-treatment decisions. In the Netherlands in 1999 a new law has been proposed to regulate the practice of euthanasia and assisted suicide. It is proposed to give legal force to advance directives concerning active life termination. A physician *may* carry out a request for active life termination in case an incompetent patient has formulated such a request in an advance directive while competent. This proposal raises a number of concerns that go beyond the scope of this article. It has met with serious criticism from nursing home physicians and other commentators. Given the analysis outlined here with regard to non-treatment decisions, it is to be hoped that this part of the law proposal will be seriously reconsidered by the Dutch government.

NOTES AND REFERENCES

1. Norman Cantor, *Advance Directives and the Pursuit of Death with Dignity* (Bloomington and Indianapolis, Indiana University Press, 1993).
2. Ronald Dworkin, *Life's Dominion: An Argument about Abortion, Euthanasia, and Individual Freedom* (London: Harper Collins, 1993); N.L. Cantor, "Prospective Autonomy: On the Limits of Shaping One's Postcompetence Medical Fate," *Journal of Contemporary Health Law & Policy*, Vol. 13 (1992), pp. 34–48; Norman Cantor, *Advance Directives, op. cit.*
3. T. May, "Reassessing the Reliability of Advance Directives," *Cambridge Quarterly of Healthcare Ethics*, Vol. 6 (1997), pp. 325–338.
4. T.E. Quill, R. Dresser, and D.W. Brock, "The Rule of Double Effect—A Critique of Its Role in End-of-Life Decision Making," *The New England Journal of Medicine*, Vol. 337, No. 24 (1997), pp. 1768–1771.
5. Norman Cantor, *Advance Directives, op. cit.*
6. R.S. Dresser and J.A. Robertson, "Quality of Life and Non-Treatment Decisions for Incompetent Patients: A Critique of the Orthodox Approach," *Law, Medicine & Health Care*, Vol. 17, No. 3 (1989), pp. 234–244.

7. A.E. Buchanan and D.W. Brock, *Deciding for Others. The Ethics of Surrogate Decision Making* (New York: Cambridge University Press, 1989); Norman Cantor, *Advance Directives, op. cit.*
8. N. Rhoden, "Litigating Life and Death," *Harvard Law Review,* Vol. 102 (1988), pp. 375–446.
9. T. Nagel, *The View from Nowhere* (New York: Oxford University Press, 1986).
10. T. May ,"Reassessing the Reliability of Advance Directives," *op. cit.*
11. M.A. Drickamer and M.S. Lachs ,"Should Patients with Alzheimer's Disease Be Told Their Diagnosis?," *The New England Journal of Medicine,* Vol. 326, No. 14 (1992), pp. 947–951.
12. N. Rhoden, "How Should We View the Incompetent?," *Law, Medicine & Health Care,* Vol. 17, No. 3 (1989), pp. 264–268.
13. J. Feinberg, *The Moral Limits of the Criminal Law. Volume III: Harm to Self* (New York/Oxford: Oxford University Press, 1986).
14. A.E. Buchanan and D.W. Brock, *Deciding for Others, op.cit.*
15. R.L.P. Berghmans, "Ethical Hazards of the Substituted Judgement Test in Decision Making Concerning the End of Life of Dementia Patients," *International Journal of Geriatric Psychiatry,* Vol. 12 (1997), pp. 283–287.
16. C. Elliott and B. Elliott, "From the Patient's Point of View: Medical Ethics and the Moral Imagination," *Journal of Medical Ethics,* Vol. 17 (1991), pp. 173–178.
17. D. Parfit, "Later Selves and Moral Principles," in A. Montefiore (Ed.), *Philosophy and Personal Relations* (London: Routledge and Kegan Paul, 1973), pp. 137–169; D. Parfit, *Reasons and Persons* (Oxford: Oxford University Press, 1984).
18. R.S. Dresser, "Relitigating Life and Death," *Ohio State Law Journal,* Vol. 51 (1990), pp. 425–437; R. Dresser,"Autonomy Revisited: the Limits of Anticipatory Choices," in R.H. Binstock, S.G. Post and P.J. Whitehouse (Eds.), *Dementia and Aging: Ethics, Values, and Policy Choices* (Baltimore/London: The Johns Hopkins University Press, 1992), pp. 71–85; R. Dresser,"Dworkin on Dementia: Elegant Theory, Questionable Policy," *Hastings Center Report,* Vol. 25, No. 6 (1995), pp. 32–38; R.S. Dresser and J.A. Robertson, "Quality of Life and Non-Treatment Decisions for Incompetent Patients: A Critique of the Orthodox Approach," *Law, Medicine & Health Care,* Vol. 17, No. 3 (1989), pp. 234–244.
19. A. Buchanan,"Advance Directives and the Personal Identity Problem," *Philosophy & Public Affairs,* Vol. 17, No. 4 (1988), pp. 277–302.
20. R. Dresser, "Dworkin on Dementia: Elegant Theory, Questionable Policy," *Hastings Center Report,* Vol. 25, No. 6 (1995), pp. 32–38.
21. Donald VanDeVeer, *Paternalistic Intervention. The Moral Bounds on Benevolence* (Princeton, NJ: Princeton University Press, 1986).
22. Norman Daniels, *Am I My Parents' Keeper? An Essay on Justice Between The Young and the Old* (New York: Oxford University Press, 1988).
23. Norman Daniels, *Am I My Parents' Keeper?, op. cit.*
24. B.A. Rich, "Prospective Autonomy and Critical Interests: A Narrative Defense of the Moral Authority of Advance Directives," *Cambridge Quarterly of Healthcare Ethics,* Vol. 6 (1997), pp. 138–147.
25. Donald VanDeVeer, *Paternalistic Intervention, op. cit.*
26. S.R. Sabat and R. Harré "The Construction and Deconstruction of Self in Alzheimer's Disease," *Ageing and Society,* Vol. 12 (1992), pp. 443–461.

The Autonomy Turn in Physician-Assisted Suicide

TOM L. BEAUCHAMP

Department of Philosophy and Kennedy Institute of Ethics, Georgetown University, Washington, D.C. 20057, USA

Prohibitions of killing and physician assistance in suicide have long been canonical in medical ethics, but their days are limited in the twenty-first century. Our moral and legal compass should and will now shift to the key moral issue driving the debate, which is the liberty to choose the means to one's death and the justification, if any, for limiting that liberty. Physician-assisted suicide in the next century will likely be about letting people alone, not about letting them die or killing them.

A powerful reformation of our views about euthanasia, physician-assisted suicide, and refusals of treatment is now under way in several countries, but I will limit my analysis to developments in the United States. I will first review the recent history of this problem, and then consider how this history reflects the unfolding of a commitment to rights of autonomy. I will suggest why certain acts that have traditionally been considered mercy killings are better framed as forms of aid-in-dying that have been requested by patients. This position secured, I turn to public policy, where I will maintain that concerns about patient autonomy are the most important, but not the sole, factors driving current controversies and changes in policy. My reason for starting with history is not to secure an ethical conclusion by historical analysis, but the converse: I believe the ethical analysis will help us understand why history is moving in the direction it is.

[Parenthetical aside: My view about the now considerable philosophical literature on this subject is that it largely evades the central context in which the distinction arises—*viz.*, medicine—and that, as a result, the analyses offered turn out to be irrelevant to that context. For example, the treatments in Jonathan Bennett, R. I. Sikora, Philippa Foot, Judy Thomson, Alan Donagan, Michael Tooley, Warren Quinn, Jeff McMahan, etc. may be profound analyses with ingenious examples and counterexamples to illustrate some theses about acting and refraining, but I have not found them helpful for understanding the medical context. James Rachels is much better, but then he fails to give an analysis of the conditions of killing and letting die. Moreover, the very considerable facility with which philosophers have generated compelling counterexamples to every analysis should give us pause.]

AN INTERPRETATION OF RECENT MORAL AND LEGAL DEVELOPMENTS

Western medical ethics and law have been slow to come to conclusions about the right to choose the time and manner of one's death. Not until the mid-twentieth century did rights to consent, to refuse, and to control one's medical fate come into prominence. However, policies, practices, and legal precedents have evolved rapidly in the last quarter of the twentieth century— from the forgoing of respirators to the use of DNR orders to the forgoing of all medical technologies, including hydration and nutrition, to the point now of legalized physician-assisted suicide in one U.S. state. The history in the United States from *Quinlan* to *Cruzan* to *Vacco* and *Glucksberg*, then to *Measure 16* in Oregon, has been as rapid as it has been revolutionary. Although primarily a history of the constitutional protection of the so-called "right to die," underlying the legal issues is a powerful moral struggle being played out in health care facilities.

Prior to the findings in 1976 of the New Jersey Supreme Court in *In re Quinlan*, few judicial cases and effectively no public policy set the contours of decision-making rights for seriously ill or injured patients. In the face of active opposition from the hospital, the physicians, state and local authorities, and a lower-court guardian ad litem, the New Jersey Supreme Court held in *Quinlan* that it is permissible for a guardian to direct a physician and hospital to discontinue all extraordinary measures and disconnect Quinlan's respirator in order to allow her to die.[1] After the respirator was removed, Quinlan lived for almost ten years.[2]

A moral issue pushed to the surface over those ten years: If it is permissible to remove a respirator, is it also permissible to remove a feeding tube? The physicians had maintained in *Quinlan* that all such judgments were *medical* in nature, but the court asserted that the patient's rights and judgment must prevail over the physician's judgment in decisions at the end of life.[3] The news from New Jersey in that case was that decision-making authority resides in the patient and family, not the physician, the medical profession, or the hospital.

The *Quinlan* case initiated a discussion about refusing respirators, but the debate quickly shifted to the use of intravenous lines, stomach tubes, and total parenteral nutrition. The main issue in the 1980s became whether all medical treatments, depending on the circumstances, can be construed as optional, rather than obligatory. These questions persisted throughout the 1980s, but were in effect already answered by the time the first relevant U. S. Supreme Court decision was handed down in 1990.[4] This case—the *Cruzan* case—held that the right to refuse[5] treatment is protected by the U. S. Constitution by virtue of the liberty interest of the patient in unwanted medical interventions.[6] Although this decision returned issues of third-party decision-making to the individual states and allowed states to impose restrictions on end-of-life decision-making for incompetents, it also recognized circumstances under which nutrition and hydration may be justifiably withheld for incompetent persons.[7]

These legal developments joined with a developing ethics literature and increasing journalistic interest to produce a social consensus in the early 1990s. Bluntly stated, the consensus was that a passive euthanasia of letting die is acceptable, but an active euthanasia of killing is not.[8] The language of "passive euthanasia" was and still is generally avoided in favor of "forgoing life-sustaining treatment," but there can be little real doubt that acceptance of passive euthanasia (intentionally letting persons die when it serves their best interest) became part of the social consensus in the United States between 1976 and 1990. Appellate decisions after *Cruzan* reaffirmed and in no respect backed away from this position; indeed, case law has shielded and expanded the consensus view.

Shortly after *Cruzan*, in 1991, Washington State's Initiative 119 was presented to the public. This Initiative proposed to legalize requests by patients for aid-in-dying from physicians. It was narrowly defeated in the November 1991 election in Washington.[9] Legal and social consensus was lacking in the state over this active-euthanasia measure, but the failure of Initiative 119 did not affect the consensus already effected over passive euthanasia. In 1991, exactly fifteen years after *Quinlan*, a rough consensus had been achieved in the U. S. over refusal of treatment and passive allowing-to-die, and the nation was poised for the next stage of the discussion, which would be about so-called *active* forms of aid-in-dying.

Chronologically, fifteen years is but a fleeting moment in the history of the subject of how to treat the dying, but morally and legally U. S. society had by 1992 experienced an extraordinary transformation in its conception of the role of patient autonomy. We migrated from a pre-*Quinlan* fear of any form of intentional hastening of death to a confidence that it is permissible under a variety of conditions to intentionally forgo life-sustaining technologies of all types. What was unthinkable, or at least bitterly contested before *Quinlan*, became routine, and protected in constitutional law by a conservative Supreme Court.

The unthinkable unravelled still further in 1996 when two favorable decisions supporting a constitutional right to limited physician-assisted suicide were handed down in successive months by the 9th and 2nd U. S. Circuit Courts.[10] Their decisions, though reversed in law by the U. S. Supreme Court's 1997 decisions, contain powerful moral and public policy arguments that the Supreme Court did not attempt to address and that American society has yet to process. The Supreme Court, in effect, said that there are no constitutional rights to physician aid-in-dying, but that each state may set its own policy. This simple decision had the effect of rendering a right to physician-assisted death in some states a virtual certainty.

Its consequences were realized almost immediately in Oregon, where voters reaffirmed what they had three years previously passed—the initiative known as Measure 16—under which physicians are legally allowed to provide lethal medication to terminally ill patients.[11] A few weeks after its decisions in *Vacco* and *Glucksberg*, the U. S. Supreme Court refused to hear an appeal in this case, and Measure 16 was shortly thereafter reaffirmed by the voters of Oregon, then becoming the law of their state.[12]

This Oregon vote allowing a limited form of physician-assisted suicide and the lower-court (circuit) opinions that preceded the Supreme Court opinion reflect the new frontier of the social and legal acceptance of expanded autonomy rights to control one's death. The cutting-edge has now shifted from *refusal* of treatment to *request* for aid. We have migrated to the next level in the evolution of the discussion, which, as I see it, is the next stage in the unfolding of autonomy rights. The frontier is now voluntary active euthanasia, assisted suicide, and various forms of third-party refusals of treatment for incompetents.

As we edge into the twenty-first century, we will recast our understanding of the rights of patients (and perhaps surrogates) to request aid in dying, to plan their deaths, and in many cases to *cause* their deaths. The right side of history, I will now argue, is the side of recasting autonomy rights to request aid and plan for death using a model analogous to the ways we have used autonomy rights to require informed consent and to allow us to control the dying process through advance directives.

CONCEPTUAL PROBLEMS OF "KILLING" AND "LETTING DIE"

Moral, legal, and institutional judgments about the acceptability of euthanasia and assisted suicide have long turned on the influential distinction between killing and letting die. In medical tradition killing is prohibited and letting die permitted under specified conditions. Despite a remarkable convergence of opinion to this conclusion, no one has yet produced a cogent analysis of the distinction between killing and letting die as it functions in medicine so that meaningful law and professional ethics can be tied to their differences.[13]

I do not exempt the philosophical literature from this judgment. The distinction between killing and letting die has there, as elsewhere, generally been treated as a particular form of a more general distinction between acting and refraining, doing and allowing, action and inaction, and the like. A commonly used strategy in this literature is to present two cases differing only in that one is a killing or a letting die (usually involving some harm or wrong done), and then to investigate conceptually what the difference is, or morally whether the difference is relevant. The hypothesis is that the apparent conceptual or moral differences in the two cases shows that the distinction either is or is not viable or is or is not morally relevant.

Of course, philosophers completely disagree as to what these cases do and do not show, and they readily produce counterexamples to show that the original examples could not possibly be correct. [I do not say that philosophical analysis fails in all contexts or for all types of cases, such as trolley cases, burning trucks, releases of toxic substances, persons stranded on desert islands, rescuing drowning persons by killing someone in our path, but these examples do usually turn out to be wholly irrelevant to showing anything about the medical context.]

Philosophers are not alone in the messy state of their literature. Society seems generally confused and diffident about these concepts and their moral relevance. In daily life, in the courts, and in medicine, many persons view certain actions as instances of justified letting-die that others, no less qualified to judge, regard as unjustified killing. Consider the example of Dr. Gregory Messenger, a dermatologist charged with manslaughter after he unilaterally terminated his premature (25 weeks gestation, 750 g) son's life-support system in a Lansing, Michigan neonatal intensive care unit. He thought he had merely acted compassionately and let his son die after a neonatologist had failed to fulfil a promise not to resuscitate the infant.[14]

Whether killing or letting-die occurred is in dispute in this and many similar cases, but not because facts are disputed. The problem is created by the vagueness and the inherently contestable nature of the concepts of killing and letting die [as well as related concepts that they may rely upon, such as doing and allowing or action and inaction]. In ordinary language (at least in medical applications), *killing* is causal action that brings about another's death, whereas *letting die* is the intentional avoidance of causal intervention so that disease, system failure, or injury causes death. These definitions are entirely unsatisfactory, however, because they allow many acts of letting die to count as killing, thereby defeating the very point of the distinction. For example, under these definitions health professionals kill patients when they intentionally let them die in circumstances in which a duty exists to keep the patients alive. It is unclear in literature on the subject how to distinguish killing from letting die so as to avoid even this simple problem of cases that satisfy the conditions of both killing and letting die.[15]

Things get less clear once we become enmeshed in the examples and counterexamples used by philosophers, allegedly to shed light on this problem. What philosophers have accomplished, I think, is a rather compelling exhibition of why it is unlikely that any general characterization of these ordinary language terms is possible, no matter how many conditions are introduced to explicate the favored beginning examples. The concepts of killing and letting die are simply not orderly, precise, or systematic in a way that would sustain what philosophers would like to achieve.

Consider how difficult it would be to perform the task that philosophers envision. An adequate general philosophical analysis of these notions would have to proceed in at least two stages: first by distinguishing inaction from forgoing in the form of letting die, and then by distinguishing letting die from killing. First, consider the contrast between inaction and forgoing (in the form of letting die, on which I will later concentrate). To refrain in order to let someone die seems to involve more than not acting at all: The doctor who sits locked in his or her office seems very different from the doctor who lets someone die. Inaction or failure to act therefore must be successfully distinguished from omission or forgoing [I here assume that forgoing always occurs in letting die].

Here is one such analysis: The conditions of forgoing are that a person with the opportunity and ability to act does not act when he or she could reasonably be expected to act (the D'Arcy/von Wright analysis). This analysis is morally neutral, in the sense that the omission or forgoing cannot be determined to be either justified or unjustified by the analysis itself.

However, this analysis of omission or forgoing is unsatisfactory. The condition "could reasonably be expected to act" is too strong for the position occupied by physicians and families when they omit or forgo treatment. It is reasonable to expect them either to act or not to act in many cases. But if we simply remove the unhelpful condition "could reasonably be expected to act," we will doubtfully have a satisfactory general analysis of omission or forgoing. We often have the opportunity and ability to act and do not act without being involved in a forgoing or omission. For example, my department chair has the opportunity and ability to play tennis several times a day, but it would seem odd to say that he has forgone or omitted such activity when he has never even thought of it.

Of course, we could add another condition to the analysis to try to patch it up, but I do not wish to pursue this game here. Somewhere in the course of the attempt to distinguish inaction from forgoing, I believe we will have to bring intention into the picture. But as soon as intention enters, it will become difficult to distinguish forgoing (or omitting) from acting—though the whole point of the analysis is ultimately to make this distinction. Even if one tries the famous dodge in double-effect theory of distinguishing between intending and merely foreseeing and allowing (e.g., allowing nature to take its course), doctors and families intentionally act to allow a person to die, which brings intentional action into the analysis.

It is not clear, then, that we can even get to the second stage of the analysis, which would show that letting die is a form of forgoing that can be distinguished from killing, understood as a form of acting. But even if we could get to this stage, it is far from clear—as I will later suggest—that the inaction-omission-act strategy is the best entree to understanding killing and letting die. I think the best entree is to say that we intentionally act to let persons die and intentionally act to kill persons. In this way we can treat both as forms of intentional action and go right to the heart of the matter, which is whether this distinction can be analyzed as it functions in medicine. In any event, this is the strategy I will adopt.

MORAL PROBLEMS OF KILLING AND LETTING DIE

I turn, then, to the *moral* problems that are directly linked to these *conceptual* problems. The first topic of interest is the excusability of some acts of killing. The term "killing" does not entail a wrongful act or a crime, and the rule "do not kill" is a *prima facie* rather than absolute rule. Standard justifications of killing include killing in self-defense, killing to rescue a person endangered by the immoral acts of other persons, and killing by misadventure (accidental, nonnegligent killing while engaged in a lawful act). To correctly apply the label "killing" or the label "letting die" to a set of events will therefore not determine whether an action is acceptable or unacceptable.[16]

Killing may often be wrong and letting die rarely wrong, but, if correct, this conclusion is contingent on the features in particular cases. This result would not be surprising inasmuch as killings are rarely authorized by appropriate parties, and cases of letting die generally are. Be that as it may, the frequency with which one kind of act is justified, by contrast to the other kind of act, is not relevant to the moral justification of either kind of act. Forgoings that let a patient die can be both as intentional and as immoral as actions that in some more direct manner take their lives, and both can be forms of killing. To recast my earlier example, if a physician is responsible for a patient's care and maleficently forgoes a treatment that should have been provided, the physician's forgoing amounts to killing, indeed to murder. Whether there is any difference—and certainly any relevant difference—between acting and forgoing or between killing and letting die here comes openly into question.

Furthermore, the killing/letting die distinction is entirely irrelevant to today's central cases of so-called physician-assisted suicide, because these cases are not ones of either killing or of letting die. For example, a physician who prescribes a lethal medication at a patient's request does not thereby cause the patient's death and neither kills the patient nor lets the patient die, whether or not the patient voluntarily ingests the medication and dies. Since the prescription of fatal medication dominates the current discussion in the United States, this problem of the irrelevance of the killing/letting die distinction is not trivial. This distinction has been at the center of the classical discussions, but no longer can claim such status.

THE PIVOTAL POSITION OF THE CATEGORY OF LETTING DIE

Writers on the subjects of euthanasia, assisted suicide, and the killing/letting die distinction typically concentrate on killing, but the notion of letting patients die is conceptually the more important. A familiar thesis is that "letting die" occurs in medicine by "ceasing useless medical technologies."[17] This account fails to capture the full range of cases of letting die. "Letting die" occurs in medicine under two circumstances: cessation of medical technology because it is *useless* and cessation of medical technology because it has been *refused*. Honoring a refusal of a useful treatment knowing of a fatal outcome is a letting die, not a killing. The type of action—a killing or a letting die—can thus depend entirely on whether a valid refusal justifies the forgoing of medical technology.

A final conceptual point deserves attention: In the medical context, "letting die" is conceptually tied to *acceptable* acts, where acceptability derives either from futility of treatment or refusal of treatment. Killing, by contrast, is conceptually tied to *unacceptable* acts. The value-neutrality of "killing" and "letting die" found in ordinary moral discourse is thereby abandoned in the medical context: Letting die is justified, killing unjustified.

PROBLEMS OF CAUSATION

I now turn to the received account of letting die in law and medicine. It relies on a certain doctrine of causation of death that I believe cannot sustain the account. The central thesis is that intentionally forgoing a medical technology qualifies as letting die, rather than killing, if and only if an underlying disease or injury causes death.[18] The thesis is that when medical technology is withheld or withdrawn, a natural death occurs, because natural conditions do what they would have done if the technology had never been initiated. By contrast, killings occur when acts of persons rather than natural conditions cause death.

Despite its venerability and wide acceptance, the received view is unsatisfactory. To obtain a satisfactory argument, it must be added that the forgoing of the medical technology is *justified*. If the forgoing of the technology were *unjustified* or a person died from "natural" causes of injury or disease, it would be unjustified killing, not justified allowing to die. Imagine two persons in a semi-private hospital room, both with the same malady and both respirator-dependent. [This is my version of the two-case analysis.] One has the refused the respirator; the other wishes to remain on the respirator. A physician now intentionally flips a master switch that turns off both respirators. They die in the same way at the same time of the same physical causes.

Though they die of the same physical causes, they do not die of the same legal causes, because the proximate cause is not the same in the two otherwise identically situated patients. The doctor unjustifiably caused the death of and killed one patient (under criteria of legal causation); but the doctor justifiably let the other patient die. Causation in the law, unlike causation in other fields of inquiry, is structured to identify *responsibility* for an outcome. Locating the "cause of death" involves inquiry into who or what is responsible for death (whereas locating the "cause of death" in medical science identifies causal facts in an inquiry controlled by causal laws and the medically relevant features of medical inquiry into death).

In law one could not assess causal responsibility and liability for negative outcomes without a preexisting system of duties. Without an assigned duty, no causal responsibility or liability exists. Therefore, if a physician has no duty to treat, forbearing to treat does not breach a duty and does not cause death. Authorized withdrawal of treatment is such a forbearance, and the physician's forbearance is therefore not causally connected in law to the death. When no duty to treat exists, preexisting disease, system failure, or injury is the cause, and the physician escapes liability.

To bring out the importance of this point, consider again our physician who maleficently removed the respirator from the patient who wanted to continue living. It would be absurd to say, "The physician did not cause the patient's death; he only allowed the patient to die of an underlying condition." By "letting" this patient die a "natural" death, he failed to discharge a duty and legally caused the patient's death—indeed, he killed the patient. Legally, the physician is the cause of death, even if a coroner's account of the death does not mention what the physician has done. The law and the coroner have different criteria controlling their causal judgments.

Thus far, I have been considering patients whose death is physically caused only by "natural" conditions of illness or injury. It deserves additional consideration that in many cases of withdrawing or withholding a medical treatment, death is not physically caused by an underlying condition of disease or injury. For example, an act of removing a nasogastric tube to abate hydration or nutrition causes death from malnutrition, even if there is an underlying condition of disease or injury that motivates and justifies the decision to forgo treatment. Here a natural condition of disease or injury that counterfactually would have caused death plays a role in the justification of causing death, but does not itself cause death.

This conclusion clearly leaves open the possibility that physicians are causal factors in death when respirators or nutrition and hydration are removed. Removing medical technology such as hydration and nutrition is a relevant causal condition of death when and as it occurs. It is a physical cause of death, and it may or may not be a proximate cause of death in law. Whether a valid refusal is present is again likely to make the critical legal difference. From both a legal and a moral point of view, one reason why physicians do not injure or maltreat patients when they withhold or withdraw medical technology and thereby physically cause death (often with the intention of bringing about death) is that a physician is morally and legally obligated to recognize and act upon a valid refusal, irrespective of the causal outcome of doing so. Since valid refusal of treatment obligates the physician to forgo treatment, it would be absurd to hold that these legal and moral duties require physicians to cause the deaths of their patients—in the legal sense of "cause"—and thereby to kill them.

However, it is not absurd to say that the physicians' actions physically cause death. More precisely, the actions of physicians are commonly necessary parts of sufficient conditions of death as it occurs. To withhold nutrition and hydration so that a patient dies of starvation is a necessary part of a sufficient condition of death at the time and in the way the death occurs. Think about it counterfactually: Had the physician's act not occurred, the death would not have occurred. The singular causal statement "Dr. X caused the death of patient Y" is therefore a true statement; more precisely, the doctor is an insufficient but necessary part of a sufficient set of conditions of death. If the patient is suffering from conditions such as severe brain damage, cancer, or quadriplegia, these conditions are neither necessary nor sufficient conditions of death in the way it comes about.

In many cases both a physician's intervention *and* a disease, system failure, or injury are joint causal conditions of death when and in the way it occurs. In a few more uncommon cases, multiple causal conditions may be relevant, each forming an independent causal sequence sufficient to cause death. That is, any one of several distinct sequences of causally linked events may be sufficient to cause death. In some cases, we can say counterfactually, "Dr. X's action would have caused patient

Y's death had it not been for the immediately prior occurrence of condition Z in the patient, which actually caused death."

I conclude that the particular form or mode of causation of death is not the material matter in moral and legal issues about the justification of assistance in dying by forgoing treatment. Moral problems about forgoing treatment and letting die in medicine are not fundamentally causal problems. As long as a refusal of medical technology is valid, there exists no problem about responsibility for the death that ensues or about the justification of the action, no matter the causal route to death. Whatever the full causal story may be, if a duty not to treat exists because of a valid forgoing of medical technology, then the physician never legally causes death or kills when forgoing validly refused treatment; the physician who honors the refusal merely allows to die.[19]

The degree of the physician's involvement in the physical causation of death is here irrelevant, as the example of starvation clearly indicates. The valid refusal carries by itself the full burden of justification for the physician's action or inaction; the refusal nullifies what would otherwise be an injury or maltreatment, thereby preventing the possibility that the act is one of killing and also rendering irrelevant whether the death is or is not caused by natural conditions.

To generalize, these problems, as moral problems, are centrally ones of authorization, not causation. If validly authorized, the act is a letting die; if unauthorized, the same act is a killing. The justification of forgoing the medical technology, not the physical condition of death, is therefore the key condition both in conceptually distinguishing killing and letting die and in the moral and legal justification of letting die. This shows the powerful conceptual and moral connection between refusal of treatment and letting die. I will now develop this thesis further.

VALID REFUSALS AND VALID REQUESTS

My account is not yet adequate to handle moral and legal problems about forms of aid-in-dying that do not rest on *refusals*. I will now consider whether a valid *request* for help likewise authorizes a physician's assistance.[20] Clearly the two types of authorization—refusal and request—are not the same or even perfectly analogous. Whereas a health professional is obligated to honor a refusal, he or she is not obligated to honor a request. Valid refusals obligate a physician to do something (or forbear from doing something) that leads to death, whereas valid requests only make it permissible for a physician (or some other person) to lend aid in dying. Refusals, from this perspective, have a moral force lacking in requests. Informed refusals are sufficient conditions of justified forbearance, whereas informed requests are necessary but not sufficient conditions of justified assistance.[21]

Even so, the physician's precise responsibilities to the patient may depend on the nature of the request made and the nature of the pre-established patient–physician relationship. In some cases of justified compliance with requests, the patient and the physician will pursue the patient's best interest under an agreement that the physician will not abandon the patient or resist what they jointly determine to serve the patient's best interests. In some cases, patients in a close relationship with a physician *both* refuse a medical technology *and* request an accelerated death in order to lessen pain or suffering. Refusal and request are parts of a single overall plan. If the physician accepts the plan, assisted suicide or euthanasia grows out of the pre-established relationship.

UNDER WHAT CONDITIONS IS KILLING WRONG?

I have thus far avoided the language of "killing" in describing actions that are justified by valid requests. Nonetheless, let us now presume that some forms of assistance in death by physicians do involve killing their patients. The question still must be asked whether these acts can be justified.

The way to decide whether killing is wrong in specific cases is to determine what makes it wrong in general. My earlier arguments suggest that causing a person's death is wrong, when it is wrong, not merely because the death is caused by someone, but because an unjustified harm or loss to the person occurs. The death is bad for the person because of the deprivation of opportunities and goods that life would otherwise have afforded.[22] If this premise is correct, a sufficient condition of the wrongness of killing is that a person unjustifiably suffers a setback to personal interests that the person otherwise would not have experienced.[23]

However, if a person chooses death and sees that event as a personal benefit, rather than a setback or deprivation of opportunities, then killing at the person's request involves no clear harm or wrong. If letting die based on valid refusals does not harm or wrong persons or violate their rights, how can assisted suicide or voluntary active euthanasia harm or wrong a person who dies? In each case, persons seek what for them is the best means to the end of quitting life. Their judgment is that lingering in life is worse than death. The person in search of assisted suicide, the person who seeks active euthanasia, and the person who forgoes life-sustaining technology to end life may be identically situated. They simply select different means to end their lives.

Killing an autonomous person at his or her request may, from this perspective, be a way of showing respect for the person's autonomous choices. Medicine and law now seem to say to many patients, "If you were on life-sustaining treatment, you could withdraw the treatment and we could let you die. Because you are not, we can only give you palliative care until you die a natural death." This position condemns some patients to live out a life they wish to abandon, an act that both disrespects the patient's autonomous choice and prevents the physician from a discretionary discharge of fiduciary duties.

JUSTIFYING LEGALIZATION AND JUSTIFYING ACTIONS

It might be objected that even if this thesis is correct, it is insufficient to justify *public policies* in support of physician-assisted suicide (such as Measure 16 in Oregon[24] as well as present Dutch physician practices). Fair enough. My goal has been to justify acts rather than policies. I have been clarifying foundational questions about the morality of physician-assisted suicide and voluntary active intervention. I shift now to questions of policy and legalization.

The problem is this: The moral justification of acts is sometimes consistent with the moral justification of public policies that prohibit the same acts. That is, it is not inconsistent to conclude that morally acceptable acts are legally unacceptable. Similarly, it is not inconsistent to maintain that the government should prohibit certain morally wrong acts. Accordingly, the judgment that active euthanasia or physician-assisted suicide is morally justified for some patients does not entail that the government should legally permit active euthanasia and physician-assisted suicide under the conditions these patients suffer. Factors such as the costs of controlling abuses and the possibility that institutional standards of health care will deteriorate are deservedly considered in assessing the merit of legalization or policy, yet they need play little or no role in judging the morality of the action.

The theoretical backbone of public resistance to physician-assisted suicide and voluntary active euthanasia has long been slippery-slope and potential-abuse arguments.[25] I agree with proponents of these arguments that it is a reasonable presumption that some acts acceptable in one type of circumstance will, if legalized, inevitably be extended to similar circumstances in which the acts are morally unacceptable. For example, particular acts of assistance in dying that occur in circumstances of a long and affectionate patient–physician relationship might, if legalized, be extended to circumstances in serious risks of abuse that would, on balance, outweigh the benefits to society.

The argument is not that negative consequences such as impairing the trust vital to the patient–professional relationship or weakening the fabric of restraints on killing will occur immediately after legalization of physician-assisted suicide, but that they will grow incrementally over time. The concern is that restrictions initially built into legislation will eventually be revised or ignored, ever increasing the possibilities for unjustified killing. Unscrupulous persons will game the system. These concerns will be magnified in importance if the medical system does not come to grips with the needs of particularly vulnerable patients, who could be ignored or encouraged to end their lives by the system's expectations.[26]

If such consequences will result from the legalization of assisted suicide or voluntary active euthanasia, we have a powerful reason for resisting legalization. Still, how good is the evidence that these dire consequences will occur. Is there a sufficient reason to think that we cannot maintain control over and even improve public policy (as is now a common view in the Netherlands)? Those who use predictive arguments in defense of legalization as well as those who use such arguments in opposition to legalization owe us a careful accounting of the basis of their predictions, yet it remains unclear that such evidence has been or could be marshalled. This is one reason why the arguments about euthanasia and physician-assisted suicide are on firmer ground when judging acts rather than policies. The justification of acts requires no such evidence (unless one adopts a strict-rule consequentialist view of ethics).

The greater concern at the present time seems to be with the protection of vulnerable patients against a system of health care delivery that encourages premature death. The elderly, the homeless, the destitute, and the disabled are all legitimate objects of concern in a system that discourages expensive care and fosters an attitude that less-aggressive treatment is appropriate.

These fears deserve consideration in the construction of social policies, but they still fail to address the principal issue of whether there is a valid reason to deny either vulnerable or nonvulnerable parties aid-in-dying. It would be a bold paternalism that stripped vulnerable persons of the right to choose on grounds that they might choose wrongly. At bottom, current social problems about euthanasia and assisted suicide should take account of the threat to the vulnerable or to the larger society, but the central issue is about the right to choose and the valid limits on the exercise of that right.

Even if slippery-slope arguments point to dangers of the most profound sort, they do not undercut the view that at least some patients who seek aid-in-dying do no wrong in requesting aid and that their physicians do nothing morally wrong in acting to help them. Slippery-slope arguments are even consistent with justified moral nonconformity to state laws and evasive noncompliance with the prohibitions on physician-assisted suicide recommended by professional associations.[27]

The enemies of autonomous choice in this domain may reply that the moral grounds that justify legal prohibitions of euthanasia and physician-assisted suicide are also morally sufficient to prohibit individual nonconforming acts. Why, these critics might ask, do individual acts, including acts of disobedience, not give rise to the same slippery-slope and abuse concerns that warrant legal prohibitions? The bare fact that an individual is not harmed by an act of euthanasia or assisted suicide will not lead us to ignore the social consequences of these acts, which are morally relevant considerations inasmuch as they create a moral climate and set of expectations within which further actions will be taken.

Although correct and important, as far as it goes, this reasoning does not come to grips with a major feature of my argument. When I speak of the morality of acts, I mean their morality independent of the social consequences of a larger group of actors either performing or not performing the acts. Many features of morality have to do with justifying interpersonal relations that cannot be adequately assessed by their broader social consequences. For example, a physician may justifiably disclose confidential information about a patient to an endangered third party, although it is the type of information whose disclosure is generally prohibited, and properly so. Only a rigid-rule consequentialist moral theory would challenge these assumptions.

CONCLUSION

I have defended the view that some acts of physician-assisted suicide can be morally justified, but that empirical uncertainties render it unclear whether legalization is morally justified. The former position is premised largely on autonomy rights, whereas the latter is primarily an issue about public utility. Now that the dust has settled in the U.S. courts, an attractive context has been created (in that country) in which to continue this controversy. We know that, at least for now, no constitutional right is recognized and that one state, Oregon, is willing to confer a limited right. We can now observe how well Oregon fares, just as we have been watching the Netherlands. From this perspective, I find appealing Sandra Day O'Connor's conclusion—extracted from *Cruzan*—that liberty interests in physician-assisted suicide should be entrusted to the "'laboratory' of the states." O'Connor rightly invites trial runs and democratic voting as a potential way out of our current controversies.

Whatever the merits of this procedure, there is this unresolved problem of public policy: We constitutionally protect the forgoing of life-sustaining technologies in the United States, whereas every state except Oregon criminally prohibits physician-assisted suicide. This social policy seems incoherent if, as I believe, there is no morally relevant difference between forgoing treatment with the goal of death and requesting assistance with the goal of death.

Under these conditions, there is a denial of equal treatment and legal protection to persons who seek help in dying. Our social policies are incoherent in allowing one group to act in a manner relevantly similar to the way another group is not allowed to act. This situation makes no sense until placed in the light of the act/policy distinction with which I began. If law had only to consider the acceptability and coherence of individual acts, we should immediately reverse our bans on physician-assisted suicide. But law must consider the larger consequences of decriminalizing physician-assisted suicide. We are struggling at the present time with how to gauge those consequences, and we have, as yet, but a primitive premonition.

In the twenty-first century I expect the following to happen: The law will prove manageable and even be improved in Oregon and the Netherlands. Similar laws will then spread to other states and countries. In the meanwhile, law, ethics, and medicine will struggle to find more conservative alternatives. One option will be the cultivation of a wider array of circumstances under which competent patients are allowed to refuse nutrition and hydration in order to end their lives. The refusal of nutrition and hydration appears to encounter no legal or moral problems in many countries, despite the fact that there is no clear distinction between starving oneself to death and suicide or between a physician's starving a patient to death at the patient's request and physician-assisted suicide. The only problem appears to be a lack of awareness in medicine and among patients that this option is medically manageable and legally acceptable.

The other option that is virtually certain to come into increased favor is a dramatically improved and more aggressive style of palliative care. There is already a consensus that better end-of-life care, including palliative care, is needed, and we can expect to see more resources and training in support of this option.

None of these three very different options—(1) administration of fatal conditions, (2) planned forgoing of nutrition and hydration, and (3) improved aggressive palliative care—is necessarily the best for all patients. This is one reason for supporting all three options. The presentation of options is also consistent with the larger argument I have presented, which is that these issues of euthanasia, physician-assisted suicide, and aid-in-dying are primarily about increased liberty of choice, not about killing and letting die.

NOTES AND REFERENCES

1. *In re Quinlan*, 70 N.J. 10. 355 A.2d 647 (1976).
2. Unable to communicate with anyone, she lay comatose in a fetal position, with increasing respiratory problems and bedsores, her weight dropping from 115 to 70 pounds. Several Catholic moral theologians advised the parents that they were not morally required to continue medical nutrition and hydration or antibiotics to fight infections. However, the Quinlans believed both that the feeding tube did not cause pain and that the respirator did.

3. *In re Quinlan,* 70 N.J. 10, 40.
4. *Cruzan v. Director, Missouri Dept. of Health,* 110 S.Ct. 2841 (1990). Twenty-five-year old Nancy Cruzan had been in a persistent vegetative state for more than three years. Her parents then petitioned for permission to remove the feeding tube, knowing that, by doing so, their daughter would die. The Missouri Supreme Court ruled that no one may order an end to life-sustaining treatment for an incompetent person in the absence of clear and convincing evidence of the patient's wishes, and this decision was upheld by the U. S. Supreme Court. The Supreme Court decision was followed by a hearing before a County probate judge at which three friends of Nancy Cruzan provided sufficient additional evidence that she had expressed a clear and convincing preference not to live "like a vegetable" connected to machines. This new evidence led the judge to accept the parents' request to remove the feeding tube, and thirteen days after removal, and after eight years in a coma, Nancy Cruzan died. The U. S. Supreme Court did not, of course, grant the Cruzan family the relief it had sought.
5. A constitutional right to die in the sense of a right of competent persons to decline life-sustaining treatments.
6. *Cruzan v. Director, Missouri Dept. of Health,* 110 S.Ct. at 2851. The protection of a liberty interest is stressed in this case.
7. The Court held that it is constitutionally permissible for states to impose procedural precautions when third parties are making decisions for incompetent patients. 110 S.Ct. esp. at 2852.
8. See Alan Meisel, "The Legal Consensus about Forgoing Life-Sustaining Treatment: Its Status and its Prospects," *Kennedy Institute of Ethics Journal,* Vol. 2 (1992), pp. 309–345.
9. Initiative 119 read as follows: "Shall adult patients who are in a medically terminal condition be permitted to request and receive from a physician aid-in-dying?"
10. United States Court of Appeals for the Ninth Circuit, *Compassion in Dying v. State of Washington,* No. 94-35534, filed March 6, 1996; United States Court of Appeals for the Second Circuit, *Vacco v. Quill,* No. 95-7028, decided April 2, 1996; 1996 U.S. App. LEXIS 6215. See, further, *Compassion in Dying v. State of Washington,* 850 F. Supp. 1454 (W.D. Wash. 1994); U.S. D. Ct., W.D. Wash., No. C94-119R, decided May 3 and overturned March 9, 1995 by the United States Court of Appeals for the Ninth Circuit in an opinion written by Judge John T. Noonan. *Compassion in Dying v. Washington,* No. 94-35534 (U.S. App. March 9, 1995) (available March 1995 on LEXIS).
11. "The Oregon Death with Dignity Act" was approved by voters in November 1994. Under its provision a patient must wish to escape unbearable suffering and must three times request a physician's prescription for lethal drugs. The doctor then must wait fifteen days after the first request before writing a prescription for the requested lethal drugs. In late December 1994, a federal judge in Eugene, Oregon, issued a preliminary injunction that prevented putting the new law into effect for an indefinite period of time. At the time, physicians' and pharmacists' groups in Oregon had not decided whether to participate under the new law.
12. On November 4, 1997, by a 60–40 margin, voters rejected Measure 51, which would have repealed Measure 16. The 9th U. S. Circuit of Appeals had, one week previously, lifted an injunction that had kept Measure 16 from going into effect.
13. See Bonnie Steinbock and Alastair Norcross (Eds.) *Killing and Letting Die,* 2nd ed. (New York: Fordham University Press, 1994); Tom L. Beauchamp (Ed.) *Intending Death* (Upper Saddle River, N.J.: Prentice Hall, 1996). See also H. M. Malm, "Killing, Letting Die, and Simple Conflicts," *Philosophy and Public Affairs,* Vol. 18 (1989), pp. 238–258; Jeff McMahan, "Killing, Letting Die, and Withdrawing Aid," *Ethics,* Vol. 103 (1993), pp. 250–279; Lawrence O. Gostin, "Drawing a Line Between Killing and Letting Die: The Law, and Law Reform, on Medically Assisted Dying," *Journal of Law, Medicine & Ethics,* Vol. 21 (1993), pp. 94–101; James F. Childress, "Non-Heart-Beating Donors: Are the Distinctions Between Direct and Indirect Effects and Between Killing and Letting Die Relevant and Helpful?" *Kennedy Institute of Ethics Journal,* Vol. 3 (1993), pp. 203–216; Susan Kowalski, "Assisted Suicide: Where do Nurses Draw the Line?" *Nursing and Health Care,* Vol.

14 (1993), pp. 70–76; Donald G. Casswell, "Rejecting Criminal Liability for Life-shortening Palliative Care," *Journal of Contemporary Health Law and Policy,* Vol. 6 (1990), pp. 127–144.
14. Howard Brody, "Messenger Case: Lessons and Reflections," *Ethics-In-Formation,* Vol. 5 (1995), pp. 8–9; "Man Acquitted in Son's Death," *New York Times* (4 February 1995), p. 10; John Roberts, "Doctor Charged for Switching Off His Baby's Ventilator," *British Medical Journal,* Vol. 309 (13 August 1994), p. 430. In February 1995, Dr. Messenger was cleared by a jury in a lower court of manslaughter charges brought in 1994.
15. Discussion of these subjects has been further thwarted by additional conceptual confusion surrounding the terms "euthanasia" and "physician-assisted suicide." The term "euthanasia" now has two general meanings and types: (1) painlessly putting to death those who suffer from terminal or severely painful conditions (active euthanasia), and (2) intentionally forbearing from preventing death in those who suffer from terminal or severely painful conditions (passive euthanasia). There are questionable features in this conception, especially the underlying distinction between the passive and the active. But I will here ignore these problems and consolidate the two meanings into a single definition, which I will use hereafter: Euthanasia occurs if and only if: (1) The death of a person is intended by at least one other person who is either the cause of death or a causally relevant factor in bringing about the death; (2) the person killed is or soon will be terminally ill, acutely suffering, or irreversibly comatose, which alone is the primary reason for intending the person's death; and (3) the means chosen to produce the death are as painless as possible, or there is a sufficient moral justification for choosing a more painful method. Finally, "physician-assisted suicide" is sometimes treated as a form of voluntary active euthanasia, on grounds that the voluntary choice of the patient makes the death a suicide and that physician-assistance is active rather than passive. However, voluntary active euthanasia and physician-assisted suicide should be kept distinct. "Euthaniasia" does not entail that a *physician* brings about the death, and "physician-assisted suicide" does not entail that the person who dies be acutely suffering or that this condition forms the reason for suicide or for assisting in suicide.. There is also no conceptual requirement in physician-assisted suicide that the means chosen be as painless as possible. Assisted suicide and voluntary active euthanasia both involve assistance in bringing about another's death, but "assisted suicide" entails that the person whose death is brought about be the ultimate cause of death (the final relevant link in a causal chain leading to death), whereas "voluntary active euthanasia" entails that the ultimate cause of one person's death be another person's action.
16. Cf. James Rachels, "Active and Passive Euthanasia," *New England Journal of Medicine,* Vol. 292 (January 9, 1975), pp. 78–80. See also his *The End of Life: Euthanasia and Morality* (Oxford: Oxford University Press, 1986); and Dan W. Brock, "Voluntary Active Euthanasia," *Hastings Center Report* Vol. 22, No. 2 (March/April 1992), pp. 10–22.
17. Willard Gaylin, Leon Kass, Edmund Pellegrino, and Mark Siegler, "Doctors Must Not Kill," *Journal of the American Medical Association,* Vol. 259 (April 8, 1988), pp. 2139–2140. It is sometimes added, as a condition, that the patients must be dependent on life-support systems. See Ronald E. Cranford, "The Physician's Role in Killing and the Intentional Withdrawal of Treatment," in Beauchamp (Ed.), *Intending Death, op. cit.*, p. 160.
18. See Daniel Callahan, "Vital Distinctions, Mortal Questions: Debating Euthanasia and Health Care Costs." *Commonweal,* Vol. 115 (July 15, 1988), pp. 397–404; Callahan, *The Troubled Dream of Life* (New York: Simon and Schuster, 1993), Chapter 2; and several articles in Joanne Lynn (Ed.), *By No Extraordinary Means* (Bloomington, IN: Indiana University Press, 1986), pp. 227–266. See also *In the Matter of Claire C. Conroy,* 190 N.J. Super. 453, 464 A.2d 303 (App. Div. 1983); *In the Matter of Claire C. Conroy,* 486 A.2d 1209 (New Jersey Supreme Court, 1985), at 1222–23, 1236; *In re Estate of Greenspan,* 558 N.E.2d 1194, at 1203 (Ill. 1990).
19. Nonetheless, the actions of physicians are commonly, from a scientific point of view, necessary parts of sufficient conditions of death as it occurs. To withhold nutrition and

hydration so that a patient dies is a necessary part of a sufficient condition of death at the time and in the way the death occurs. If the patient is suffering from conditions such as severe brain damage, cancer, or quadriplegia, these conditions are neither necessary nor sufficient conditions of death as it occurs. In some circumstances, both physician action *and* a relevant causal condition of disease, system failure, or injury are present. In a few cases, multiple causal conditions may be relevant, each forming an independent causal sequence sufficient to bring about death. That is, any one of several distinct sequences of causally linked events may be sufficient to cause death.

20. On the importance of the refusal-request distinction, see James L. Bernat, Bernard Gert, and R. Peter Mogielnicki, "Patient Refusal of Hydration and Nutrition," *Archives of Internal Medicine,* Vol. 153 (1993), pp. 2723–28; Gert, Bernat, and Mogielnicki, "Distinguishing Between Patients' Refusals and Requests," *Hastings Center Report,* Vol. 24 (July/August 1994), pp. 13–15; and B. Gert, J.L. Bernat, and R.P. Mogielnicki, "The Distinction Between Active and Passive Euthanasia," *Archives of Internal Medicine,* Vol. 155 (1995), p. 1329.

21. A physician who in principle accepts the permissibility of assistance in bringing about death may still refuse to honor any particular request for assistance on grounds that the patient's condition has not reached the point of last resort or on grounds that standard measures of palliative support and supportive help should be sufficient to relieve the patient's suffering at this stage. For example, a sympathetic physician willing to assist a patient at a crisis point may refuse a patient's request for lethal medication at a premature stage.

22. See Thomas Nagel, "Death," in *Mortal Questions* (Cambridge: Cambridge University Press, 1979). For criticisms and extensions, see F. M. Kamm, *Morality, Mortality,* Vol. I (New York: Oxford University Press, 1993), chapt. 1.

23. Cf. Allen Buchanan, "Intending Death: The Structure of the Problem and Proposed Solutions," in Beauchamp (Ed.), *Intending Death,* pp. 34–38.

24. Oregon Legislature. Measure No. 16. *Oregon Death with Dignity Act* (1994), approved by voters in a 1994 referendum. Under this act, terminally ill adults are allowed to obtain lethal drugs from physicians in order to hasten death and escape unbearable suffering. This initiative, once scheduled to become law, was permanently enjoined by a Federal district court until the U.S. Supreme Court decision.

25. Cf. James Rachels, *The End of Life: Euthanasia and Morality,* chapt. 10; John Arras, "The Right to Die on the Slippery Slope," *Social Theory and Practice,* Vol. 8 (1982), pp. 285-328; Wibren van der Burg, "The Slippery Slope Argument," *Ethics,* Vol. 102 (October 1991), pp. 42–65; Ruth Macklin, "Which Way Down the Slippery Slope? Nazi Medical Killing and Euthanasia Today," in Arthur L. Caplan (Ed.), *When Medicine Went Mad: Bioethics and the Holocaust* (Totowa, NJ: Humana Press, 1992), pp. 173–200, 343–345; J.A. Burgess, "The Great Slippery-Slope Argument," *Journal of Medical Ethics,* Vol. 19 (1993), pp. 169–174; Douglas Walton, *Slippery Slope Arguments* (Oxford: Clarendon Press, 1992); Frederick Schauer, "Slippery Slopes," *Harvard Law Review,* Vol. 99 (1985), pp. 361–383.

26. Joanne Lynn, "The Health Care Professional's Role When Active Euthanasia Is Sought," *Journal of Palliative Care,* Vol. 4 (1988), pp. 100–102; Susan Wolf, "Holding the Line on Euthanasia," *Hastings Center Report,* Vol. 19 (January-February 1989), S13–S15.

27. Compare James F. Childress, "Civil Disobedience, Conscientious Objection, and Evasive Noncompliance: A Framework for the Analysis and Assessment of Illegal Actions in Health Care," *Journal of Medicine and Philosophy,* Vol. 10 (1985), pp. 63–83. For a contrasting view that rests on a form of slippery slope argument, see Daniel Callahan, *The Troubled Dream of Life, op. cit.,* chapt 3.

A Circumscribed Plea for Voluntary Physician-Assisted Suicide

RAPHAEL COHEN-ALMAGOR

The University of Haifa, Mount Carmel, Haifa 31905, Israel

INTRODUCTION

The concept of "death with dignity" does not automatically imply a desire to die; it certainly does not mean to put someone to death in a dignified way. Organizations that support euthanasia speak of the "right to die with dignity," and this terminology became a euphemism that promotes euthanasia. I believe in the concept of death with dignity, and recognize that some prefer death over the continuation of tormented living. Some organizations are so dedicated to the idea, however, that they conceive of themselves as missionaries whose role is to educate and "advance" society in the "right" direction, and sometimes they do not make judgements and decisions carefully.[1] They become too eager and their strong motivation overshadows the need for utmost caution. After all, this is a matter of life and death. We cannot be simplistic or ambiguous with this delicate issue.

I recall a discussion with an Israeli attorney who specializes in representing patients who wish to die, and who is active in the right-to-die organization in Israel. I asked him what his prime concern is. His answer was the patient's expressed will to die. I further pressed the issue and questioned him about different scenarios: What if your client needs some emotional support? What if he or she is unaware of all the relevant considerations relating to his or her disease? I wanted to understand to what extent the attorney was sensitive and cognizant of the possibility that some of the patients/clients might change their mind if things were explained to them in a different manner. The attorney's answers clearly showed that he did not care. For him the client's desire to die was sufficient. His attitude lacked compassion for the clients.

Our first obligation is to place the issue in its proper context and to emphasize that most patients seek to preserve life. With this proviso in mind, my opinion supports the right to die with dignity in certain cases, which will be clarified. I will do my best to describe these cases clearly, without being overzealous, and without offending the people involved. Life should not be seen as a virtue to be preserved at any cost, regardless of the patient's will; at the same time euthanasia should not be supported without reservation. In this context I shall criticize Dr. Jack Kevorkian's campaign for euthanasia and the utilization of his "Mercitron." Kevorkian himself may not be considered seriously by bioethicists, but his deeds deserve serious consideration. From 1990 until his arrest in 1999 Dr. Kevorkian has helped dozens of people to die. Kevorkian recognized a need of people facing or enduring illness that has not been addressed adequately by society, and he employed a missionary vigor in trying to close this lacuna. His campaign is the result of failures of the medical system in caring for patients with intractable or chronic problems. It forces society to think harder than before about medical mercy and assistance at the end of life, and to find suitable answers so that Jack Kevorkian's ministrations may be made redundant.

The *Eyal* case, which took place in Israel in 1990, serves as an illustration to show that on some occasions physician-assisted suicide may be allowed. I assert that in instances such as this one, patients' autonomy would be sustained and their dignity better served by helping them to die. It is not always true that keeping a person alive is to treat her as an end. In some incurable situations we respect agonizing patients and their dignity when we help them to cease living. My justification for helping such patients fulfil their request rests on the assumption that they freely and genuinely expressed their will to die, and that they persist in expressing that desire.

THE *BENJAMIN EYAL* CASE

In 1990, the magistrates' court of Tel Aviv received an appeal made by a patient named Benjamin Eyal. Mr. Eyal suffered from the same disease that attacked Sue Rodriguez in Canada,[2] amyotrophic lateral sclerosis (ALS). Mr. Eyal, aware of the expected progress of the disease, asked not to be attached to a respiratory machine when he could no longer breathe spontaneously, but to be allowed to die. He expressed this wish in an affidavit, in a video cassette, and verbally as well. The specialist who testified before the court said that his commitment to care for Mr. Eyal "does not include a duty to prolong life of unimaginable suffering by committing an intrusive act that could be avoided by following the will of the patient."[3]

In considering Mr. Eyal's motion, Judge Uri Goren emphasized two principles: the "sanctity of life" principle, and the "decent death" principle. As for the "sanctity of life" principle, Judge Goren articulated that this principle should be employed when medical treatment could save life or improve the medical state of patients. (However, Jewish law does recognize the need not to *afflict* dying people, taking into consideration human suffering and pain.[4])

Judge Goren explained that in this case, no doubts arose with regard to the wishes of the patient. Mr. Eyal clearly manifested his wish not to be connected to a respirator when the time came and no other alternative was available to keep him alive. In addition, there were no doubts that Mr. Eyal was competent and clear-minded upon voicing his request, knowing its obvious consequences. In his testimony before the court, the Director of Lichtenstaedter Hospital, Dr. Nachman Wilensky, explained that Mr. Eyal was a senior patient, well known to the hospital officials, and that he was thoroughly convinced that Eyal's intentions were sincere and freely chosen.

Judge Goren decided to accept the appeal. He emphasized that such a decision concerning life and death should be made by a senior director, either by the Director of the Hospital or by the Head of Department. This was because the decision involved expertise, moral values, religion, and ethics.[5]

The *Eyal* case stimulated much debate in Israel. Rabbinical authorities were asked their opinion regarding this situation. I should first reiterate that the major difference between the *halachic* view and the liberal view is that many *halachic* commentators do not endorse the autonomy principle. According to their perspective, persons are not masters of their lives. Life is given to us as a deposit by the Creator, and we should not destroy it.[6] Human life is intrinsically good, irrespective of its condition. Rabbi Elyashiv, a well known *halachic* decider (*Posek Halacha*), said that when medical treatment may only prolong transient life and involved additional suffering, a patient may refuse to accept it. The physicians were allowed to terminate treatment when the last stages of Mr. Eyal's disease were reached. Rabbi Israel Meir Lau, currently the Ashkenazi Chief Rabbi in Israel, also endorsed this view.

In a letter concerning the *Eyal* case, Rabbi Lau wrote that his discretion was limited to the case in hand, and to the specific circumstances as described to him. He contended that the *halacha* did not require, and sometimes prohibited, the performance of exceptional treatment that only prolonged the patient's suffering without healing the cause of the pain. Mr. Eyal's disease was said to be incurable and the disputed treatment would not sustain his life in any meaningful sense. So, when the time came, the attending physicians should be allowed to act upon Mr. Eyal's request, and refrain from connecting him to a respirator. Rabbi Lau maintained that, in any event, regular medical treatment should be sustained. That is, Mr. Eyal should be provided with nutrition and all means should be taken to relieve his pain.[7]

Benjamin Eyal died of disease complications before the disease had reached its final stage and before a respirator was necessary. Thus, the physicians at Lichtenstaedter did not have to act upon the court's decision. For the sake of argument, however, let us suppose that the final stage had been reached, and the physicians refrained from connecting Benjamin Eyal to the respirator machine. Would it be humane to witness Mr. Eyal suffocating to death? I asked one of Mr. Eyal's senior doctors if it would be possible for him to stand idly by while his patient was choking to death. The doctor's replied: "I would 'give Eyal something' to shorten his suffering."

I think that this is a humane answer, in harmony with the morals of humane medicine. Any other answer, principally opposed to active intervention, would be inhumane and cruel. Under such circumstances, there are strong reasons to consider physician-assisted suicide. When the patient is obviously suffering and expresses his or her will to die, and the doctors admit that they are unable to cure the illness and all they can do is to ease the physical and not the emotional pain, then there is no substantial difference between voluntary passive euthanasia and voluntary physician-assisted suicide.[8] The term "voluntary" refers both to the request of the patient and to the act of the doctor. The patient should have the right to decide for himself/herself about his/her fate, and the doctor should not be compelled to abide. The doctor should abide only if he/she feels that physician-assisted sucide is the appropriate, dignified, and kind medical measure.

Those who oppose assisted suicide will say that there is no need to reach the stage where we have to consider such termination of life. Benjamin Eyal could have been given medicine to stop him from suffering. The responsibility rests with the doctor to give medicine to patients, even if the medicine shortens their lives. This is allowed because the purpose is to care for the patients and decrease their suffering, not to bring about their death.

I discussed the double-effect doctrine in another essay.[9] This doctrine serves both spiritual leaders and careful healers as a way out of dealing directly and sincerely with the question of mercy termination of life. Undoubtedly the doctrine provides a better solution than letting people like Benjamin Eyal die slowly in agony. In the everyday medical practice in hospitals there are many instances in which doctors perform double-effect interventions: their intention is to alleviate pain and suffering, not to kill the patient, but the result is the death of the patient. However, I suspect that there are enough cases in which partisan interests, and not the patients' best interests, are first and foremost before the doctor's eyes, and the double-effect doctrine serves as a convenient guise for pursuing those partisan interests.

The reader should not infer from the ongoing discussion that allowing merciful medical assistance to end life in cases where the patient's condition is irreversible, and the patient lacking autonomy seeks assistance to fulfil his or her desire to die, entails the killing of patients in other instances. Sometimes a patient whose human life is reduced to a phantom or chimera of human life might progress and his or her situation might improve. It is only when we are certain that no progress may be made (as in the cases of severe, irreversible damage to the brainstem described as brain death) that we can speak in definite terms of a shadow of life rather than of a life. Physicians are convinced that, for all practical purposes, the identification of brain death means that the patient is dead (see Truog's essay in this volume). As things stand now, when confronted with brain-dead patients, human dignity must prevail to bring about at least a dignified death.

THE DOCTOR'S ROLE

A troubling question is whether or not it is within the doctor's responsibility to terminate life. Obviously, when patients are competent and able to commit suicide they can assist themselves and seek death in various ways without having the need to involve doctors. The case is different when the patients are unable—physically or mentally—to commit suicide. These patients seek the doctors' assistance.

Doctors who are opposed to active euthanasia and physician-assisted suicide find no dignity in killing a patient, and express anxiety about the character of a society in which doctors assume such a responsibility.[10] Charles Sprung describes doctors' consent to perform euthansia as "unethical."[11] Avraham Steinberg writes in his criticism of this essay that the doctor's role does not include killing. If society accepts the need for active euthanasia then such an act can be committed by any person. The doctor's role is to heal, to help patients, and to relieve their suffering. Society must not assign its doctors the additional task of execution.

Although my plea is a circumscribed one in favor of physician-assisted suicide and not active euthanasia, let me first demur and say that I resent the use of the term "executioner" in this context. Support for active euthanasia is not necessarily associated with the acceptance of execution in society. One of the doctor's roles is, indeed, to ease patients' suffering. The daily practice in hospitals demonstrates that sometimes the only way to achieve this objective also shortens the patient's life. We are dealing with a population of patients with reasons, drives, and wills of their own. Failing to listen to those reasons, drives, and wills would lead to gross paternalism: an unjustified action that takes the responsibility from the patient. Such behavior is unjustified because (*a*) the person for whom the doctor acts paternalistically is competent, and (*b*) the conduct in question is involuntary and coercive. Is it the task of a doctor to keep a person alive against that person's will? How do we answer that small group of patients who have lost their will to live and plead to their doctors for help? Steinberg and others think that it is not among the doctor's responsibilities to perform mercy killings. The question is whether another professional body exists in society that could take responsibility for this troubling task. Is it conceivable to ask another association (trained paramedics) or social group (the patient's beloved people) to assume this responsibility? My answer is conclusive. It is impossible to act on matters of health without qualified medical opinion. While I see no escape from including doctors in the decision-making process, Steinberg wishes, in his words, "to keep the doctor outside the killing circle," and does not want to consider active intervention as an option. While I seek an answer for *all* patients, including those who wish to die, Steinberg ignores those patients who suffer from incurable diseases and express their wish to die. Obviously Dr. Steinberg and others who are opposed to physician-assisted suicide should not be expected to commit an act that contravenes their conscience; that would be as paternalistic as ignoring the patient's will. However, there are doctors who might agree with this line of reasoning and who would not necessarily regard such medical intervention as contrary to their medical and moral conscience.

One major objection to the circumscribed argument evinced here for physician-assisted suicide holds that the action is irreversible in the sense that it curtails the possibility of medical "miracles." Medicine is not a precise science and doctors do not know all. Often when the body responds differently from what was expected, contrary to the prognoses, contrary to the statistics and to recorded probabilities, explanations are given in a vocabulary that expresses humility regarding human knowledge and ability to comprehend. The popular press often terms such positive responses as "miraculous." Physician-assisted suicide precludes any chance for such "miracles" and the possibility of re-diagnosing a misdiagnosis. There is also the fear of abuse, of killing patients against their will; thus there is a need for safety valves and for installing mechanisms of control. In the next sections I shall further circumscribe my reasoning in an effort to provide answers to these fair challenges.

THE NEED FOR SAFETY VALVES

Preliminaries

The above warnings are well founded and we should therefore strive to minimize the possibility of errors taking place. Because most patients wish to live almost regardless of their condition, this discussion is relevant for a small number of cases, like that of Benjamin Eyal and Sue Rodriguez.

To minimize the danger of misdiagnosis, a separate prognosis should be provided by at least two *independent* experts. One should be the patient's attending physician, who is in charge of her treatment and knows her case better than the other doctors in her surroundings. Where none of the attending doctors really knows the patient well, the decision-making process should involve the entire medical team. Competent patients should be advised of the doctors' doubts and hesitations about the nature of the illness, if such doubts exist. The patients should be informed, in language and terms they are able to understand, of the existing knowledge about their illnesses, to what extent it is based on data or speculations, and the margins of error. When the patients are incompetent, their family members and beloved people should be told about the prognoses and thoughts of the doctors.

As to the claim that physician-assisted suicide unnecessarily shortens life we should bear in mind that many of the patients who ask to die do so not because they want to live another day, another week, another month, but because life has become a burden they are better off without. People like Benjamin Eyal no longer wish to explore just how constrained such a life might be. Let me further stress that the circumscribed argument that I am making in favor of physician-assisted suicide relates only to people at the end of their lives, when their medical situation is diagnosed as incurable, and when patients reiterate their request to die several times over a certain period of time. This formulation would exclude physician-assisted suicide for patients who enjoy having helpful medicine that could improve their condition. The argument would also exclude physician-assisted suicide for patients who might suffer depression and who might come to re-enjoy life after the depressive period is over.

Fear of Sliding Down the Slippery Slope

A serious objection to both active euthanasia and physician-assisted suicide concerns sliding down the slippery slope, toward total disrespect and contempt for human life. The argument holds that it is preferable to keep active euthanasia and physician-assisted suicide illegal so as to raise a clear voice regarding the value and importance of human life, and to force physicians to think hard when they assume the responsibility of shortening life. This argument contains several warnings: first, the weak populations who are unable to protect themselves would be severely harmed once active euthanasia and physician-assisted suicide would be allowed. Sweeping interpretations of allowing active intervention to terminate life could bring about the ending of lives of the poor, the neglected, the unwanted. Justice Menachem Elon's decision in the *Scheffer* case is germane to this discussion:

> When we begin to estimate and to consider the *worth* of human life, these "evaluations" and "weightings" will lead firstly to permission to kill people whose minds and bodies are severely defective, then to the killing of those who are defective a bit less, and with time there will be no measure as to how limited the defect would have to be...[12]

Second, there is a danger of applying pressure on patients to die. This pressure could stem from various causes. There might be exploitation of the patient by family members who are after money and consequently would welcome the patient's death. In fact, this claim raises suspicion about doctors who do not always act in accordance with the best interests of the patient and hence allow room for family exploitation.[13] There is also a danger of exploitation by the establishment—that is, by hospitals and medical centers, which often operate under circumstances of scarce resources and budget cuts. The argument is that, in an atmosphere permitting active intervention to end life, human life might become less important, and thus it might be in jeopardy when there are serious budgetary pressures and long lines for beds.

Warnings against a slippery slope process that might result in the deaths of some who wish to continue living are valid. The rationale for creating ethical directives for doctors, from the Hippocratic Oath to hospital ethics committees, arises out of a recognition that doctors might abuse the power they possess. Such fears can be avoided by paying careful attention to the fine details when formulating concepts and regulations, and by using explicit wording that does not allow abusive interpretations. The fear of abuse, and the desire to grant patients control over their lives until the very last moment were the prime motivations to restrict my plea to physician-assisted suicide and to refrain from advocating active euthanasia as well. From the Netherlands and Oregon we learn that most patients who opted for death were cancer patients. It can be assumed that they were capable of activating a lethal needle administered by a qualified doctor. The claim made by some Dutch physicians that active euthanasia is preferable to physician-assisted suicide can be rebutted.[14] In the Netherlands, unsuccessful physician-assisted suicide happened because physicians administered oral drugs that were not always effective. In the scheme offered here, the lethal medication will be provided by injection and it is the patient who operates the suicide mechanism.

Fear of the slippery slope should not lead to a *tout court* rejection of active involvement of physicians in the termination of lives, but to a commitment to create clear and definitive guidelines. We must examine the will of the patient, her condition, the extent of her suffering, and the doctors' prognoses regarding the possibility of improving her condition.[15] At the same time we should punish the abusers in order to prevent them from committing further wrong-doing, and to deter others who might contemplate abuse. But the fear of abuse in itself does not constitute a strong moral ground that overrides the autonomy interests of patients.

Conscientious commentators, while aware of the possibility of the slippery-slope argument, that allowing mercy killing in some cases might lead to allowing this act in other cases, nevertheless argue that in specific circumstances mercy killing (often times active euthanasia and physician-assisted suicide are lumped together) does not go against the patient's interests but conforms to them.[16] Such an act is conceived as not offending against the intrinsic value of human life but rather affirming its convictions, its sense of integrity, and its dignity.

I now turn to the warnings concerning possible negative ramifications for society at large. There are those who claim that licensing mercy killing and physician-assisted suicide in certain cases will lead to an increase in violence and in indifference to human life in general.[17] Note that the slippery-slope argument does not state that active euthanasia and physician-assisted suicide are wrong or immoral, but that permitting them might have negative consequences. The argument emphasizes what could happen to society if we indulge a request of a certain patient, but to a certain extent it disregards the *patient*. My claim is that we should not ignore the individual in need, and that each case should be considered in its own right. Moreover, the slippery-slope argument focuses the attention on what might happen in society as a result of granting a certain patient her wish, but it ignores the misery of the patient *now*. In the center of the ensuing analysis lies the individual. I believe that voluntary physician-assisted suicide conducted out of an honest and true motivation to provide relief from suffering is a humane act that respects the patient. There is reason to think that allowing physician-assisted suicide under the specified terms could increase sensitivity to human suffering and dignity, and not contribute to the devaluation of human life. The consequences of voluntary physician-assisted suicide for society may be positive.

Furthermore, we may be sliding down the slippery slope if we allow the present situation to continue. It is my feeling that we have been sliding down the slope. Through the "simple" concepts of "terminal" patients, life "devoid of *quality*," "*futile*" treatment, "*vegetative*" patients (or simply "*vegetables*") and the double-effect doctrine, shortening of life—not always for sincere motives geared to serve the best interests of the patients—is a common practice in hospitals.[18] The patients would be better off if those key concepts were replaced by long sentences describing their diseases and by elaborate discussions about their medical prognosis and the available knowledge to help them cope with their illnesses. Single-word vocabulary and obscure Latin words serve the interests of doctors, not of the patients. They facilitate an atmosphere that does not really help to relieve patients' insecurities and anxieties.[19] In addition, physicians are often hard to reach, not sufficiently attentive to patients and their families, impatient about explaining things in detail, and rushed to do other things. As Anspach shows, this unattentive attitude leads the medical staff to refrain from using the *consent* model; rather, they obtained *assent*, or agreement to decisions to terminate life support already made by the staff.[20] Passive euthanasia, invoking the double-effect doctrine, and discrimination against weak groups like aging patients and patients in prolonged unawareness are taking place in hospitals around the globe without sufficient mechanisms of control ascertaining that the patients' best interests are being served.[21]

Many of the fears that are voiced against allowing active euthanasia and physician-assisted suicide are concerned with the possible misbehavior of doctors, yet the people who express these fears are content with the present situation with its "grey" areas for doctors' maneuvering. Grey areas will apparently always remain. The question is whether we should be content with the present situation or look for ways to reduce these grey areas. It is time to change the present situation because it does not address the genuine needs of some patients who raise a clear and agonizing voice to die, and because we should not consent to the amount of abuse that is already taking place. What is suggested is a two-tier process: (*a*) to open a public debate about patients' rights and doctors' duties, educate the citizens about the existing state of affairs, put the abovementioned key conceptions on the public agenda, speak openly about the conflicting considerations, and mobilize the media to address these issues; and then (*b*) ask the public whether the institution of guidelines is preferable to the present situation. It might be the case that the public would feel that clear and specific guidelines would limit the doctors' maneuverability and better serve the interests of all patients, those who wish to live and those who wish to die. Society should address these troubling questions in a common endeavor to specify the roles and duties of doctors, and the rights of patients, including their right to ask for a dignified death. This two-tier process is preferable to leaving the situation as it is where various people around the patient's bed might act in ways that may not coincide with the best interests of the patient.[22]

Fear of Overzealousness

Overzealous promoting of medical active termination of life may create the impression that dying with dignity is more important than living with dignity. The guiding rule must be to preserve and maintain life. The termination of life must be the exception. Caution is necessary, both morally and professionally. The prime example of overenthusiasm for the shortening of life concerns the innovation called the "Mercitron."

The Mercitron is a suicide machine invented by an American doctor, Jack Kevorkian, who has lead the campaign for assisted suicide and has become a folk hero in the United States and throughout the world.[23] From 1990 until September 1998, Dr. Kevorkian has helped sixty-five women and twenty-eight men to die.[24] During the 1990s, in a nine-year battle against the medical, legal, and religious communities in Michigan, Kevorkian had been acquitted three times by juries in Oakland

and Wayne counties in the assisted-suicide deaths of five people. A fourth trial in Ionia County ended in a mistrial. In those trials, Kevorkian relied on evidence about the pain and suffering of people he was charged with helping to die.[25]

On 4 August 1993, Thomas Hyde, age 30, of Novi, Michigan, who suffered from amyotrophic lateral sclerosis, inhaled carbon monoxide. He was the 17th (some say the 20th) person to die in Kevorkian's presence. In May 1994, Kevorkian stood trial for the first time for his involvement and was acquitted. After the trial, a juror commented: "He convinced us he was not a murderer, that he was really trying to help people out." A second juror said, "Dr. Kevorkian had acted principally to relieve Mr. Hyde's pain, not to kill him, and that is an action within the law."[26] One month later, Dr. Kevorkian's medical license was revoked on the grounds that he had been disciplined by the Michigan Board of Medicine, and that he had assisted five patients to commit suicide.[27]

In March 1996, Kevorkian stood trial for the second time on the charge of causing the deaths of Mrs. Merian Frederick, who suffered from amyotrophic lateral sclerosis (also known as Lou Gehrig's disease), and of Dr. Ali Khalili, who suffered from bone cancer. Kevorkian said that Frederick and Khalili had caused their own deaths by removing the clip on the tubing to allow poisonous gas to flow from a small, black tank into their plastic masks. Kevorkian further claimed that he encouraged both of them to remove the mask if they changed their mind at the last moment. Frederick and Khalili's relatives testified that they appreciated Dr. Kevorkian's help and compassion in ending their loved ones' suffering. The prosecutors suggested that Kevorkian did not fully explore other options with Frederick and Khalili and made hasty decisions about their conditions without consulting their doctors. The jury, however, was not convinced; they felt that Kevorkian's purpose was merely to relieve the patients' suffering, not to cause their death, and hence he was found not guilty.[28]

One of the first patients who asked for Dr. Kevorkian's assistance to die was Janet Adkins, an Alzheimer's patient in the first stages of the disease. Aware as she was of the deterioration of human characteristics as a result of this terrible disease, Mrs. Adkins wished to die while she was still competent and able to be in charge of her actions. Dr. Kevorkian assisted her suicide although Mrs. Adkins apparently had quite a few months left to live during which she could have functioned more or less autonomously. Her private doctor thought that Mrs. Adkins had at least another year before losing her ability to think clearly, and Dr. Kevorkian agreed that she was not a "terminal patient."[29] He estimated that Mrs. Adkins had four to six months before becoming incompetent.[30] If Mrs. Adkin's mental health was intact and she "was not the least depressed over her impending death," as Dr. Kevorkian testifies,[31] the question arises: Why the rush? The criticism concerns the doctor's neglecting his obligation to preserve life. Clearly it would have been possible to perform this assisted suicide at a later more advanced stage of the disease. Similar charges were brought against Kevorkian at his second trial.

The case of Janet Adkins exhibits the need to change the legal system to accommodate physician-assisted suicide. If patients knew that physician-assisted suicide would be available to them as an option, they would not need to seek physicians like Kevorkian to end their lives prematurely. The existing situation brings patients to forgo life earlier than they should in fear of helplessness and degeneration into a prolonged, painful, and degrading dying process.

Kevorkian's third trial was concerned with assisted suicide of Marjorie Wantz and Sherry Miller. Mrs. Wantz (fifty-eight years old) suffered from excruciating pelvic pain; Mrs. Miller (forty-three years old) suffered from multiple sclerosis. Chief prosecutor Larry Buntig characterized Kevorkian as a "reckless agent of death." Referring to Wantz, whose subsequent autopsy showed she was unlikely to die from her illness, Buntig said she "needed mental health treatment, not a bottle full of poison."[32] Here as in the previous trials the jury remained unconvinced and acquitted Dr. Kevorkian.

In December 1997, Dr. Kevorkian challenged Michigan lawmakers to pass a law banning assisted suicide, declaring at a news conference he will no longer "sneak around" in his assisted-suicide campaign, and that he would starve himself to death in prison if convicted of the offense. Kevorkian vouched that "We shall not submit to that tyranny." At a news conference with his associate to the latest killings, Dr. Georges Reding, a retired psychiatrist, Kevorkian maintained that a ban on "patholysis" (Kevorkian's term for assisted suicide) "is sorely needed to clear the air.... The ban itself will then be put on trial, because we fully intend to challenge it to facilitate a so-called trial—so-called because any trial mandated by an immoral law is nothing if not a lynching."[33] Kevorkian also said that the conviction of him and his colleague will help future, more enlightened societies gauge the darkness of our plutocratic and theocratic age.[34] When repeatedly pressed by reporters to name the number of people whose suicides he has attended, Kevorkian would not be specific. But he did place the number at "somewhere between 80 and 100."[35]

My impression from an examination of Dr. Kevorkian's deeds is that his acts are tainted with overenthusiasm. In his book, *Prescription: Medicide*, Kevorkian describes in detail his obsession with assisted suicide: how he came to the decision to help patients end their lives; his efforts to convince his colleagues that his conduct is justifiable; the process of building his suicide machine; and the efforts to receive recognition for his newly adopted profession ("obitiary," in his words, a term derived from the Latin word *obitus* and from the Greek word *iatros,* meaning a doctor who helps patients meet death).[36] The efforts to find a place to perform Mrs. Adkins' suicide were described as "Herculean."[37] Dr. Kevorkian states that he does not help patients who are confused and are not of sound and coherent mind.[38] The first patient that Dr. Kevorkian considered treating lost his ability to think clearly before the appointed date for treatment. Kevorkian described what had happened as a "near miss": "...the patient unexpectedly slipped into babbling incoherence. That eliminated him as the first candidate for my services."[39]

Dr. Kevorkian's acquaintance with most of those patients who sought his help and his suicide machine, which he called "Mercitron," was superficial. He did not know the patients who approached him, nor did he take pains to study their medical history. He knew Janet Adkins for only two days. The decision to nominate her as the first candidate for his suicide machine was made after a few phone calls and reading through her medical file, without ever having met her face to face.[40] Mrs. Adkin's doctor strongly opposed her killing and refused to cooperate with Dr. Kevorkian. Kevorkian himself coldly describes their meeting in a businesslike manner. He writes, "After getting acquainted through a few minutes of conversation, the purpose of the trip was thoroughly discussed."[41] Kevorkian did not invest effort in convincing those who turn to him to reconsider their situation, and perhaps to opt for life.

He did not insist that the request to die be consistent, expressed several times over a certain period of time, so as to make sure that the patients were convinced they reached the right decision. For him, like for the Israeli attorney I mentioned before, the important thing was the expressed will of the autonomous patients to die. The doctor supplied a service that honors their request.

However, the emphasis in Dr. Kevorkian's book is not on the patient who asks to die but upon the doctor who takes the action. Janet Adkins, Thomas Hyde, Sherry Miller, Marjorie Wantz, Merian Frederick, Ali Khalili, and the other dozens of patients whom Dr. Kevorkian helped to die are but a means to convey his message to the world. The pioneer to experience the Mercitron, Janet Adkins, serves in his book as no more than a secondary actress in a tragedy he wishes to mount on any possible stage to diffuse his cold ideas, which lack human compassion. I confess: I found it difficult to read his book. The concept of the right to die with dignity, which is, in my opinion, a concept worthy of the most serious and painstaking consideration and study, becomes distorted in Dr. Kevorkian's book.[42] His book is an easy target for those who oppose euthanasia and assisted suicide; a butting tool against those who side with the right to die with dignity.

Dr. Kevorkian's respect for the individual's right to decide autonomously about his or her destiny (for some reason Kevorkian mainly helped women) was extreme. He posed the virtue of respect for the patient's autonomy as the most important consideration, overshadowing other concerns. Because he was unqualified and apparently disinterested in examining his patients and verifying their cause of illness, he assisted the suicide of some patients who were misdiagnosed. Kevorkian did not care very much. These people wanted to die and all he did was help them fulfil their desire.

Kevorkian and his attorney, Geoffrey Fieger, insisted that the retired pathologist had assisted in the suicides only of people with terminal illnesses—including, by Kevorkian's definition, the late stages of Alzheimer's disease and multiple sclerosis —or severe, chronic pain. But of the 44 people Kevorkian had acknowledged helping die in Oakland County, Dr. Ljubisa J. Dragovic said 11 were terminally ill, 29 had chronic conditions, and *four others had no signs of disease.* Dragovic, the coroner who examined the bodies, has classified nearly all of the 44 deaths linked to Kevorkian as homicides.[43] Among the controversial deaths I would mention the death of Margaret Garrish, 72, of Royal Oak (26 November 1994), who suffered from rheumatoid arthritis—Kevorkian kept his promise to help her die if doctors did not provide better pain medication; Judith Curren, 42, of Pembroke, Mass (15 August 1996), who had chronic fatigue syndrome and suffered from depression[44]; Loretta Peabody, 54, of Ionia (30 August 1996), who had multiple sclerosis. Her husband remarried shortly after her death; Janet Good (26 August 1997), who was Kevorkian's assistant—she had pancreatic cancer, but the coroner said there were no visible signs of cancer, maintaining that she would have lived at least six months before eventually succumbing to the disease[45]; Deborah Sickels, 43, of Arlington, Texas (7 September 1997), who suffered from multiple sclerosis and other medical ailments—her family said she was mentally unstable and accused Kevorkian of being irresponsible for helping her die[46]; and Roosevelt Dawson, a 21-year-old quadriplegic college student from Southfield, Michigan (26 February 1998)—he was paralyzed from the neck down and relied on a ventilator to breathe since a virus infected his spinal cord.[47]

The assisted suicide of young Dawson has energized Kevorkian's critics. They charged that the retired pathologist has slowly evolved his practice from terminal patients to all comers. Not Dead Yet, a national disabled-rights group fighting the legalization of assisted suicide, contended that Kevorkian was slowly conditioning people to view death as the logical alternative to life with a disability. During an August 1990 court proceeding in Oakland County, Kevorkian made the following chilling statement: "The voluntary self-elimination of individual and mortally diseased or crippled lives, taken collectively, can only enhance the preservation of the public health and welfare." Dr. Georges Reding, Kevorkian's associate who attended Dawson's death, was quoted saying that anyone can choose assisted suicide because "we are all terminal."[48]

However, this case was not a case of assisted suicide. Dawson was completely incapacitated before his death and could not have operated the Mercitron. No wonder that right-to-die activist groups distanced themselves from Kevorkian. Carol Poenisch of Merian's Friends, a Northville-based group working to legalize assisted suicide, said that according to Kevorkian "we are cowards because we want to document things and do it in a proper fashion... [Dawson's] case would need much more careful study before he would qualify under Merian's Friends' guidelines. He may not have qualified."[49] Indeed, for Kevorkian a person's choice to live or die should depend on how they view their "quality of life."

In June 1998, Dr. Kevorkian harvested the kidneys of Joseph Tushkowski, a Nevada man who died with his help. By this act he wanted to attract more media attention and to inflame the debate. The medical authorities refused to accept the organs. National transplant organizations and area hospitals said that Kevorkian's conduct did not meet their criteria. Dave Wilkens, a spokesman for the University of Michigan Medical Center in Ann Arbor, commented that Kevorkian's act was nothing that any kind of responsible institution would participate in. Joel Newman, spokesman of the United Network for Organ Sharing—a private company in Richmond, Virginia under federal contract to match organ donors with recipients—said regulations require detailed medical and social histories and that procedures are carried out by surgeons in a hospital setting.[50]

In November 1998, Dr. Kevorkian further radicalized his campaign. Throughout his crusade he was dictating the moves, provoking public debate, pressing harder and harder the issue of assisted suicide, and the right of persons to choose the time of their death, forcing the legal authorities to address the question and calling upon them to prosecute him. On 22 November 1998, the *Detroit News* reported that Kevorkian actively euthanaised Thomas Youk, who was suffering the advanced stages of Lou Gehrig's disease and would have been unable to inject himself with the lethal dose. By that time, it was estimated that Kevorkian was responsible for more than 130 deaths.[51] On this occasion, Kevorkian publicly admitted that he administered the lethal poison and, furthermore, submitted a videotape to CBS's show *60 Minutes*.[52] Derek Humphry commented on this development by saying:

> I think that Dr. Kevorkian was absolutely right, in human terms, to help Mr. Youk to die by lethal injection. Not to have helped him die just because he could not do it himself would have been the worse kind of discrimination. But I part company with Kevorkian in that active voluntary euthanasia should only take place under a new law, with strong guidelines. He seems to think the medical profession can be trusted, and be willing to hasten deaths in this manner; I think the people should—if a majority want it—pass a careful law permitting both physician-assisted suicide and active voluntary

euthanasia for a competent, terminally ill adult. But he's made the point very effectively. I have been making the same arguments (accompanied by a plea for a new law) for the past 20 years. Kevorkian—and CBS TV—have moved the educational process forward hugely this Sunday evening.[53]

After the showing of the *60 Minutes* episode that documented Kevorkian administering a lethal injection to Thomas Youk,[54] a poll of the public was conducted asking, *inter alia*: "Did the experience of watching tonight's *60 Minutes* segment on Jack Kevorkian influence you to be more supportive of assisted suicide or more opposed to assisted suicide?" The results were:

6% Much more supportive of assisted suicide
31% Somewhat more supportive of assisted suicide
13% Somewhat more opposed to assisted suicide
38% Much more opposed to assisted suicide
12% Undecided/Don't know.[55]

The majority of the people in the poll testified that the program made them feel more opposed to assisted suicide. So Kevorkian's initiative granted him huge publicity and served his interest in provoking public debate, but it did not further public support for his mission.

Ellen Goodman, a *Boston Globe* Columnist, wrote that Thomas Youk was little more than a prop for Kevorkian's act, a dead body he could use in challenging authority. There is little surprise that Kevorkian upped the ante, moving to active euthanasia. Assisted suicide no longer caught the spotlight. Goodman expressed the opinion that Kevorkian was the wrong role model to cast for the lead in the movement for a more merciful death. Kevorkian forced the issue of assisted suicide and euthanasia onto the public stage, but he also polarized that public audience. Goodman maintained: "Nor would I wish him at my deathbed offering these last words of comfort: 'We're going to inject in your right arm. OK? Okey-doke.'"[56]

By videotaping himself giving a man a lethal injection, bringing the tape to the CBS News program *60 Minutes*, and daring prosecutors to charge him with murder, Kevorkian was trying to move the legal system further and faster than most Americans were ready to accept. The Michigan prosecutor could not remain indifferent to this blunt breach of the law. Kevorkian stood trial on charges of first-degree murder and delivering a controlled substance for injecting Youk with lethal drugs. This time, the jury could not ignore the explicit videotape and the language of the law. A "not guilty" verdict would have nullified the law on murder and left Kevorkian free to continue his death campaign with a quick-to-inject syringe. Kevorkian was found guilty of second-degree murder, and of delivering a controlled substance.[57] He was given a jail sentence of 10 to 25 years on the second-degree murder conviction, and 3 to 7 years on the "controlled substance" conviction. Judge Jessica Cooper emphasized in her verdict that the trial was not about the political or moral correctness of euthanasia. Instead, it was about lawlessness: "It was about disrespect for a society that exists because of the strength of the legal system. No one, sir, is above the law. No one," Judge Cooper told Kevorkian: "You had the audacity to go on national television, show the world what you did, and dare the legal system to stop you. Well, sir, consider yourself stopped."[58]

Kevorkian's deeds put the issue of death with dignity on the public agenda and compel the American authorities to invest efforts in finding a solution to the problem he poses. If adequate solutions will not be found, then one should not be surprised to find more Kevorkian-like doctors who will come to the help of patients. Indeed, the Reuters Agency in Pontiac, Michigan, reported that Dr. Georges Reding, who began an apprenticeship under Kevorkian in December 1997, helped a 35-year-old woman from San Francisco suffering from AIDS to die.[59] Reding became an active participant in some other cases of assisted suicide until he was charged with first-degree murder in the August 1998 death of Donna Brennan, a 54-year-old multiple sclerosis patient who died of an overdose of the sedative pentobarbital. In January 2000 it was reported that Reding fled to Europe, and that the authorities do not know for sure where he is.[60]

Kevorkian's missionary vigor, like any unqualified vigor, betrays the best interests of patients and ill-serves the interests of society. The United States should devise ways to stop Kevorkian-like-minded doctors, and to think creatively to answer the genuine wills of *all* patients in this modern, technologically advanced era of medicine.

CONCLUSIONS

The right to die with dignity includes the right to live with dignity until the last minute and the right to part from life in a dignified manner. There are some adult patients who feel that the preferable way for them to part from life is through physician-assisted suicide. We must ponder the following considerations on their behalf:

Guideline 1. The physician should not suggest assisted suicide to the patient. Instead, it is the patient who should have the option to ask for such assistance. Initiation by the physician might undermine trust between the patient and his/her physician, conveying to the patient that the doctor gave up on him/her, and values his/her life only to the extent of offering assistance to die. Such an offer might undermine the will to live and to explore further avenues for livelihood. Many Dutch physicians do not see this issue as a significant one. Some of them think it is important for them to raise the issue when it seems that the patient does not dare to raise the issue upon his or her own initiative.[61] However, undoubtedly all people in the Netherlands are aware of the availability of active euthanasia and physician-assisted suicide in their society. The reluctance the patients show with regard to this issue should be honored and respected.

Guideline 2. The request for physician-assisted suicide of a patient who suffers from an incurable and irreversible disease must be voluntary.[62] The decision is that of the patient who asks to die without pressures, because life seems the worst alternative in the current situation. The patient should state her wish several times over a period of time. We must verify that the request for physician-assisted suicide does not stem from a momentary urge, an impulse, a product of passing depression. This emphasis of enduring request was one of the requirements of the abolished Northern Territory law in Australia,[63] and is one of the requirements of the Oregon *Death with Dignity Act*,[64] and of the Dutch guidelines.[65] We must also verify that the request is not the result of external influences. It should be ascertained with a signed document that the patient is ready to die now, rather than depending solely on directives from the past. Section 2 of the Oregon Act requires that the written request for medication to end one's life be signed and dated by the patient and witnessed by at least two individuals who, in the presence of the patient, attest to the best of their knowledge and belief that the patient is capable, acting voluntarily, and is not being coerced to sign the request.[66]

A person can express general attitudes regarding euthanasia in an informal discussion made in a social setting. She might say that she would not want to live if she had to rely on the mercy of others, depend on them, and if she were unable to function alone. Such hypothetical observations do not constitute reliable evidence of the patient's current desires once an actual illness is in progress. This is especially true if the wish was stated when young and healthy. The younger people are, and the further they are from serious disease, the more inclined they are to claim that in a hypothetical hopeless state, painful and degrading, they would prefer to end their lives. On the other hand, there is a tendency to come to terms with suffering, to compromise with physical disabilities, to struggle to sustain living, and this tendency grows as the body weakens. Many people change their minds when they confront the unattractive alternatives. Many prefer to remain in what others term the "cruel" world, and continue the Sisyphean struggle for their lives.

Guideline 3. At times, the patient's decision might be influenced by severe pain. In this context, the role of palliative care can be crucial. The World Health Organization defines palliative care as the "active, total care of patients whose disease is not responsive to curative treatment," maintaining that control of pain, of other symptoms, and of psychological, social, and spiritual problems, is paramount.[67] The medical staff must examine whether by means of medication and palliative care it is possible to prevent or to ease the pain.[68] If it is, then we may not fulfil the patient's wish, but instead prescribe the necessary treatment. This is provided that the educated patient (i.e., the patient who was advised by the medical staff about the available palliative-care options) does not refuse to receive the painkillers, and that when the pain goes, so does the motive (or one of the main motives) that caused the patient to ask for assisted suicide. If the patient insists on denying all medication, doctors must try to find first the reasons for this insistence before they comply.

At times, coping with pain and suffering can demand all the patient's emotional strength, exhausting her ability to deal with other issues. In cases of competent patients, it must be determined that the decision is based on ability to make decisions. The assumption is that the patient understands the meaning of her decision. A psychiatric assessment of the patient could confirm whether the patient is able to make such a meaningful decision concerning her life. A meeting with a psychiatrist should confirm that the decision is truly that of the patient, expressed consistently and of her own free will. The Northern Territory *Rights of Terminally Ill Act* required that the patient meet with a qualified psychiatrist to confirm that he or she is not clinically depressed.[69] It is worthwhile to hold several such conversations, separated by a few days. The patient's beloved people and the attending physician should be included in at least one of the conversations.

Guideline 4. The patient must be informed of her situation and the prognoses for both recovery and escalation of the disease and the suffering it may involve. There must be an exchange of information between the doctors and the patient.[70] Bearing this in mind, we should be careful to use neutral terms and to refrain from terms that might offend patients and their beloved people.

Guideline 5. It must be ensured that the patient's decision is not a result of familial and environmental pressures. At times, the patient may feel that she constitutes a burden to her beloved people. It is the task of social workers to examine the motives of the patient and to see to what extent they are affected by various external pressures (as opposed to a true free will to die). A situation could exist in which the patient is under no such pressure, but still does not wish to be a burden on others. Obviously, we cannot say that the feelings of a patient toward her beloved people are not relevant to the decision making.

Guideline 6. Verification of diagnosis. To minimize misdiagnosis, and to allow the discovery of other medical options, the decision-making process should include a second opinion provided by a specialist who is not dependent on the first doctor, either professionally or otherwise.[71] The patient's attending physician, who supposedly knows the patient's case better than any other expert, must be consulted. All reasonable alternative treatments must be explored. The Oregon *Death with Dignity Act* requires that a consulting physician shall examine the patient and his/her relevant medical records and confirm, in writing, the attending physician's diagnosis that "the patient is suffering from a terminal disease," and verify that the patient is capable, is acting voluntarily, and has made an informed decision.[72] The Dutch guidelines require that the physician consult a colleague.[73] The Northern Territory *Rights of Terminally-Ill Act* required that the patient be examined by a physician who specializes in treating terminal illness.[74]

Guideline 7. Some time prior to the performance of physician-assisted suicide, a doctor and a psychiatrist are required to visit the patient, examine him or her, and verify that this is the genuine wish of a person of sound mind who is not being coerced or influenced by a third party. A date for the procedure is then agreed upon.[75]

Guideline 8. The patient can rescind at any time and in any manner. This is granted under the Australian Northern Territory Act,[76] and is granted under the *Oregon Death with Dignity Act*.[77]

Guideline 9. Physician-assisted suicide may be performed only by a doctor and in the presence of another doctor. The decision-making team should include at least two doctors and a lawyer, who will examine the legal aspects involved. Insisting on this demand would serve as a safety valve against possible abuse. Perhaps a public representative should also be present during the entire procedure—the decision-making process and the actual performance of the act. This extra caution should ensure that the right to die with dignity does not become a duty. The doctor performing the assisted suicide should be the one who knows the patient best, has been involved in her treatment, taken part in the consultations with her and with her beloved people, and has verified through the help of social workers and psychologists that euthanasia is the wish of the patient.

Guideline 10. Physician-assisted suicide may be conducted in one of two ways, both of them discussed openly and decided by the physician and his/her patient: (*1*) oral medication; (*2*) self-administered lethal injection. After a physician inserts an intravenous needle, the patient could press a button to begin the flow of medication. Research in Oregon showed that oral medication may be difficult or impossible for many patients to ingest because of nausea or other side effects of their illnesses.[78] In the event that oral medication was provided and the dying process lingers on for long hours, the physician is allowed to administer a lethal injection by himself/herself.

Guideline 11. Doctors may not demand a *special fee* for the performance of assisted suicide. The motive for physician-assisted suicide is humane, so there must be no financial incentives and no special payment that might cause commercialization and promotion of the death operation.

Guideline 12. There must be extensive documentation in the patient's medical file including the disease diagnosis and prognosis; attempted treatments; the patient's reasons for seeking physician-assisted suicide; the patient's request in writing or documented on a video recording; documentation of conversations with the patient; documentation of discussions with her beloved people; and a psychological report confirming the patient's condition. This meticulous documentation is meant to prevent exploitation of any kind: personal, medical, or institutional.[79] Each physician-assisted suicide report should be examined by a coroner.[80]

Guideline 13. Pharmacists should also be required to report all prescriptions for lethal medication, thus providing a further check on physicians' reporting.

Guideline 14. A doctor must not be coerced into taking actions that contradict her conscience and her understanding of her role. This was provided under the Northern Territory Act.[81]

Guidelines 15. The local medical association should establish a committee whose role will be not only investigating the underlying facts reported in the reports, but to investigate whether there are "mercy" cases that were not reported and/or that did not comply with the guidelines.

Guideline 16. Licensing sanctions will be taken to punish those health-care professionals who violated the guidelines, failed to consult and to file reports or who engaged in involuntary euthanasia without the patient's awareness or consent, or euthanized patients who lacked decision-making capacity. Physicians who failed to comply with the above guidelines will be charged and procedures to sanction them will be opened by the disciplinary tribunal of the medical association. The maximum penalty for violation of guidelines should be the revoking of the medical license.

What is presented here is a circumscribed reasoning for physician-assisted suicide to help a designated group of patients who require help in departing from life and who deserve to get such help from the medical profession to meet their wish. The detailed procedure is required to prevent abuse. After all, it is human life at stake. At first I suggest adopting this reasoning for a trial period of one year and examine whether the consequences justify implementation of the policy for a lengthier period of time. During this one-year trial period, feedbacks from physicians, ethicists, and the public at large in reviewing the policy and practice of physician-assisted suicide should be welcomed and encouraged. If the proposal fails (for instance, physicians do not adequately report incidents of physician-assisted suicide), all the data should be brought before a reviewing committee to closely study the policy and practice. Members of the committee will issue a report recommending whether they wish to continue the practice, to amend the guidelines, or to abolish physician-assisted suicide. Preferably, the final decision should be made by the people via referendum.

With regard to more complicated situations that do not satisfy the criteria presented above (free, voluntary, persistent and enduring requests for assisted suicide made by a competent patient who suffers from an incurable and irreversible disease), I urge expanding the circle involved in the decision-making process, discussing these cases in ethics committees and in the courts. The issue is urgent and real and people from different walks of life and with different perspectives—those of medicine, law, philosophy, psychology, social work, religion—should take part in the decision-making process, enriching the discourse with their insights.

Lastly, although the above guidelines refer *only* to competent patients, I would like to note that in the case of minors, their parents serve as their guardians. The parents decide on behalf of their child after consulting the attending physicians. As Justice Ariel stated in the *Scheffer* case, the minor's parents do not serve only as her mouth. Because Yael Scheffer was unable to construct an opinion regarding her future, her parents did so for her.[82] Keeping that in mind, we must insist, as Justice Elon did in the same case, that the decision must be made by both parents (assuming that the minor has two parents), and not only by one of them.[83]

NOTES AND REFERENCES

1. Notorious among them are the Hemlock Society in the United States, and the corresponding association in Vancouver, British Columbia. Sue Rodriguez disassociated herself from the British Columbia association after she felt they used her and betrayed her trust. For further discussion see http://www.FinalExit.org/world.fed.html; e-mail: <ergo@efn.org>, and Death Net http://www.island.com/~deathnet/. In November 1999, a weekend conference was held in Seattle dealing with methods of self-deliverance from a terminal illness using new equipment. Only those with "hands-on" experience with assisting death were invited, and the conference location was kept secret. Derek Humphry, whose Euthanasia Research and Guidance Organization sponsored the two-day meeting, explained that they did not want "observers, moralists, philosophers or protesters." See the *Seattle Times,* http://www.seattletimes.com/news/local/html98/suic_19991115.html and http://www.finalexit.org/practice.html
2. *Sue Rodriguez v. The Attorney General of Canada* , File No. 23476 (September 1993).
3. Opening Motion (Tel-Aviv) 1141/1990. *Benjamin Eyal v. Lichtenstaedter Hospital.* P.M. 1991 (3), 194.
4. Fred Rosner, *Modern Medicine and Jewish Law* (New York: Yeshiva University Press, 1972); A. Carmi, "Live Like A King: Die Like A King," in Amnon Carmi (Ed.), *Euthanasia* (Berlin: Springer-Verlag, 1984), pp. 3–28; Haim David Halevi, "Disconnecting a Patient Who Has No Chance of Surviving from an Artificial Resuscitation Machine," *Tchumin* (Alon Shevut, 1981), Vol. 2, pp. 297–305 [in Hebrew].
5. Opening Motion (Tel-Aviv) 1141/1990. *Benjamin Eyal v. Lichtenstaedter Hospital.* P.M. 1991 (3), 187. For further deliberation on similar cases see 1030/95 *Israel Gilad v. Soroka Medical Center and Others,* Beer Sheva District Court (23 October 1995); Opening Motion 2339 + 2242/95 *A.A. and Y. S. v. Kupat Holim and State of Israel,* Tel Aviv District Court (11 January 1996); Opening Motion 2242/95 *Eitay Arad v. Kupat Holim and State of Israel,* Tel Aviv District Court (1 October 1998). Judge Talgam emphasized in the *Arad* case that the starting point must be the dignity of the patient, and not of the hesitant doctor.
6. See David Novak, *Jewish Social Ethics* (New York: Oxford University Press, 1992), esp. p. 17; David Novak, *Jewish-Christian Dialogue* (New York: Oxford University Press, 1989), pp. 8, 142–151. For a contesting view see Justice Elon in Civil Appeal 506/1988 *Yael Scheffer, through Talila Scheffer v. The State of Israel*, para. 20.
7. I thank Dr. Nachman Wilensky for showing Rabbi Lau's letter to me.
8. For an opposing stance see Avraham Steinberg, "The Terminally Ill—Secular and Jewish Ethical Aspects," *Israel J. Med. Sci,* Vol. 30, No. 1 (January 1994), pp. 130–135, esp. 134.
9. "Can Life Be Evaluated? The Jewish Halachic Approach vs. the Quality of Life Approach in Medical Ethics: A Critical View" (with Merav Shmueli), *Theoretical Medicine and Bioethics* (2000). See also Timothy Quill, Rebecca Dresser, and Dan Brock, "The Rule of Double Effect—A Critique of Its Role in End-of-Live Decision

Making," *New England Journal of Medicine*, Vol. 337 (11 December 1997), pp. 1768–1771.
10. Will Gaylin, Leon Kass, Edmund Pellegrino, and Mark Siegler, "Doctors Must Not Kill," *Journal of the American Medical Association,* Vol. 259 (1988), 2139; Edmund D. Pellegrino, "Doctors Must Not Kill," in Robert I. Misbin (Ed.), *Euthanasia: The Good of the Patient, the Good of Society* (Frederick, MD: University Publishing Group, 1992), pp. 27–41; Charles L. Sprung, Leonid A. Eidelman, and Avraham Steinberg, "Is the Physician's Duty to the Individual Patient or to Society?," *Critical Care Medicine*, Vol. 23, No. 4 (1995), pp. 618–620. For a contrasting view see Fredrick R. Abrams, "The Quality of Mercy: An Examination of The Proposition 'Doctors Must Not Kill,'" *in* Robert I. Misbin (Ed.), *Euthanasia: The Good of the Patient, the Good of Society, op. cit.,* pp. 43–51.
11. Charles Sprung, "Changing Attitudes and Practices in Forgoing Life-sustaining Treatments," *Journal of the American Medical Association,* Vol. 263, No. 16 (25 April 1990), p. 2214.
12. Civil Appeal 506/88 *Scheffer v. The State of Israel*, P.D. 48 (1) 87, at 172–173.
13. Sprung *et al.* present data showing that doctors see the CPR treatment as "useless," even when the patients' chances are 5 to 10 percent. They further note that the chances for giving such treatment drop when the patients are black, and that many life-and-death decisions are made without the consent of the patients or their family members. See Charles L. Sprung *et al.*, "Changes in Forgoing Life-Sustaining Treatments in the United States: Concern for the Future," *Mayo Clin Proceedings,* Vol. 71 (1996), pp. 512–516, at 513–514.
14. Interviews with Dr. George Beausmans (Maastricht, 26 July 1999), and Dr. Gerrit K. Kimsma (Koog 'aan de Zaan, 28 July 1999).
15. Those opposed to my view will say that the Netherlands exemplifies a state in which the defining guidelines for mercy killings are often crossed, resulting in many patients' being killed against their will. See David Orentlicher, "The Legalization of Physician Assisted Suicide: A Very Modest Revolution," *Boston College Law Review,* Vol. XXXVIII, No. 3 (May 1997), pp. 459–462.
16. The anxiety over the slippery-slope syndrome was probably foremost in the minds of the participants of the 39th World Medical Assembly, held in Madrid in October 1987. In the *World Medical Association Declaration on Euthanasia* it was contended that euthanasia, "that is, the act of deliberately ending the life of a patient, even at the patient's own request or at the request of close relatives, is unethical. This does not prevent the physician from respecting the desire of a patient to allow the natural process of death to follow its course in the terminal phase of sickness." For critical discussion of the slippery-slope syndrome see R. G. Frey, "The Fear of a Slippery Slope," *in* Gerald Dworkin, R.G. Frey, and Sissela Bok (Eds.), *Euthanasia and Physician-Assisted Suicide* (New York: Cambridge University Press, 1998), pp. 43–63; Ronald Dworkin, "When Is It Right to Die?," *The New York Times* (17 May 1994), at A19; Bernard Williams, "Which Slopes Are Slippery," in Michael Lockwood (Ed.), *Moral Dilemmas in Modern Medicine* (Oxford: Oxford University Press, 1985), pp. 126–137.
17. See, for example, Yale Kamisar, "Some Non-Religious Views against Proposed "Mercy Killing Legislation'" *Minnesota Law Review,* Vol. 42, No. 6 (1958), pp. 969–1042; Yale Kamisar, "Against Assisted Suicide—Even a Very Limited Form," *The University of Detroit Mercy L. Review* Vol. 72 (Summer 1995) pp. 736–739; Sissela Bok, "Death and Dying: Euthanasia and Sustaining Life," *Encyclopedia of Bioethics,* edited by Warren T. Reich (New York: The Free Press, 1978), Vol. 1, pp. 268–267; Sissela Bok, "Euthanasia" in Gerald Dworkin *et al. (*Eds.), *Euthanasia and Physician-Assisted Suicide, op. cit.,* esp. pp. 112–118; Peter A. Singer and Mark Siegler, "Ethaniasia—A Critique," *New England Journal of Medicine,* Vol. 322 (June 1990), pp. 1881–1883; Charles J. Dougherty, "The Common Good, Terminal Illness and Euthanasia," *Issues in Law and Medicine*, Vol. 9, No. 2 (Fall 1993), pp. 151–166; Carl Elliot, "Philosopher Assisted Suicide and Euthanasia," *BMJ*, Vol. 313 (26 October, 1996), p. 1088.

18. See R. Cohen-Almagor, "'Muerte con dignidad', 'calidad de vida,' 'estado vegetativo,' 'doble efecto' y otras expresiones empleadas por los medicos," *Perspectivas Bioeticas,* No. 5 (1998), pp. 26–44 [Spanish].
19. One of Swigart and colleagues' findings on the role of families in the critical care setting is that explanations should be made in language clearly understandable to family members. They note overuse of medical terms or presentations of medical minutiae that may be overwhelming and confusing for family members. Valerie Swigart, Charles Lidz, Victoria Butterworth and Robert Arnold, "Letting Go: Family Willingness to Forgo Life Support," *Heart and Lung,* Vol. 25, No. 6 (1996), p. 492.
20. R. Anspach, *Deciding Who Lives* (Berkeley: University of California Press, 1993), pp. 85–163. Quoted in Swigart *et al.,* "Letting Go: Family Willingness to Forgo Life Support," *op. cit.,* p. 484.
21. R. Cohen-Almagor, "Some Observations on Post-Coma Unawareness Patients and on Other Forms of Unconscious Patients: Policy Proposals," *Medicine and Law,* Vol. 16, No. 3 (1997), pp. 451–471.
22. In March 1998, Justice Antonin Scalia declared that Congress, not the Supreme Court, should decide such vexing questions as abortion rights, the death penalty, and physician-assisted suicide. Scalia said: "It is not supposed to be our judgment as to what is the socially desirable answer to all of these questions. That's supposed to be the judgment of Congress, and we do our job correctly when we apply what Congress has written as basically and honestly as possible." Glen Johnson, "Scalia: Let Congress, not court, decide abortion, assisted suicide," *The Associated Press* (9 March 1998, 2:14 PM EST). http://www.nytimes.com
23. Songs were written about Jack Kevorkian. For instance, Detroit rocker Mitch Ryder dedicated his song "Mercy" to "Dr. Jack" Kevorkian. The lyrics are straightforward: "Cast your spell, Dr. Jack/ I am willing, I can't wait/ End my pain/ No one else/ seems to understand my fate." Dr. Kevorkian himself released a CD with 12 songs, 11 of which he wrote. The liner notes say that Kevorkian wants to be remembered as a doctor who help relieve human suffering.
24. These are the documented cases. See http://www.finalexit.org/kevorkian.htm. I have checked this site for updates in December 1999 and then the requested URL / kevorkian.htm was not found on this server.
25. Cf. *People v. Kevorkian,* No. 90003196 (Oakland County, Mich., 14 December 1990); *People v. Kevorkian,* No. 90-390963-A2 (Oakland County, Mich., 5 February 1991); Jim Persels, "Forcing the Issue of Physician-Assisted Suicide," *Journal of Legal Medicine,* Vol. 14 (1993), pp. 95–100.
26. Stephen Vicchio, "Death's logic" (4 April 1999), in URL: http://www.sunspot.net
27. *Jack Kevorkian and John Doe v. Arnett,* No. CV-94-6089 CBM (Kx), 939 F.Supp. 725 (11 September 1996), at 351.
28. *State of Michigan v. Kevorkian,* Michigan CirCt (Oakland City), verdict 8 March 1996. See http://www.courttv.com/verdicts/kevorkian.htm
29. Jack Kevorkian, *Prescription: Medicide* (New York: Prometheus Books, 1991), p. 222.
30. *Ibid.,* p. 226.
31. *Ibid.,* p.227.
32. 2 April 1996: Pontiac, Mich: Kevorkian: Trial or witch-hunt?, from ERGO's electronic mailing list. e-mail: <ergo@efn.org>
33. Orlando Sentinel Online, "Kevorkian responds to new allegations" (31 December 1997). URL: http://www.orlandosentinel.com/
34. Brian Harmon, "Kevorkian: I'll put law on trial. Suicide advocate says he'll fight attempts to rein him in," *The Detroit News,* Metro (1 January 1998). URL: http://detnews.com
35. Orlando Sentinel Online, "Kevorkian responds to new allegations" (31 December 1997). URL: http://www.orlandosentinel.com/
36. Kevorkian explains his guiding rationale in his book *Prescription: Medicide,* especially in chapters 13 and 14.
37. *Ibid.,* p. 223.
38. *Ibid.,* p. 215.
39. *Ibid.*

40. *Ibid*, p. 225.
41. *Ibid*.
42. Compare Kevorkian's cold and detached descriptions to Quill's caring and humane train of thought in *Death and Dignity*, especially his depiction of the stories of Diane, Mark, Wendy and Mrs. J. There are stark differences between the two. See Tomothy E. Quill, *Death and Dignity* (New York: W. W. Norton, 1993), esp. pp. 9–16, 52–56, 84-–91, 167–175, 177–179.
43. *The Detroit News* Metro (6 September 1997). URL: http://detnews.com/1997/metro/9709/06/09060039.htm
44. Kevorkian had no training to detect or to treat depression. For further discussion see Paul R. McHugh, "The Kevorkian Epidemic," *The American Scholar* (Winter 1997), pp. 15–27.
45. "Coroner: Janet Good would have lived more than 6 months," *The Detroit News*, Metro (6 September 1997), URL: http://detnews.com/1997/metro/9709/06/09060039.htm
46. Brian Harmon, "Critics: Kevorkian taking all comers. They claim terminal illness no longer only standard for suicides," *The Detroit News* (Sunday, 1 March 1998). http://detnews.com; http://www.oregonian.com
47. Brian Harmon, "Paralyzed man fulfills death wish: Kevorkian assists 21-year-old hours after leaving hospital," *The Detroit News* (Friday, 27 February 1998). See http://detnews.com; Free Press URL: http://www.freep.com; *The Associated Press*, "Kevorkian speaks out against police" (28 February 1998, 4:38 PM EST).
48. Brian Harmon, "Critics: Kevorkian taking all comers. They claim terminal illness no longer only standard for suicides," *The Detroit News* (Sunday, 1 March 1998). See also http://www.oregonian.com
49. *Ibid*.
50. David Goodman, "Kevorkian has kidneys available to donate from suicide," *The Associated Press* (7 June 1998). Article is available from URL: http://www.nytimes.com. See also Joe Swickard and David Crumm, "Kevorkian harvests kidneys," *The Free Press* (8 June 1998) http://www.freep.com/news/extra2/index.htm
51. For chronology of events involving Kevorkian see http://deathnews.com/TDNHOME/kevo
52. Opinion Editorial, "Kevorkian's Needle," *The Detroit News* (Sunday, 22 November 1998).
53. Derek Humphry (22 November 1998), e-mail: dhumphry@efn.org, circulated via ergo@efn.org
54. *60 Minutes*. Death by Doctor (22 November 1998).
55. URL source: Kevorkian *60 Minutes* poll results, http://www.freep.com/news/extra2/kevo_poll.htm (24 November 1998). See also URL source: Killing not murder, most say, http://www.freep.com/news/extra2/qpoll24.htm. For discussion on the ethics of showing Kevorkian's killing on television see Fritz Wenzel, "Media are ripped at U of M forum on assisted-suicide coverage" *The Toledo Blade* (23 February 1999); Brian Murphy, "Wallace rethinks suicide episode" (23 February 1999). URL: http://www.freep.com/news/metro/qdeath23.htm
56. Ellen Goodman, "Kevorkian has punctured the ethical gray zone where most of us live," *Boston Globe* (3 December 1998). URL: http://www.boston.com/dailyglobe2/337/oped/
57. See Julie Grace, "Curtains for Dr. Death," *Time* (5 April 1999), p. 50.
58. *Associated Press* report, "Kevorkian Gets 10 to 25 Years," Pontiac, Mich. (13 April 1999); *New York Times* (14 April 1999), p. A23. For further deliberation see http://www.freep.com/news/extra2/index.htm; and http://www.freep.com/news/extra2/qkevo14.htm
59. "Kevorkian Assistant helps AIDS patient die" (Monday, 19 January 1998, 6:50 AM EST), Pontiac, Michigan (Reuters).
60. "Reding believed hiding in Europe," *The Albuquerque Journal*, New Mexico (26 January 2000).
61. Interview with Dr. Gerrit K. Kimsma (Koog 'aan de Zaan, 28 July 1999).

62. See the Dutch requirements of careful practice *in* John Griffiths, Alex Bood and Heleen Weyers, *Euthanasia and Law in the Netherlands* (Amsterdam: Amsterdam University Press, 1998), p. 66.
63. See, for instance, Section 7, *Rights of the Terminally Ill Act (1995)* (NT).
64. In Australia, the law required a "cooling off" period of nine days. In Oregon, the Act requires a waiting period of fifteen days. I do not wish to suggest an arbitrary time period of waiting, saying instead that the patient should state his or her wish several times "over a period of time." I concur with Miller and colleagues ,who think that a fifteen-day waiting period may be highly burdensome for patients who are suffering intolerably and may preclude access to assisted death for those who request it at the point when they are imminently dying. Franklin G. Miller, Howard Brody and Timothy E. Quill, "Can Physician-Assisted Suicide Be Regulated Effectively?," *Journal of Law. Medicine & Ethics,* Vol. 24 (1996), p. 226. See also Oregon *Death with Dignity Act, Oregon Revised Statutes,* Vol. 8, 1998 Supplement, at 982.
65. John Griffiths *et al., Euthanasia and Law in the Netherlands, op. cit.*, p. 66.
66. Oregon *Death with Dignity Act, Oregon Revised Statutes,* Vol. 8, 1998 Supplement, at 980.
67. World Health Organization, *Cancer Pain Relief and Palliative Care: Report of a WHO Expert Committee* (Geneva, Switzerland: World Health Organization, 1990), at 11.
68. Directive 7 in *The General Manager Circular*, Israel Ministry of Health, no. 2/96 (31 January 1996) holds: "Doctors must concentrate their efforts on easing the pain, torment, and suffering of the patient, a subject of highest priority in medical treatment, especially where terminal patients are concerned," p. 12 [in Hebrew]. In order to institute effective consultation, new programs for the training and certification of palliative care consultants need to be developed and implemented. See Franklin G. Miller, Timothy E. Quill, Howard Brody *et al,* "Regulating Physician-Assisted Death," *New England Journal of Medicine,* Vol. 331, No. 2 (14 July 1994), pp. 119–123; Timothy E. Quill, Bernard Lo, and Dan W. Brock, "Palliative Options of Last Resort," *JAMA,* Vol. 278, No. 23 (17 December 1997), pp. 2099–2104; P. Anne Scott, "Autonomy, Power, and Control in Palliative Care," *Cambridge Quarterly of Healthcare Ethics,* Vol. 8, No. 2 (1999), pp. 139–147; Janet L. Abrahm, "The Role of the Clinician in Palliative Medicine," *Medical Students JAMA (MSJAMA),* Vol. 283 (5 January 2000), p. 116. URL: http://www.ama-assn.org/sci-pubs/msjama/articles/vol_283/no_1/jms90047.htm. For further discussion on making palliative care decisions for *incompetent* patients see Jason H.T. Karlawish, Timothy Quill and Diane E. Meier, "A Consensus-Based Approach to Providing Palliative Care to Patients Who Lack Decision-Making Capacity," *Annals of Internal Medicine,* Vol. 130 (18 May 1999), pp. 835–840.
69. Section 7, *Rights of the Terminally Ill Act (1995)* (NT).
70. On this issue see Oregon *Death with Dignity Act*, Section 3: Attending Physician Responsibilities. See also Section D: Consent to Medical Treatment of The Israel *Patients' Rights Law*, 1992, Law Proposal 2132 (16 March 1992); The *Patients' Rights Law*, 1996, *Israel Book of Laws*, 1591 (12 May 1996), at 329-331; and *The General Manager Circular*, The Ministry of Health, no. 2/96 (31 January 1996), at 10–11 [in Hebrew].
71. The first practical recommendation stated in *The General Manager Circular*, Israel Ministry of Health, no. 2/96 (31 January 1996), is that the diagnosis and evaluation that a patient's condition is "irreversible and terminal" shall be made by two independent doctors. At least one of them is required to be a head of department, p. 9 [in Hebrew].
72. Oregon *Death with Dignity Act, Oregon Revised Statutes,* Vol. 8, 1998 Supplement, at 981–982.
73. John Griffiths *et al., Euthanasia and Law in the Netherlands, op. cit.*, p. 66.
74. Section 7, *Rights of the Terminally Ill Act (1995)* (NT).
75. This Guideline is somewhat similar to the guidelines of the Swiss EXIT protocol. See South Australian Voluntary Euthanasia Society, DID YOU KNOW ? Assisted Suicide in Switzerland–SAVES Fact Sheet No. 20, issued February 1997. Correspondence with:

Hon. Secretary, SAVES, PO Box 2151, Kent Town, SA 5071, Australia–Fax + 61 8 8265 2287. URL: http://www.finalexit.org/
76. Andrew L. Plattner, "Australia's Northern Territory: The first Jurisdiction to Legislate Voluntary Euthanasia, and the First to Repeal It," *De Paul Journal of Health Care Law,* Vol. I (Spring 1997), p. 648.
77. 13 Or. Rev. Stat. § 3.07 (1998).
78. See Arthur E. Chin, Katrina Hedberg, Grant K. Higginson and David W. Fleming, "Legalized Physician-Assisted Suicide in Oregon: The First Year's Experience," *New England Journal of Medicine,* Vol. 340, No. 7 (18 February 1999), pp. 577–583; Melinda A. Lee, Heidi D. Nelson, Virginia P. Tilden *et al.,* "Legalizing Assisted Suicide—Views of Physicians in Oregon," *New England Journal of Medicine,* Vol. 334, No. 5 (1 February 1996), pp. 310–315. See also http://www.ohd.hr.state.or.us/cdpe/chs/pas/pas.htm
79. For further deliberation see the Dutch guidelines *in* John Griffiths *et al., Euthanasia and Law in the Netherlands, op. cit.,* p. 66; Oregon *Death with Dignity Act, Oregon Revised Statutes,* Vol. 8, 1998 Supplement, Section 3, at 983. Rebecca Cook pointed out to me that such a bureaucratic procedure might discriminate against minorities who will not find it easy to cope with the described demands. However, the demand for detailed documentation is meant to prevent abuse, not to discourage people from getting the help they want. We should be sensitive to cultural differences and strive to meet special needs that arise from cultural norms, but not at the expense of opening the door wide for "eliminating" unwanted people.
80. Directive 6 in *The General Manager Circular,* Israel Ministry of Health, no. 2/96 (31 January 1996) states: "The decision to respect a patient's objection to a life-prolonging treatment shall be documented in the medical statutes, expressing maximum reasons for the decision and the discussions with the patient," p. 12 [in Hebrew]. See also Israel *Patients' Rights Law* (1996), 1591, Chapter E: medical documentation and medical information, p. 331.
81. Andrew L. Plattner, "Australia's Northern Territory: The First Jurisdiction to Legislate Voluntary Euthanasia, and the First to Repeal It," *op. cit.,* p. 648.
82. 506/88 *Scheffer v. The State of Israel,* Vol. 48 (1) 87, paragraph 7 of Ariel J.'s opinion (198–199).
83. 506/88 *Scheffer v. The State of Israel,* Vol. 48 (1) 87, paragraph 65 of Elon J.'s opinion. For further discussion on incompetent patients and minors see Edmund D. Pellegrino and David C. Thomasma, *For the Patient's Good* (New York: Oxford University Press, 1988), pp. 148-161; Winifred J. Pinch and Margaret L. Spielman, "The Parents' Perspective: Ethical Decision-Making in Neonatal Intensive Care," *Journal of Advanced Nursing,* Vol. 15 (1990), pp. 712–719; American Academy of Pediatrics Committee on Bioethics, "Guidelines on Forgoing Life-Sustaining Medical Treatment," *Pediatrics,* Vol. 93, No. 3 (March 1994), pp. 532–536; S. Saigal, B.L. Stoskopf and D. Feeny, "Differences in Preferences for Neonatal Outcomes among Healthcare Professionals, Parents, and Adolescents," *JAMA,* Vol. 281, No. 21 (2 June 1999), pp. 1991–1997; Norman Fost, "Decisions Regarding Treatment of Seriously Ill Newborns," *JAMA,* Vol. 281, No. 21 (2 June 1999), pp. 2041–2043.

Peter Singer's Theories and Their Reception in Germany

JAN C. JOERDEN

Europa-Universität Viadrina, Institut für Strafrecht, Grosse Scharrnstrasse 59, 15230 Frankfurt (Oder), Germany

THE "SINGER DEBATE" IN GERMANY

There are people and groups (especially) in Germany (and Austria) who dispute the right of Peter Singer to publicly deliver his theories on euthanasia and abortion. By using quotes taken out of context many associations for the handicapped and politically left-wing students have equated Singer with a national socialist. The following quotes from Singer, for instance, especially raised much public attention: "The Nazis committed terrible crimes; but that does not mean that everything which the Nazis did was terrible. We cannot condemn euthanasia just because the Nazis carried it out, just as we cannot condemn the new roads simply because they were built by the Nazis."[1] Another such quote is: "Nevertheless the main point is clear: Killing a disabled infant is not morally equivalent to killing a person. Very often it is not wrong at all."[2] Or a last example: "It is the sense we have in mind when we say that an infant born without a brain is more like a vegetable than like a human being."[3] The public use of these quotes led to a situation in which students, and others, physically prevented Peter Singer from delivering his planned lectures. As a result most universities withdrew their invitations to him in order to avoid public disorder on their campuses.

One can understand that Peter Singer is sensitive to such attacks, considering that the right to freedom of speech and freedom of teaching are guaranteed in the German constitution. In an article written for *the New York Review of Books* entitled "On Being Silenced in Germany" Singer comments on this situation. He describes how attacks, sometimes violent, have hindered him from delivering his lectures in German cities: "Meanwhile Germans and Austrians, both in academic life and in the press, have shown themselves sadly lacking in the commitment exemplified by the celebrated utterance attributed to Voltaire: 'I disapprove of what you say, but I will defend to the death your right to say it.' No one has, as yet, been asked to risk death in order to defend my right to discuss euthanasia in Germany, but it is important that many more should be prepared to risk a little hostility from the minority that is trying to silence a debate on central ethical questions."[4]

There can be no doubt that Peter Singer quite rightly calls on his right to freedom of speech and freedom of teaching. A large number of philosophers at German universities affirmed this at the beginning of the so-called "Singer debate."[5] It is also clear that Peter Singer must have the possibility of publishing his theories. In this respect the publishers Harald Fischer Verlag (Erlangen) played an important role by publishing the German edition of the book *Should the Baby Live?*, after the publishers Rowohlt, who had planned to publish the book, felt that the affair had become too controversial.[6] It was rumored that Rowohlt came to its decision not to publish after receiving bomb threats. I myself had the opportunity in Erlangen, a small university town close to Nuremberg, to participate in a workshop with Peter Singer and his co-author Helga Kuhse, where we were able to discuss his theories. The workshop was organized by Harald Fischer Verlag to present the German edition of the book. Only a few guests were personally invited and the meeting was not made public in order to avoid provocation from groups opposed to Peter Singer. It was thus possible to pursue a controversial but fair discussion of Peter Singer's theories.[7]

Regardless of all the attacks on Peter Singer's right to freedom of speech, it should, in my opinion, be expected that he is sensitive and careful when dealing with such difficult questions as the possibility of abortion and euthanasia. For here the concern is with the right to *life* and not some other less important right, such as the right to free speech. The care and sensitivity which can be expected of Peter Singer should begin with the choice of words. Choosing such a bold title as *Should the Baby Live?* (or even the German title *Muß dieses Kind am Leben bleiben?*) leads one to question whether this was not done with an eye on the circulation figures of the book, an unfortunate practice which is detrimental to an objective discussion of the issues Peter Singer raises.

My objection to the choice of title is that it is ambiguous and thus leaves room for misinterpretation. It is difficult to believe that the author did not know this when deciding upon the title, while banishing the actual problem he wants to deal with to the subtitle ("The Problem of Handicapped Infants," or, in the German edition, "Das Problem schwerstgeschädigter Neugeborener"). Some would call this a question of taste, which one clearly cannot argue over. However, he who so vehemently defends the safeguarding of his own rights, as Peter Singer does concerning his right to free speech, should have understanding for those who could feel their right to life threatened, even if it is not his intention to question their right to life. That fear should be respected by employing clear and unequivocal formulations, even if they have a disadvantageous effect on the sales figures of a publication. It seems evident to me that the handicapped *could feel* threatened when the theory is presented that it is ethically justifiable to kill certain handicapped babies shortly after birth,[8] even if in the same breath it is said, as Peter Singer does, that this clearly does not apply to those handicapped who are already "persons."[9] Which women, for the sake of argument, would not have a strong tendency to feel threatened if in an academic discussion it was questioned whether female babies have the right to life during the first month after birth, even if it was added that naturally this right was not at issue for already grown women.

OBJECTIONS TO PETER SINGER'S ARGUMENTS

1. On the right to life

In the following I shall address some of the problems in Peter Singer's arguments, mainly in relation to his discussion of early euthanasia. One of the central problems with Peter Singer's theory in this context is not that he raises the question of under which specific circumstances the life of a seriously disabled newly born infant can be ended, in as far as a life of terrible suffering is to be expected, but rather, it is his opinion, that the "solution" to all such tragic "cases" is to dispute the right to life of newly born infants up to a certain time period. In the words of Peter Singer: "But we have now concluded that new born infants do not have a right to life."[10] One must keep this dimension of his solution-concept in mind when discussing Peter Singer's theories because it is this dimension that allows the selecting of (in his words) "life that is not worth living."[11] In my opinion Peter Singer's solution is too excessive. For clarification of the cases in which a life of suffering may be ended there is absolutely no need for the far-reaching theory of Peter Singer, because this applies to *all* newly born infants. Moreover, in the already mentioned "cases" it is possible to think of a special regulation containing concrete requirements bound by a justificatory norm.[12]

In my opinion an excusatory norm may be preferable because this does not question the *right* to life of any newly born child. Parents and doctors may then have an excuse, if after careful consideration and the fulfillment of certain, yet to be discussed and legally determined, precise requirements, they come to the conclusion that the suffering of the child appears to make the compulsion to carry on living no longer endurable. Comparable is the much-discussed case of a car-driver trapped inside a burning car begging for a mercy-shot.[13] In this case the driver's *right* to life may not be questioned (which is especially the case if the driver rejects, say because of his religious beliefs, the killing via a mercy-shot); at best the person who kills the driver upon his express demands (thus fulfilling the requirements of the offence "killing upon consent"[14]) has an excuse.

2. On the slippery slope argument

Apart from this central objection, the argumentation of Peter Singer strikes me partly as problematic and even sometimes quite inconclusive. In one place in his works he deals with one of the arguments against early euthanasia. The argument is that such measures must be rejected because this would be the start of a "slippery slope" which could finally lead to the killing of adults. Peter Singer, however, rejects this argument and takes the position that every one agrees that some lives are not worth living. For whoever decides that certain handicapped children should not receive medical treatment ascribes less worth to the life of those children with a "severe handicap" than to the life of "normal" children. If we are prepared not to extend such a life then we must admit that we consider some lives not worth living. Then follows the core of Peter Singer's objection to the slippery slope argument: "So if the judgement that some lives are not worth living were enough to put us on the slippery slope to Nazism, we would already be well down that slope."[15] This objection is, however, unconvincing. His argument is comparable to the clearly false "argument" of a thoughtless mountaineer who, hesitating because of the danger while climbing down a risky way, calls to his companions that he could continue to descend, for he has already started climbing down. In other words, one cannot reject the "slippery slope argument" by arguing that one is already on the slippery slope and therefore one can freely slip further down. The only demand that can be derived is that one should leave the slope at once.

3. On the acceptance of infanticide

In other places Peter Singer points out that there are examples throughout history, as well as in present societies, in which infanticide has been accepted. This then leads him to the sub-conclusion: "The preceding pages have shown that we live in an unusual society. We reject infanticide...Why do we take a view so different from that of the majority of human societies?"[16] It is quite astonishing that Singer uses such research, interesting though it may be, to further an *ethical* discussion. For hardly anyone (at least it is to be hoped) would have the idea of justifying torture by referring to the fact that it is practiced in a number of countries in the present. The aim here is clearly to play an (alleged) majority off against a minority. Arguments of this kind have never been of interest to a serious ethical discussion.

Peter Singer further points out that some peoples have adopted infanticide as a practical and prudent attempt to combat overpopulation.[17] This is, however, in my opinion, irrelevant to an ethical discussion. Similarly, one would not argue in favor of waging war that it is good means of solving the problem of overpopulation. There are obviously other more humane methods of solving population crises. In any case it does not reassure me when Peter Singer gives an (endorsing) account of Jeremy Bentham's criticism that in his time infanticide was too harshly punished, and Bentham's further statement that this was a crime that did not disquiet even the most timid of natures. Peter Singer adds to this: "Infanticide threatens none of us, for once we are aware of it, we are not infants."[18] With such an argument even the killing of other races could quite easily be, falsely of course, "justified," though I in no way wish to suggest that *this* is Peter Singer's intention. In fact Peter Singer clearly states that he is against such consequences[19]; this does not, however, eliminate the reproach against using arguments that would allow such consequences. Peter Singer has emphasized the "equanimity with which many other cultures have accepted"[20] infanticide, but there have also been many "cultures" that have killed other races with comparable equanimity, and this equanimity is also easy to comprehend because the members of these "cultures" felt themselves to be "ethnically pure." Again, however, I assume, that this is in no respect valid as an ethical argument.

4. *On the speciesism argument*

In many places in his works Peter Singer utilizes the so-called "speciesism" argument.[21] This argument suggests that, insofar as the right to life is only conceded in connection with the biological element of being a human, there is an unjustifiable disadvantaging of those life forms that, although from a moral perspective are equal, are not treated equally. The term *speciesism* is thus parallel to the terms *racism* and *sexism*.[22] Peter Singer employs this argument to question the right to life of the unborn and the newly born infant. He argues that it is "speciesistic" to forbid abortion, yet on the other hand to allow the killing of animals when their mental development is equal to, if not higher than, that of a fetus. For Peter Singer the only morally convincing criteria for drawing a temporal limit for granting the right to life is the ability to experience oneself as identical in the past, present, and future. Further, on the basis of this experience there must be an ability to form future wishes, especially the wish to live.[23] It then follows that human beings who have not yet reached this status (such as fetuses and newly born infants) do not have the right to life.[24] Meanwhile, certain apes can quite clearly be described as having the characteristics that Peter Singer reserves for the term *person*. Peter Singer thus states: "Not just chimpanzees but also the animals we commonly kill for food—pigs, cows and chickens—would compare favorably with anencephalic infants, or those who have suffered massive brain haemorrhages."[25] Only a legal regulation that also forbids the killing of such "persons" would not be criticized by Singer as speciesistic.

This line of argument also does not seem convincing to me. Peter Singer's position is that only those who can develop present and future wishes, and accordingly have an awareness of themselves, should be called *persons*. From this *only* follows that protection and the right to life must be granted not only to all those "persons" who are human beings but also to those "persons" that are animals possessing this quality. The speciesism-objection would not, however, necessarily lead to permitting the killing of future lives, and even newly born infants, which do not yet have the characteristic "personhood." For, there is nothing to speak against giving preferential treatment to members of ones own species over and above *the minimum legal-ethical position* to which they—together with other species—are entitled. Such favoring *over and above* what can be demanded based on legal-ethical considerations does not constitute *reprehensible* discrimination of another.

There is also, for example, no reprehensible discrimination, when I feel under a higher degree of duty towards the members of my family than I owe to other people. Similarly, it does not seem to be reprehensible discrimination if a state, alongside granting a legally-ethically required minimum of human rights to everyone, grants its citizens further rights (e.g., the right to vote). Peter Singer takes the position that in relation to the granting of the right to life there is an ethical minimum in the sense that only "persons" (as understood by Singer) can claim this right. However, the speciesism-objection does not exclude favoring human life forms (e.g., fetuses) over the ethical minimum by granting a right to life, even though this is not (strictly speaking) ethically compelling.

There is no doubt that by granting "yet to be persons" a right to life certain animals are discriminated against. This, however, is a form of *positive* discrimination of the "yet to be persons," which is at least easier to ethically accept than *negative* discrimination. In his book *Practical Ethics* Peter Singer describes another case of "positive discrimination," which we all know as "affirmative action." In his words: "If affirmative action is open to objection it must be because the goals it seeks to advance are bad, or because it will not really promote these goals."[26] Insofar as such positive discrimination is not arbitrary, it is, in principle, acceptable. In support of the positive discrimination of "yet to be persons" it should especially be mentioned that they *could* become "persons," which is indeed never the case with most animals. At best one could argue that the embryos of some apes should not be killed because they could become "persons" in the sense of Singer's definition of the term. Speciesism is thus not a suitable argument against granting the right to life to "yet to be persons," even if one adopts Peter Singer's definition of a person (which, I must point out, I do not).

CONCLUSION

In the midst of all these objections it should not be forgotten that Peter Singer delivers quite a degree of stimulating ideas and arguments. He also presents interesting analyses of some very intense case descriptions. And many of the arguments that Singer raises against other ethical models are indeed noteworthy. For instance, he criticizes the common differentiation in our legal systems between active killing and passive allowing-to-die. Maybe our continental European moral beliefs are here and elsewhere too concerned with formal terminology. The theory based on Thomas

Aquinas's "doctrine of double effect" is quite correctly criticized. Peter Singer is also to be agreed with in his criticism of the often superficial and basically pragmatic character of "ethical" discussions in the field of medicine.

Finally, to Peter Singer's credit, it must at least be emphasized that he has addressed this extremely sensitive and highly problematic issue. If there were no stimulation of discussion and presentation of possibly incorrect theories, medics would concern themselves alone *nolens volens* with these problems and "muddle on" without any ethical concept—a tendency not only limited to this area of medical ethics.

ACKNOWLEDGMENTS

I am grateful to Thomas Crofts, LL.B. (London), LL.M. (Würzburg), for the translation of this paper.

NOTES AND REFERENCES

1. Peter Singer, *Praktische Ethik* (Stuttgart: Reclam, 1984), p. 210 [not in the original English edition].
2. Peter Singer, *Practical Ethics*, 2nd ed. (Cambridge: Cambridge University Press, 1993), p. 19; see fn. 1 in the German edition.
3. Helga Kuhse and Peter Singer, *Should the Baby Live? The Problem of Handicapped Infants* (Oxford: Oxford University Press, 1985/87), p. 121. German edition: *Muß dieses Kind am Leben bleiben? Das Problem schwerstgeschädigter Neugeborener* (Erlangen: Harald Fischer Verlag, 1993). Cf. also my discussion of the book in *Jahrbuch für Recht und Ethik/ Annual Review of Law and Ethics* (Berlin: Duncker & Humblot) Vol. 2, 1994, p. 529. In this paper I only deal with the arguments of Peter Singer; however, it should be remembered that the book *Should the Baby Live?* was co-written by Helga Kuhse.
4. Reprinted in *Practical Ethics*, 2nd ed., p. 359. A German translation of this article can be found in Helga Kuhse and Peter Singer, *Muß dieses Kind am Leben bleiben?*, pp. 283–297.
5. Cf. "Erklärung der deutschen Philosophen zur sog. 'Singer-Affaire,'" *in* R. Hegelsmann/R. Merkel (eds.), *Zur Debatte über Euthanasie* (Frankfurt am Main: Suhrkamp, 1991), pp. 327 ff. For a description of the problems in relation to the "Singer debate" cf. Christoph Anstötz, Reiner Hegselmann, and Hartmut Kliemt (Eds.), *Peter Singer in Deutschland. Zur Gefährdung der Diskussionsfreiheit in der Wissenschaft* (Frankfurt am Main: Peter Lang Verlag, 1995). For further discussion of Peter Singer's (and Helga Kuhse's) theories in Germany see *Analyse & Kritik*, Vol. 12., No. 2 (December 1990; special edition on Peter Singer's theories); Bernward Grünewald, "Peter Singer's Objektivismus und seine versteckte Subjektstheorie," *Jahrbuch für Recht und Ethik/ Annual Review of Law and Ethics*, Vol. 3 (1995), pp. 403–414; Norbert Hoerster, *Abtreibung im säkularen Staat*. Argumente gegen den §218 (Frankfurt am Main: Suhrkamp Verlag, 1991); Joachim Hruschka, "Zum Lebensrecht des Foetus in rechtsethischer Sicht," *Juristenzeitung* 10 (1991), 508 ff; Anton Leist, *Eine Frage des Lebens. Ethik der Abtreibung und künstlichen Befruchtung* (Frankfurt am Main: Campus Verlag, 1990); Uwe Scheffler, "Die 'Heiligkeit des Lebens' in der Philosophie. Eine juristische Kritik," *Jahrbuch für Recht und Ethik/Annual Review of Law and Ethics*, Vol. 5 (1997), pp. 481–487; Roland Wittmann, "Metaethische Überlegungen zu dem Diskurs über P. Singers 'Praktische Ethik'," in: R. Hegselmann/ R. Merkel, *ibid*., pp. 249 ff; for more references see Christoph Anstötz "Einschlägige deutsche Buchveröffentlichungen," *in* H. Kuhse and P. Singer, *Muß dieses Kind am Leben bleiben?*, pp. 303–306. Verlag, 1990).
6. Cf. the author's account of this in *Muß dieses Kind am Leben bleiben?*, pp. 24–25

7. I do not at all suggest that the appearances of Peter Singer in Germany should in future only take place in private circles. Rather it should once again be possible to publicly discuss his theories at universities without being hindered by violent demonstrators.
8. Cf. *Should the Baby Live?*, p. v; cf. the problems that the translator had with this passage in the German edition (fn., p. 25).
9. Cf. *Muß dieses Kind am Leben bleiben?*, pp. 20–21.
10. Cf. *Should the Baby Live?*, p. 140.
11. *Should the Baby Live?*, p. 96.
12. For a discussion of this point cf. Reinhard Merkel, "Teilnahme am Suizid, Totung auf Verlangen, Euthanasie, Fragen an die Strafrechtsdogmatik," *in* R. Hegselmann/R/ Merkel, *Zur Debatte uber Euthanasie*, pp. 71–127, especially pp. 88–112.
13. Cf. for a similar case Harro Otto, "Recht auf den eigenen Tod?," Gutachten D zum 56. Deutschen Juristentag, Berlin 1986 (München: C. H. Beck Verlag, 1986), p. D 60; see also Merkel *ibid.*, p. 86; and Ulfrid Neumann, "Die Moral des Rechts," *Jahrbuch für Recht und Ethik/ Annual Review of Law and Ethics*, Vol. 2 (1994), pp. 81–94.
14. Regulated in § 216 of the German Criminal Code; for a discussion of this issue in Germany see Wolfgang Mitsch, "Euthanasia and Modern German Criminal Law," *Tel Aviv University Studies in Law*, Vol. 13 (1997), pp. 63–73.
15. *Should the Baby Live?*, p. 94.
16. *Should the Baby Live?*, p. 111.
17. *Should the Baby Live?*, p. 103 *et seq.*
18. *Should the Baby Live?*, p. 138.
19. *Should the Baby Live?*, p. 91 *et seq.*
20. *Should the Baby Live?*, p. 138.
21. Cf., e.g., *Practical Ethics*, pp. 55 *et seq.*, 62 *et seq.*
22. *Should the Baby Live?*, pp. 121 et seq.
23. The author relies here especially on the thoughts of John Locke and Michael Tooley. See in this context also Norbert Hoerster, *Abtreibung im säkularen Staat*, Argumente gegen den § 218 (Frankfurt am Main: Suhrkamp, 1991, 2nd ed. 1995), and, in relation to the latter, my review in *Juristenzeitung*, Vol. 47 (1992), pp. 456–458.
24. For a certain modification of the limit drawn by the author, which responds to the objections of Hoerster, *ibid*, cf. *Muß dieses Kind am Leben bleiben?*, pp. 251 *et seq.* However, no change is made to the core of the argument regarding the "intrinsic right to life of newly born infants" (p. 251).
25. *Should the Baby Live?*, p. 122.
26. *Practical Ethics*, p. 49.

Problems Involved in the Moral Justification of Medical Assistance in Dying

Coming to Terms with Euthanasia and Physician-Assisted Suicide

EVERT VAN LEEUWEN AND GERRIT KIMSMA

Faculteit der Geneeskunde, Section of Philosophy and Medical Ethics, Free University of Amsterdam, 1081 BT Amsterdam, the Netherlands

> At best, the cult of rationality, institutionalized as modern science, proved impotent to prevent the state from turning into organized crime; at worst, it proved instrumental in bringing the transformation about.
>
> (ZYGMUNT BAUMAN, *MODERNITY AND THE HOLOCAUST*, P. 110)

INTRODUCTION

The Dutch practice of euthanasia and physician-assisted suicide has been followed by several political proposals to legalize medical assistance in dying. Short of legalization, the 1995 report of van der Wal and van der Maas has been especially-used to broach a discussion about the possibility of an intermediate "solution" midway between criminalization and decriminalization of physician-assisted suicide. This solution involved inaugurating regional committees intended to supervise and check these acts with respect to their conformity to legal and medical conditions. These committees would serve as an intermediate position between the law and the physicians. It is expected that this procedure will bridge the gap between legal and medical ethical perspectives, stimulating and inviting physicians to report the active ending of lives.

In this paper the inauguration of regional committees will be discussed with respect to the legal and moral issues of the practice of actively ending lives within the context of care. In the final part corollary philosophical issues will be analyzed.

REGIONAL COMMITTEES

In November 1997 the Secretaries of Justice and of Healthcare, Well Being and Sports, published their intention to inaugurate five regional committees that would supervise the involvement of physicians in the active ending of the lives of their patients.[1] These committes have been functioning since December 1998. The task of the committees is to evaluate retrospectively reported cases of euthanasia and physician-assisted suicide. The committees comprise a physician, a lawyer, and an ethicist, and their area of oversight encompasses all cases where a voluntary request has been made by a competent patient. Cases of physician-assisted death without such a request are directly sent to Office of the Prosecution. The government intends to inaugurate a Central Euthanasia Evaluation Committee for these cases, but this has not yet been established.

In 1999, before even one year of experience with the regional committees has been atttained, the Government introduced a proposal to legalize physician-assisted death, intending to decriminalize these acts even further. According to this proposal, the regional committees will remain in function and their conclusions will be binding for the legal authorities, meaning that a separate evaluation by local prosecutors will be out of the question.

With the policy of 1998 the government partly followed a proposal issued by the Royal Dutch Medical Society (RDMA) of March 1997, responding to the results of the 1995 study of van der Wal and van der Maas. The figures in this last study provide an opportunity to get some indication about the workload and the possible task of the committees. Using the 1995 figures as a reliable index, about 3,200 cases of voluntary active euthanasia (VAE) occur yearly in the Netherlands, while 9,700 explicit requests are made. Physician-assisted suicide (PAS) occurs in about 400 cases, and active ending of life without a request of a patient occurs in about 900 cases. Intensive treatment of pain and symptoms, presumably hastening the death of the patient, occurs in about 25,000 cases, while stopping treatment or not starting treatment occurs in about 27,000 cases.[2] Taken together this implies that in almost 58,000 cases, or 42.6% of all deaths in a particular year in the Netherlands, physicians have been involved in making some decision about the time and occurrence of the death of their patients.

The amount of 58,000 indicates a total possible workload of 11,600 cases in each committee, if we presume an equal distribution over all the regional committees in the Netherlands. On a weekly schedule of 50 weeks a year, this will boil down to 232 cases a week, or about 34 each day. We may infer from these figures that it is impossible to check all the cases in detail. Criteria will have to be set in order to make a selection. The government proposes to restrict the workload of the committees to those cases reported in which an explicit request is followed by VAE, when PAS has been performed, or when a physician has ended a life without a request.[3] This would still amount to 4,500 cases, 900 for each committee, or 18 on a weekly basis.

What sort of evaluation will a committee be able to perform, given this workload? Active consultation and investigation on site will be out of the question if we consider two or three cases each day and if we do not expect that committee members will have full-time jobs. Thorough investigation of all the relevant information will also be very difficult and requires a well-equipped bureau support staff. The investigation on site is relegated to the physician who has to be consulted before the act is performed. So we can expect that the committees will restrict themselves to examining the questions about the ways in which procedures have been followed or directives have been executed. In this way the danger of a rather bureaucratic public policy becomes realistic, with all the side effects that attend bureaucracy. Moreover, the committees will send all their conclusions to the national Medical Inspection Agency and to the judicial authorities, in both cases for further investigation. In the first event the intention is to evaluate the medical procedures and in the second case to evaluate the legal aspects.

THE POSSIBLE GOALS TO BE REACHED BY INAUGURATING REGIONAL COMMITTEES

The main goal of inaugurating regional committees is to evaluate the prudence of the practice of physician-assisted death, with the intent of public control of a highly sensitive medical practice and moral issue. The secondary goal is to increase the number of reported cases and thus to make public control more effective. According to van der Wal and van der Maas, 41% of the cases of VAE and PAS have been reported in 1995.[4] Although from 1991 to 1995 reports increased from from 18% to 41%, the majority of cases are still not being reported to the judicial authorities. The reasons given by van der Wal and van der Maas to report or to abstain from reporting are not completely clear, however:

The reasons of physicians for *reporting* are:

   I always report (75%)

   One ought to report (18%)

   Policy of the institution (13%)

   To be accountable to society (13%)

   Risk of prosecution is small (7%)

   To avoid aggravation of mourning of surviving relatives (4%)

   Not reporting is impossible (2%)

   At the request of family (2%)

   Other (2%)

The reasons for *not-reporting* VAE and PAS are given as follows:

   Wish to save oneself and the family the burden of judicial inquiry (55%)

   Wish to save surviving relatives from judicial inquiry (30%)

   Fear of prosecution (36%)

   Wish of relatives to be saved from judicial inquiry (31%)

   Not all the requirements were met (30%)

   The act is something between physician and patient (12%)

   There has been no explicit request (5%)

   Fear of the reaction of relatives (5%)

   Other (6%)

When asked in what kind of circumstances they would have reported, physicians answered:

   Never (7%)

   According to the present judicial procedure (15%)

   If there had been more time (26%)

   If relatives should ask for it (20%)

If the judicial procedures were more clear (11%)
If it would be secure that settlement would be fair (10%)
If the environment would make it public (5%)
If the requirements had been met (7%)
If VAE and PAS were removed from criminal law (1%)
Other (0%)

According to van der Wal and van der Maas the patient-characteristics of reported cases do not differ much from the not-reported ones. Moreover, they assert that 50% of the physicians who do report have also not reported in the past. They suggest that the physicians involved usually are older and more experienced in VAE and PAS.[5]

If we compare, however, the reasons for reporting and not reporting, it strikes us that those who do report do so because they feel an obligation, while those who do not report wish to save themselves or others from judicial inquiry. Moreover, van der Wal and van der Maas also assert that the procedural requirements in the not-reported cases were not fulfilled as meticulously as were the reported cases. If the cases are indeed comparable with respect to patient-characteristics, one might conclude that not-reporting occurs mainly because of emotional objections to judicial bureaucracy. Non-reporting sometimes occurs, too, because the procedural requirements were not fulfilled, meaning that either a written documentation of the request was absent, consultation with a colleague had not taken place, or a written report had not been produced. All these events feed the fear of prosecution. Sometimes physicians appear to have objections in principle against reporting, but the legal procedure itself is not mentioned as a reason for resistance to report.

On the basis of this conclusion the main goals to be reached by the committees are to remove the objections of physicians to the red tape of judicial bureaucracy and to diminish the fear of being involved in the time-consuming process of legal inspection. It can be argued that as a secondary goal the establishment of regional committees would have the effect of decriminalizing VAE and PAS as much as possible. This argument led the Royal Dutch Medical Society in the first place when its executive board made a plea for regional committees.[6]

A REALISTIC EXPECTATION?

Will the goals be reached by inaugurating these committees? The answer to this question will be positive if the checks made by the committees will convince physicians to subject their actions to public control. It is possible that physicians will feel safer and more secure if committees investigate on a collegial basis. On the other hand, the committees will relay their reports to the judicial authorities. They will therefore have to check whether all requirements are fulfilled. If a protocol or a report contains flaws or if some steps are difficult to understand and thus to evaluate adequately from a distance, one might expect that physicians will continue to shy away from reporting. For instance, the time-span between a first explicit request and the final act of VAE or PAS is sometimes limited because of a fast deterioration of the medical situation of a patient, finally resulting in a request for assisted death. In those cases a distant view (that is, an evaluation at a distance, as opposed to on site) of the condition of a durable request cannot necessarily be assessed adequately. A similar situation can occur with respect to the adequacy of consultation: in a given situation there can be adequate clarity about the nature of a request, but this assessment may be difficult for a consulting physician to make, again because the medical situation may have deteriorated so fast as to preclude an adequate evaluation of the request. In both instances, an evaluation made at a distance without adequate additional description may lead to further investigations, in which case the expected increased reporting may not materialize at all. And when this experience becomes common knowledge, the effect of decriminalization will be only cosmetic: by softening the reporting procedure, physicians may be doubly alarmed if they become aware of the fact that a committee will have to report flaws or obscurities to the judicial authorities. These authorities can be expected to be more meticulous in their research if they are advised to do so by a regional committee.

It might therefore be concluded that the foundation of regional committees will mean a faster and more collegial procedure than the present judicial inquiry. On the other hand, the effects of their establishment on the percentages of reporting and non-reporting will continue to depend mainly on the positive attitude and careful actions of the physicians who perform VAE and PAS.[7] In cases where there is no request, or when other flaws are clear, one can expect that physicians will be even more hesitant to report, while the procedure might be even more time-consuming and threatening than at present, as one physician already has described in a Dutch medical journal.[8] Natural death—the alleged cause of death in 44% of the deaths in the Netherlands—will then become the usual stated cause of death in more cases.

Behind the emotional objections and the fear of being prosecuted an even more fundamental issue is visible: the question whether judicial rules and principles are adequate instruments *per se* to evaluate moral issues of assistance to death and dying. Our contention is that the gap between medical morality and the morality of the law is not incidental but fundamental. The establishment of the regional committees does not consciously intend to close this gap, but to circumvent it practically. From a philosophical point of view this circumvention is highly interesting because it reveals a struggle between basic values underlying law and medicine in a contemporary, relatively small Western country. Although the systems of law and medical morality will be different in other countries, this gap most likely will also be present in those societies, albeit with different contours. Therefore our focus shall be on this gap, this friction, these different moralities, in order to unravel some of its complexity through reflection issues of law and regulations.

A first indication of the effects of the Euthanasia Evaluation Committees may be gleaned from the first Annual Report to the Dutch Authorities, published in May 2000. The numbers of reported cases warrant the conclusion that an increase in cases has not been substantial. Neither have there been cases that did not fulfill the conditions for physician-assisted death. None of the cases thus far have lead to an investigation. Where the Committees did have questions, physicians were able, in writing or at an invited discussion, to clarify the complexity of a case and the decisions they had to make. Noteworthy was the tendency to provide limited direct information in the written reports of the consultants, suggesting that there was little understanding of their intervention with respect to the Evaluation Committee in stead of the perceived function in relation to their medical colleagues. All in all, the experience of one year does not justify sweeping conclusions. It is obvious, however, that even though there seem to be indications of an increase in reported cases, there is still a large segment of underreporting. And the fundamental questions we put forward in this section on the functionality of legal evaluation of medical care decisions have not lost their critical intent.

MEDICAL ETHICS AND THE LAW

VAE and PAS are illegal and part of the penal code in Dutch law. According to the present state of medical ethics, VAE and PAS are permissible and can be considered as acceptable medical actions if certain requirements are met. An acceptable moral good is realized when VAE or PAS are performed when there is a repeated, durable, and explicit request; if durable, hopeless suffering is present; if a collegial consultation has taken place; and an extensive report has been written. These are the official criteria of the medical profession. Under present law, VAE and PAS are to be considered as justifiable only when there is a conflict of duties. In all other cases they are considered potentially murder and necessarily lead to prosecution.

The main reason not to legalize VAE and PAS, thus exempting it from regular scrutiny, is the perceived and considered necessity of public control. Ending someone's life does not belong to the "normal" arsenal of medicine, and the reasons for performing VAE and PAS cannot be standardized in terms of objective clinical science. Nor can these actions be justified in terms of conveying a good to a patient. Death cannot be a more desirable good than staying alive, as far as the law is concerned. As in the Canadian *Latimer* case,[9] the law has no means to express the intended good in ending the life of someone, and we might even say that this good is beyond human judgment. From the perspective of law then, life is considered to be a continuous process of equally high value, while the result of ending it is a corpse. The law is, in other words, based on a binary scheme: one is either dead or alive. And, life can only end due to some external cause. If nature is the external cause, then there is no need to investigate. But if death is caused by the actions of some other human being, then there is a suspicion and the possible claim of murder. Furthermore, all human life is equal in the eye of the law, whether it be physically or mentally deficient or diseased. This resistance to any type of discrimination between several qualities of life is deeply engraved in Dutch law and the Dutch constitution. This black-and-white perception creates the persistent gap between medical observations of diminishing life and the legal perspective. Any attempt to formulate a legal definition of dying will result in formally degrading some phase of life against other phases. Medical morality does recognize that life itself can lose its human value both according to both cultural and biological standards. A situation "worse than death" makes sense in this respect while it comes down to nonsense within the legal perspective. Within medical morality life is not considered a continuous process that will come to a dead stop at some point in time. Some remarks on Dutch law can exemplify the concepts that are at stake here.

PRINCIPLES IN DUTCH LAW

Dutch law, established in the nineteenth century, is derived from Roman statutory law. The fundamental principles are laid down in the Dutch constitution. With respect to issues of death and dying, the articles 10 and 11 are especially relevant, together with the principle of equality.

The following issues are to be mentioned in this respect:

(1) the integrity of the human body and the preservation of life;
(2) protection by the state of weak and vulnerable persons;
(3) principle of equality;
(4) relation between the power of the state and individual rights; and
(5) delegation of specific authorities to certified physicians in matters of health care.

With respect to topic 5, physicians have specific rights and duties, prescribed by law. Surgery, for example, if performed in a medical setting, does not constitute a crime, because the purpose served by the physician is deemed higher than the integrity of the body. This is called the provision of "the medical exception." The act of putting a knife into someone's body is considered to be a medical act or intervention and should be evaluated, if necessary, by disciplinary jurisdiction. The medical profession judges itself by setting the standards and norms of appropriate interventions.

With respect to death and dying, VAE and PAS are explicitly mentioned in the penal code as cases in which the cause of death is unnatural. Within the frame of the law, this implies that an investigation should follow to answer questions about the possible degree of murder. VAE and PAS are not considered to be types of "normal" medical treatment and consequently cases of VAE and PAS have to go to court.

Philosophically speaking, the integrity of the body and the necessity of investigating cases of unnatural death, are connected in the system of law. There is no possible intermediate between the protection of the integrity of the body and the unnatural ending of a life. A physician has the legal duty to protect the life of his patients as part of his delegated authority.

MEDICAL REALITY AND MORALITY

As mentioned above, a medical decision is involved in about 42.6% of all deaths in the Netherlands. This does not imply that these deaths are "caused" by medical decision-making, but it underscores the medical supervision and the power to control the end of life. One might say that the passage from life to death has been subjected to medical dominion, implying specific decisions of (palliative) care, including starting, withholding, or stopping treatment. The physician in these cases is considered to be the legally recognized caretaker in the process of dying.

The role of the physician is not restricted in these cases to technical matters. In matters of morality, physicians are often the persons of trust to whom patients turn themselves if they worry about the medical conditions of their passing away. In these circumstances the physician, especially the general practitioner or the family physician, may become a central figure of trust and support.[10] This bond of trust has a long history in the Netherlands. In the Code Civil of 1809, during the French occupation, the relation between patient and physician was already considered to be a *contract mandatum*, a mandatory contract in stead of a service contract or *locatio conductio*.[11] The contract between patient and physician could then be considered to be a contract *sui generis*.[12]

During the patient's process of dying, the physician has mainly to deal with two types of legal values: the legal protection of the integrity of the body as well as the protection of privacy. These values function in relation to the human aspects of the dying process, including the physical aspects. In principle, the physician has a duty to hold to secrecy anything he knows within the bond of trust. As far as non-medical matters are concerned, the right to privacy and the integrity of the body continue to stand firm. But as far as medical matters are involved, the privacy and the integrity of the body are protected as a function of the medical treatment. Measures of alleviating pain may, for instance, lead to hospital admission and probably to a watering down of the privacy of dying. Or the treatment or palliative measures taken may cause irremediable damage to the integrity of the patient's body, even though they are necessary to relieve the patient's suffering.

The present practices of VAE and PAS in the Netherlands originate in this relationship of personal trust and care.[13] They are not based on any constitutional right (to die). The fact that 71–74% of the 1995 cases of VAE took place within general practice, compared to 26–27% in hospitals and 0–2% in nursing homes,[14] supports the impression that the trusting relationship is still highly valued, sometimes even above the possible option of prolonging life in a hospital. From the perspective of physicians who oppose reporting VAE and PAS under any condition: the 7% of physicians who stated that they would never report a case of euthanasia to the judicial authorities[15] can be seen as remaining faithful to that relationship of trust with their patients. This implies that these physicians consider their contract with their patients as a contract *sui generis*, suggesting that they always act in the best interest of their patient according to the professional standards of medicine.

COMPARISON OF LAW AND MEDICAL MORALITY

Let us start with summing up the main differences between law and medical morality as encountered up to this point:

1. The law treats every case of unnatural death according to the principle of equality, regardless of whether an accident, a criminal event, or a medical event has taken place. Within the law it is impossible to define dying as a process of decline towards death.

2. The law makes an exception for physicians only when it is evident that the medical actions are performed according to professional standards and in the interest of the health and well-being of the person involved. In all other cases a conflict of duties is recognized. The law cannot approve of the actions.

3. Medical morality takes its starting point in the best interests of the patient with regard to his medical condition.

4. Medical morality has developed a view on the dying process that takes into account the integrity of a human being and the particular medical circumstances: the measures taken to preserve life and dignity are viewed as a function of the dying process.

The first and last points especially need careful consideration. During the last twenty years, physicians, ethicists, and lawyers have attempted to develop criteria by which each dying process could be defined or objectified. Terms like "unbearable suffering," the "terminal phase,"and the "imminence of death" have been brought forward, but have all subsequently been abandoned. They proved to leave too much room for different interpretations and/or were impractical from a legal point of view. The Chabot case, in which a psychiatrist assisted a woman in suicide who did not suffer from a somatic disease, but who deeply felt a desire to die, based on her unbearable mental suffering, provides an excellent illustration. Although the professional society of psychiatrists expressed severe reservations with respect to the professional and moral aspects of the case, within the court of law there were no subtle semantics to express the differences between mental and physical suffering. Therefore the case was treated in a similar vein as other cases of euthanasia that had been brought to trial, using autonomy and unbearable suffering as the guiding criteria to assess adequacy of conditions.

The concepts of best interest, health, and well-being point out another fundamental difference between law and medical morality. Every general discussion on the question of whether or not death is in the best interest of someone will inevitably end in abstract concepts that are not generally applicable in clinical practice. Serious legal problems will emerge when it is stated that death can never be in the interest of a patient, even when a patient begs to have his life ended. Such serious legal problems will also arise when general categories are developed in which death is considered to be in the best interest of the patient. Then, of course, the debate will turn into the question of the possible medical *duty* to end a life that falls in one of the categories. The Chabot case reminds us of the possible mistakes in that respect: although physicians make a sharp distinction between somatic and mental suffering, formally spoken, every kind of suffering continues to be a mental experience. The category of unbearable suffering should apply therefore also in mental cases, even if there is no external, somatic cause.

Finally, if the law should recognize that VAE and PAS belong to a special form of contract, in which trust and not service plays a crucial role, then it would lose its potential to check the circumstances in which the event took place. VAE and PAS would be exceptions to criminal law, comparable to surgical cutting or to isolation treatment in psychiatry. Such a procedure would treat VAE and PAS as instances of normal medical acts, suggesting that general professional standards could be developed by which physicians are held publicly responsible. Then the intrinsic aspect of the principle to preserve life would be lost, namely that human life constitutes a good beyond any type of instrumental thinking and doing. The bond of trust between patient and physician does not sufficiently warrant this intrinsic aspect, simply because that bond has no necessary grounds and cannot be taken for granted.

The present legal procedure in the Netherlands tries to circumvent these problems by establishing a prudent procedural control, first by colleagues, then by judicial authorities. The conceptual differences are diluted in this way, but not solved. In the end the gap between the law and medical morality remains. Regional committees again dilute this dilemma a bit more, but will not resolve the issue. This observation forces us to look further into the philosophical issues at hand.

PHILOSOPHICAL PROBLEMS I: HUMAN ACTION, NATURE, AND MEDICINE

The Dutch developments in the field of VAE and PAS are one possible answer to the problems of all highly industrialized societies that possess well-equipped health care systems. The Dutch answers to these struggles are representative of the cultural conditions, standards of economy, and the relation between the law and the medial profession. Instead of trying to be a protagonist or an antagonist to the specific Dutch development, it is more fruitful to focus on the fundamental issues. They have to do with:

(1) the concept of free will in issues of life and death;
(2) the medical arguments supporting interventions in the process of dying; and
(3) the concept of natural death.

Within the Dutch situation both the voluntary request and the medical judgment of the patient's suffering have been accepted as primary and indispensable criteria that have to be fulfilled if VAE and PAS are to be allowed. As Capron and Callahan have argued, these two criteria cannot be separated, although their union is "jerry-rigged," since each belongs to a different domain of moral and professional evaluation and each could be used by itself to justify VAE. Capron continues to quote Callahan by stating that "the logic of each could not long remain suppressed 'by the expedient of arbitrary legal stipulations.'"[16] In other words, each criterion can be morally sufficient by itself, although both are necessary in order to establish a legally controllable practice.

Capron points to a problem that has implications for physicians in any type of assistance in dying. The problem consists in balancing two incompatible criteria: the voluntariness of the request and the degree of suffering. With respect to the latter: should an incompetent patient be kept alive, even if his medical condition would urge other patients who would be competent to ask for assistance in dying? And to the first: the Chabot case shows that a patient who repeatedly asks for assistance in dying, while her suffering is acute and heavy, poses severe problems to medical justification. But also in ordinary cases, physicians often need time in order to evaluate the medical condition. While doing so they implicitly reassure the patient that they will not abandon him. The time-span between the first request and the act has gained in this way a considerable moral weight.

The incompatibility of the two criteria inevitably causes problems when a situation does not allow that both can be evaluated independently and at the same time. Dutch reports show that when competence is compromised, as seen within psychiatric care, nursing home care, and neonatology, active assistance in dying only rarely occurs. This reveals that physicians are extremely prudent in making judgments only based on their professional judgment. Still one might wonder whether or not this prudence has to do more with a fear for legal repercussions or with their moral point of view. At least in some cases, physicians feel that they have to obey the rules, leaving their patient in distress.

The necessity of the linkage between the two criteria while each could be morally sufficient therefore needs more clarification from the perspective of the law. However, as stated above, it is not possible to produce legal definitions of the medical conditions allowing for VAE and PAS without *ipso facto* defining legal categories that will allow physicians to end the lives of patients, regardless of their wishes. The necessity of the linkage and the possibility of separation cannot be founded in general terms of medicine, but have to be based on the circumstances of the patient. This leads Capron to defend the maintenance of a general prohibition, and yet allowing for morally acceptable exceptions and violations.[17] Following this option, the law will stay clear from the debate, keeping its general principles intact and distant from the changes in morality and medical perspectives. At the same time it prohibits the medical profession from developing a consistent and reliable attitude towards death and dying, forcing it to adopt concepts and procedures that may be clear from a legal perspective but that stay muddled from a medical perspective. The first philosophical problem can thus be formulated as follows: Is there a possible way to integrate the clinical findings of physicians, based on science and experience, into the human perspective of a dying person in such a way that it allows for public control of medical assistance?

Another problem is the well known distinction between letting die and actively assisting in dying. From an American legal point of view this distinction, "widely recognized and endorsed in the medical profession and in our legal traditions," is "both important and logical." It "comports with fundamental legal principles of causation and intent."[18] From a medical point of view this distinction is, however, far from clear and has even been abandoned in the Netherlands. If there is a clear intention to cause somebody harm by knowingly allowing a bad event to happen that could have been prevented by using professional means or by actively withdrawing professional support, the moral distinction between non- or active participation in the event seems unclear. Moreover, if a physician is allowed to withdraw medical support in one case, while letting a patient die without inducing harm or suffering, is he equally permitted to do so if the withdrawal would induce harm and suffering? This as well as other questions can be raised with respect to the practical morality of the distinction.

A more philosophical objection has to do with the concepts of cause and intent. Withdrawing treatment does not make the physician the cause of death, while active assistance does. Thus it would seem that every death occurs as the result of one single cause that has to be located outside the living being. Either the physician or something else, like "disease" or "nature," is the cause. It must be questioned, however, whether death ever occurs by singular causation; certainly in medical practice a singular cause of death seems rarely to be the case.[19] Frequently, many different causes can be identified, while most of them have to do with the condition of the living being itself. By assigning a singular cause to the event of death, the law neglects, in other words, the fact that dying is an inevitable event of life in all its varieties. Apart from the connection with principles like the integrity of the body or the preservation of life, this neglect refers to a conception of nature and of natural law, forged in the days of Enlightenment philosophy, that clearly disregards the power of medical technology. Within that technology, nature plays a small part in the context of controllable and uncontrollable factors, making the outcome of treatment and prognosis uncertain. If the set of controllable factors, for example, is strong enough, death by a natural cause can be prevented for an estimated lapse of time. If the set of uncontrollable factors dominates, as in cases of AIDS or cancer, death will be imminent in spite of all the means available to support the patient. To speak of a natural death in both these cases has almost no relevant normative or descriptive meaning. It merely tells us that nothing more has been or could have been done. The control on this matter lies, however, not within the bounds of nature, but totally within the perimeter of medicine. The use of the legal phrase "natural death" is therefore concealing and describes a myth rather than a fact.

PHILOSOPHICAL PROBLEMS II: MEDICINE, NATURE, AND HUMANITY

The problems involved in discussing "natural death" and "natural human life" have been paramount within the realm of moral philosophy in the twentieth century. We should not only be reminded of Nazism or racism in this respect, but also of the histories of eugenics, sterilization, and tribal wars. The abuse of medical power and technology has a prominent place in these discussions, but the exclusion of people from necessary health care can be mentioned as well. In law, in philosophy, and in the public debate, nature is often still considered to have an intrinsic meaning. With the advancement of technology in genetics as well as in agriculture, the conception of the intrinsic meaning of nature seems even to gain new strength. In its essence this intrinsic meaning dates back to the Romanticism of the eighteenth and nineteenth century, when Nature was discussed either as a threat to human culture or as the original state of purity which has been violated and forsaken by human culture.

Within this tradition nature and culture are considered to be dichotomous. Nietzsche criticized this dichotomy as a lack of courage to appreciate the human powers to control nature. The power of society has superseded that of nature, especially in medicine:

> *Moral für Ärzte*. Der Kranke ist ein Parasit der Gesellschaft. In einem gewissen Zustande ist es unständig, noch langer zu leben. Das Fortvegetieren in feiger Abhängigkeit von Ärzten und Praktikern, nachdem der Sinn vom Leben, das Recht zum Leben verloren gegangen ist, sollte bei der Gesellschaft eine Tiefe Verachtung nach sich ziehn.[20]

> [*Moral for physicians*: The patient is a parasite of society. In a certain situation it is incorrect to live much longer. The continued vegetative life in cowardly dependence of doctors and practitioners, after the meaning of life, the right to life has been lost, should draw a deep disgust from society.]

It would be wrong to conclude from this quote that Nietzsche tried to restore a natural life of physical strenghth. Instead he continues by stressing the personal dimension of death and dying:

> …Hier gilt es, allen Feigheiten des Vorurteils zum Trotz, vor allem die richtige, das heißt physiologische Würdigung des sogenannten *natürlichen* Todes herzustellen: der zuletzt auch nur ein "unnatürliche," ein Selbstmord ist. Man geht nie durch jemand anderes zugrunde, als durch sich selbst….[21]

> […Here we should, against all cowardice and prejudice to resurrect the physiological dignification of the so-called *natural* death; that finally only also an "unnatural" is, a suicide. One never perishes because of someone else, but only because of himself….]

Nietzsche is here critical that society takes an interest in biological life instead of valuing personal life.[22] In *Menschliches, Allzumenschliches* the same argument can be found. He then compares human life with a machine that has done its work and becomes superfluous. He continues by saying that natural death is irrational and represents the destruction of the rational being. He concludes then that outside of religious thinking natural death cannot be praised.[23] In this peculiar way Nietzsche seems to have argued in favor of a human approach towards death without invoking a meaning of life and death that would be given by some external cause.

It has been essentially this struggle for a humane death that characterizes the development of palliative care and the questions of VAE and PAS. On the one hand, it is recognized that a purely "natural death" without any kind of medical intervention can be horrible and inhuman. On the other hand, the dominion of medical technology in matters of life and death is not accepted and is even considered to alienate mankind from its origin. Ivan Illich, for instance, has criticized the medical developments of the last forty years sharply by stating that "industrialized humanity needs therapy from crib to terminal ward."[24] He continues by arguing that the medicalization of death ends up in a commercialization of the death-image. "In its extreme form, 'natural death' is now that point at which the human organism refuses any further input of treatment.... Socially approved death happens when man has become useless not only as a producer but also as a consumer.... Dying has become the ultimate form of consumer resistance."[25] To these sentences a note is attached in which Illich criticizes Brims *et al.* and their book *The Dying Patient*. Illich describes their 1960 professional attitude towards palliative care as "the macabre turns into a new kind of professionally conducted obscenity."[26]

From these quotations two things become clear: first, the philosophical criticism stays within the dichotomy, without evaluating medical support as a necessary cultural complement to human nature. Illich aims at general moral conclusion in which medicine is responsible for the alienation from nature: "Health, or the autonomous power to cope, has been expropriated down to the last breath. Technical death has won its victory over dying.... Mechanical death has conquered and destroyed all other deaths."[27] This conclusion could be compared to fragments in the philosophy of Heidegger, who also considered technology as a threat to the depth of human experience. Second, Illich interprets culture in a sociological way: within culture economic forces determine what people will experience and do. Instead of the external powers of nature or religion, economy has gained the authority to determine the meaning of life and death.

Illich repeats in this way the same type of argument Nietzsche already made a century ago: medical technology has no value in itself, and the dependence on medical assistance is considered to be some kind of treason to the essence of humanity. In fact, this comes down to a fundamental misconception of medical technology and assistance. Every type of medical care should be a function of a human goal that has to be reached by using technology. Otherwise there is no meaning to it at all. The demand that technology should be subjected to human goals and purposes has produced the practices of VAE and PAS in the Netherlands as means to transcend or overcome the dominion of medical assistance.[28] It also produced the quandary between the voluntary request and the medical condition. Is medical assistance really becoming a species of dehumanized technology making it impossible to transcend the medical facts in the encounter with patients? If we are to deny this question, then we must be ready to explain the human values inherent in the use of medical technology and clinical science.

PHILOSOPHICAL PROBLEMS III: LAW, MEDICINE, AND HUMANITY

The preservation of life serves more than one purpose as a legal principle. The verdict in June 1997 by the Supreme Court of the United States made clear that besides protecting individuals from being harmed by their fellow men, the State has its own interest. Indeed, the preservation of life has become an economic factor of importance, not only in the industry of health care, but also in terms of ecology and the continuity of labor.[29]

The way in which people can contrast their personal interests in life on an individual basis nowadays primarily rests in their fundamental human rights. Philosophers like Ronald Dworkin and others have therefore tried to contrast the individual interests in the preservation of life from the interests of the State by stressing the right to die.[30] In itself this right constitutes an awkward phenomenon. It presupposes that the law has the first and last word to say in matters of life and death[31] as if the law had been there before human life and decided that it would come into existence. The traditional prohibition of suicide in many countries of the world supports this legal opinion. The law in this frame of thought is given the final authority that used to be part of metaphysics and religion.

In medicine the seat of the last authority has been given to the individual patient. During the last decades of this century, this seat became vacant when "nature" withdrew itself in favor of technology, but the law still seems willing to take it. Instead of following the rules of nature, physicians will in the future have to obey the law, both in research and in clinical practice. The question then becomes urgent: Whose interests is the law is going to serve? The interests of persons or those of society? The Supreme Court of the United States has chosen the latter option, prohibiting individuals to govern their own death. Dutch society continues to try and find an approach in which the law follows the interests of individual human beings. The law restricts itself then to the investigation of possible wrongful or harmful doings by physicians, allowing them otherwise to follow the wishes of their patients. The Dutch approach can only succeed, however, if it can settle the relationship between the law and the phenomenon of dying in establishing sufficient public control. Medical assistance then becomes a socially recognized moral action in a relationship between human beings. Until this moment it is recognized that the morality of that relationship might escape legal reasoning, forcing the law to make exceptions to what otherwise would be murder. The idea behind this argument is based on the authenticity of the trust between patient and physician. This trust is considered to transcend the server–provider relationship in situations of death and dying and could be evaluated by a special committee. But will this trust last in the future?

Like every other relationship, caring relationships are nowadays subjected to the rules of economy and the marketplace.[32] Palliative care, for instance, can be available in some circumstances only on a commercial basis. It may therefore be assumed that economic considerations will pervade the care during the process of dying, especially as the number of elderly dying patients continues to grow in the coming decades. Then it will become necessary to uphold fundamental concepts of human dignity and sanctity of life before the law and economy take their seat. Bauman rightly warns modernity of the dangers looming in such circumstances.[33]

Are we able to develop such concepts of human dignity and value outside the law, without making use of religious ideas of moral authority? According to sociological research in the Netherlands, the majority of the population thinks that traditional norms and values maintain their validity and force outside religion.[34] The civil society will continue to use traditional moral concepts in a secularized way. Dworkin has made a contribution to this perspective by trying to define a secularized concept of the sanctity of life. Arguing that sanctity of life does not so much have to do with a nature external to human life as with the ways in which human beings value their own life and that of others, he tries to establish a moral standard that can be accepted by the law. By discerning experiential and critical interests in life, Dworkin tries furthermore to define the human sanctity of life as a set of norms that everybody develops during his course in life.[35] Proposals like this might bring us a step further in developing ways to settle the unique, finite human aspects according to general legal criteria. Furthermore, we have to admit that these norms and values are of an intrinsic metaphysical nature. They transcend our regulations and general rulings by their biographical and time-bound character. In return, they pervade the social rules with their meaning if their relational nature is taken seriously.

CONCLUSION

The Dutch practice of VAE and PAS can be considered as one of the answers to the issues of dying at stake in Western civilization. The present state of medicine requires every welfare state to redefine basic questions that have to do with the preservation of life in general and the respect of the finitude of personal life in particular. The value of personal life, as developed over time in specific circumstances, has especially to be taken into account in general considerations. These considerations include the medical aspects of the person involved. Not as a score on some general scale of quality of life, but by integrating those aspects into the subjective life-story. This means that general standards to judge whether or not VAE and PAS can be performed will only have limited value. One of the most serious dangers to any solution of this problem lies in the dehumanizing effect of economic and bureaucratic considerations. Relying on statistics as well as distanced measures of control can easily result into the opposite of what was intended. Human beings live and die within their own history, which includes their physical development, and to forget this would reiterate basic Romantic failures both in palliative care and in VAE and PAS.[36]

NOTES AND REFERENCES

1. Brief aan de Voorzitter van de Tweede Kamer der Staten Generaal (24 November 1997)
2. G. van der Wal and P. van der Maas, *Euthanasie en andere medische beslissingen rond het levenseinde.* (Den Haag: Sdu. 1996), pp. 90–92.

3. Cases concerning minors and incompetent patients also fall into the last mentioned category.
4. G. van der Wal and P. van der Maas, *ibid.*, p.110.
5. G. van der Wal and P. van der Maas, *ibid.*, p. 114
6. KNMG, "Meldingsprocedure euthanasie: Reactie van het Hoofdbestuur van de KNMG op het Kabinetsstandpunt uit januari 1997," *Medisch Contact,* Vol. 52 (1997), pp. 420–425.
7. The RDMA runs a pilot project on consultation and support in Amsterdam (SCEA) aiming to establish this attitude.
8. B.V.M. Crul, "Melding en toetsing vooraf, daar had ik wat aan gehad. [Reporting and prior evaluation, that would have been useful], *Medisch Contact,* Vol. 54 (1999), pp. 1038–1039.
9. *R. v. Latimer,* Can. S.C.R. LEXIS 2803; 1 Can. S.C.R. 217 [1997].
10. According to recent research findings, the Dutch turn more easily to their physician (14%) in questions of personal conscience than to a clergyman (9%). Most people turn, however, to a friend (62%). Cf. G. Dekker, J. De Hart, and J. Peters, *God in Nederland* (Amsterdam: Anthos, 1997), p. 16
11. D.P. Engberts, *Met Permissie* (Dordrecht: Kluwer, 1997), p. 26. Cf. A.K. Huibers and W. van der Burg, "De arts: heilige of koopman? De arts-patient relatie en de Wet Geneeskundige Behandelovereenkomst," in W. van der Burg and P. Ippel (Eds.) *De Siamese tweeling.* (Assen: Van Gorcum, 1992), p. 106.
12. Engberts, *Ibid.*, pp. 23 and 33.
13. This trust can be seen as a particular cultural phenomenon. In other countries the physician seems not to feel obliged to stay with his patients to the end. In the Netherlands one can also expect differences between several types of medical specialty. Cf. E.D. Pellegrino, "The Place of Intention in the Moral Assessment of Assisted Suicide and Active Euthanasia," in T.L. Beauchamp, *Intending Death* (New Jersey: Prentice Hall, 1996), p. 174.
14. G. van der Wal and P. van der Maas, *ibid..*, p.52
15. G. van der Wal and P. van der Maas, *ibid.*, p. 121
16. A.M. Capron, "Should Some Morally Acceptable Actions of Killing and Letting Die Be Legally Prohibited and Punished?," in T.L. Beauchamp (Ed.), *Intending Death* (New Jersey: Prentice Hall, 1996), p. 197.
17. Capron, *ibid..*
18. Supreme Court of the USA. No 95-1858, Rehnquist, Westlaw (1997), at 3
19. It does not suffice, as Capron argues, that cause and intent can no longer constitute valid arguments, while a distinction between refusal of treatment and wrongful taking of a life, as probably would be the case in PAS or VAE, does. In that way the problems of the discrepancies between the legal concepts of intent and cause and the medical concepts are pushed aside instead of scrutinized. A rhetorical use of the experience of ethics committees does not help much.
20. *Götzen-Dammerung*, 36 K. Schlechta II, 1010.
21. *Götzen-Dammerung*, 36 K. Schlechta II, 1011
22. Willems M. Kluizenaar, *Zonder God* (Amsterdam: Duna, 1996), p. 121
23. *Menschliches Allzumenshliches,* II, 185. K. Schlechta, I, 949.
24. I. Illich, *Medical Nemesis* (New York: Bantam Books, 1976), p. 202.
25. I. Illich, *ibid.,* p. 203.
26. I. Illich, *ibid.,* p. 204
27. I. Illich, *ibid.,* p. 204
28. J.H. Van den Berg, *Medical Power and Medical Ethics* (New York: WW. Norton, 1978).
29. The relationship between social values and personal values in issues of life and death has to be clarified. Arguments like "fundamental dignity is not a purely individual matter, it is the common moral currency of the community" need to be clarified with respect to those who are vulnerable to society's neglect or dismay. At this point it is striking that against empirical evidence, the Dutch practice of VAE and PAS is still commented upon as proving that mentally handicapped, comatose, and Alzheimer's patients are at risk in Dutch medical practice. See M.C. Kaveny, "Assisted Suicide,

the Supreme Court, and the Constitutive Function of the Law," *Hastings Center Report*, Vol. 27, No. 5 (1997), p. 32.
30. R. Dworkin, R. Nozick, J. Rawls *et al.*, "Assisted Suicide: The Philosophers' Brief," *New York Review of Books*, XLIV, 5 (March 22, 1997).
31. Dworkin's preface to *Law's Empire (*London: Fontana Press, 1986) p.vii: "We live in and by the law. It makes us what we are."
32. Quality of life programs are already commercialized as interesting targets for investing money in the Netherlands. Cf. ING money funds (December 1997).
33. Z. Bauman, *Modernity and the Holocaust* (Oxford: Polity Press, 1989), pp. 100–105
34. G. Dekker, J. De Hart and J. Peters, *God in Nederland* (Amsterdam: Anthos, 1997), p. 25
35. R. Dworkin, *Life's Dominion* (New York: Knopf, 1993), pp. 81–84, 200–204.
36. Z. Bauman, *Modernity and the Holocaust, op. cit.,* pp. 200–203.

Euthanasia
Reflections on the Dutch Discussion

GOVERT DEN HARTOGH

Faculty of Philosophy, Nieawe Doelenstraat 15, 1012 CP, Amsterdam, the Netherlands

INTRODUCTION: THE IMPORTANCE OF CONTEXT

In philosophy, and particular in ethics, all of us are anti-foundationalists these days. Well, almost all of us are. We do not believe that there are any absolute beginnings, in Hegel's sense, true beliefs that do not need any justification themselves and are capable of justifying other beliefs. However, we do not always realize the consequences of this position. For example, if justification has to be understood in a holistic way, as a process of connecting the beliefs under investigation to others we already hold, it is inevitable that some conceptions which we used to state in quite abstract and general terms derive part of their meaning and relevance from a particular context of discussion. If you forget this, if you implicitly assume that all the world is America (or perhaps even Massachusetts), you will end up with an approach that is virtually indistinguishable from foundationalism, and also rather parochial. It reminds one of the remark of a Frenchman reported by Wittgenstein: it may be the case that people speak different languages, but everyone thinks in French.

It doesn't follow that we should stop doing moral theory in abstract and general terms, only that we should make its contextual embeddedness explicit, in order to enable others to recover the meaning and relevance of what we say in terms of their own framework of relevant conceptions. It is in this spirit that I want to present some reflections on the Dutch discussion concerning euthanasia. If you consider what has been written on this topic in different countries, it is clear, on the one hand, that the same concerns tend to recur everywhere: the exact nature of the value of life, the doctrine of double effect, the importance of self-determination, conditions of competence and the question to which extent they can be satisfied by a person who wants to be dead, and the probabilities of mistake and abuse. But on the other hand, even arguments that are couched in these general and common terms are used to different effects within different frameworks of discussion.[1] For instance, if you look at the Dutch discussion, you will find most of the arguments elsewhere used as arguments against euthanasia as such used by people who don't dispute its possible moral legitimacy, but only feel that the present scope of its recognition should not be extended. Obviously the same arguments can be used within different spectrums of possible positions. Other aspects that differentiate the contexts of discussion, are matters of institutional fact, such as the important role of general practitioners in the Dutch health care system—family doctors are responsible for 70% of all cases of euthanasia and assisted suicide—and, perhaps most fundamentally, the basic fears that motivate people. The Dutch people, rightly or wrongly, seem to be hardly afraid of doctors killing them too early, either intentionally or by mistake. Their primary fear is that their life, mainly as a result of the exercise of medical power, will be lengthened in ways that involve severe suffering and slow decay.

It will be clear from what I have said that I will leave it to my readers entirely to determine the possible relevance of my argument for their own or any other non-Dutch context. I am not trying to sell anyone Dutch euthanasia.

THE DOMINANT VIEW: RESPECT FOR AUTONOMY

The Dutch debate on euthanasia began in earnest during the 1960s. And the most striking fact about it from the very beginning is the extent to which explicit moral argumentation for the legalization of euthanasia relied on one single principle, the principle of respect for individual self-determination. Medical ethics made a radical break with its past at the end of the decade, when two books were published, both by psychiatrists, which strongly attacked the predominant paternalistic attitude of physicians, warning that, with the rapid growth in medical power, the life of individuals would become dependent on medical direction to a fully unknown extent. One of those books, by J.H. van den Berg, explicitly pleaded for permitting euthanasia in this context.

This anti-paternalistic thrust has since been characteristic for patients' organizations, which have more and more succeeded in making their voice heard over the last decades. "Health ethics," as the new medical ethics called itself to mark its discontinuity from the old, largely had the same agenda for a time, and still occasionally comes in for criticism for its onesidedness on this account, even though it has become far more diversified in its tendency in the meantime. "Health law," on the other hand, which was created as a identifiable discipline by H.J. Leenen almost single-handedly, continues to be strongly characterized by its insistence on patients' autonomy. As such, it has in general been very influential on the development of the law in the anti-paternalistic direction advocated by the patients' organizations. The culminating point of this development is a recent law that requires the explicit consent of the patient (if he is able to give it) for all forms of medical treatment, including life-saving treatment.

This historical background is reflected in the dominating arguments for the legalization of euthanasia. The Dutch Society for Voluntary Euthanasia during its 28 years of existence has never wavered from the path of self-determination. Statements of moral principle it issues are seldom longer than one or two sentences, for the Society tends to believe that the principle of respecting autonomy is fully clear in its meaning and self-evident in its justification. In his manual of health law, Leenen sets out to explain the existing law as an embodiment of basic human rights.[2] In his view, all relevant rights can be seen as specifications of the right to self-determination. This is also true for the right to life and the right to bodily integrity: they are protective shields against the state and against others, but what they protect is not really the goods of life and of bodily integrity, but the possession of these goods, in particular the power to dispose of them. Because they are means to protect freedom, they cannot restrict it. As far as these liberty-rights are concerned, in Leenen's view there really is only one relevant basic good, which could be called self-ownership. (That does not make him a libertarian, for he also recognizes welfare rights like a right to health care). Given these fundamental rights Leenen believes that it cannot be impermissible for a physician to comply with a competent person's unambiguous wish to have his life ended. The only further restriction he makes is that the person should be a patient. He should have come to the doctor for medical care, not for euthanasia; otherwise the doctor has no business to be involved. It is also stressed by health lawyers that an assessment of a person's competence should exclusively be based on the way his decision is reached, not on its outcome.[3]

The ethicists are more sophisticated. Perhaps the most influential defense of the moral acceptability of euthanasia has been given by the theologian, H.M. Kuitert.[4] He starts by saying that the physician is not in the service of the patient's self-determination, he has his own job to do, serving the well-being of the patient in as far as this is threatened by illness and untimely death, and he has to make up his own mind about what doing this job requires. If the patient's illness makes his suffering unbearable, it may be the case that the suffering can only be ended by ending the life of the patient. In that case the physician's basic motive is compassion.

However, when Kuitert discusses the question under which conditions the patient's suffering is to be considered unbearable, he insists that the patient himself is the final arbiter on this matter.[5] But of course this makes him the final arbiter on the question whether it is in his overall interest to die as well, and the original insistence on the necessity of the doctor's independent judgment becomes vacuous. The situation is analogous to the present legal regime on abortion in the Netherlands and many other European countries: abortion is only justified by the pregnant woman's "need," but whether she is in need in the relevant sense is up to her to decide. No wonder that hardly anyone knows what the law really says; Dutch people commonly believe abortion to be available on request.

LAW AND MEDICAL PRACTICE

The appeal to the principle of respect for autonomy has been contested, of course, by opponents of the legalization of euthanasia, most interestingly by some Catholic theologians.[6] Among the defenders of euthanasia it has only been rejected explicitly in a few writings by medical doctors.[7] These authors go on at the point at which Kuitert draws back. If the basic reason for accepting the patient's request is compassion, the doctor should form an independent judgment that the patient is right in considering his suffering to be unbearable and hopeless. Significantly, these authors now belong to the top echelon of representatives of the Royal Dutch Society of Medicine, the most important organization of the medical profession.

This is significant because the dominant view on the morality of euthanasia has never been accepted by the law or by medical practice. About the behavior of doctors we are informed by the recent report on life-shortening actions: of patients' requests for euthanasia only one in three is finally agreed to.[8] (A datum to which the president of the Society for Voluntary Euthanasia responded by saying that his organization had still a long way to go.) The reasons, in order of importance, for denying the patients' wishes include the following: there was no unbearable suffering, alternative options for treatment were available, the presence of mental disturbance, in particular depressive states, defective understanding of diagnosis and prognosis, and undue pressure by third persons. A recent study by an anthropologist who for two and a half years observed the decision-making process on euthanasia requests in a Dutch hospital confirms this view. Doctors receiving such a request invariably take a reserved attitude to begin with. They start negotiating for time, sometimes by minimizing communication with the patient. Their discussions with the patient and their use of information from the nursing staff and from others aim at establishing that the wish of the patient is unambiguous and well considered, and whether the condition of the patient makes his wish understandable. Contrary to the reigning legal doctrine of competence these criteria turn out to be strongly connected with each other. Doctors in the anthropologist's report say things like "it really is an unacceptable life," "so many other patients in her condition are able to cope." When an AIDS-patient tells a nurse that it is not the pain that motivates his request, but his general condition and prospects, the doctor on hearing this calls out: "that is what we want to hear."

What about the law?[10] The Dutch criminal code has two separate articles, which forbid killing someone on his earnest request and assisting suicide, and threaten these crimes with maximum penalties of 12 and 4 years, respectively. However, the system of penal law contains some general justifying grounds for actions which are covered by its provisions, and one of these grounds is necessity. One of the forms necessity can take (since an earlier Supreme Court decision to that effect) is that of a conflict of duties, the one duty being to do what the law requires, and the other duty following from norms that are generally recognized as defining the duties of one's profession. (So an appeal to one's conscience is not sufficient, or, rather, is irrelevant.) In a path-breaking decision of 1984 the Dutch Supreme Court has established that an appeal to necessity can justify euthanasia if a number of conditions of careful action have been satisfied. As the relevant notion of conflict of duties would lead one to expect, these conditions reflect the criteria that the Royal Dutch Society for Medicine had developed in the preceding years. So it is not accidental that the present legal regime reflects medical practice more than the reigning ideology, even if this ideology is strongly supported by the dominant trend in health law. Some of these conditions aim at making the decision controllable, but their main point is to announce the two criteria that we found Dutch doctors to use in practice already: the patient's wish should be steadfast, unambiguous, and well-considered, and he should be in a state of unbearable and hopeless suffering.

It is not only the fact that this second criterion is added that is significant. For what exactly is this professional duty which is supposed to conflict with the duty not to kill? Oddly enough, the Supreme Court didn't state this explicitly in its 1984 decision. However, it cannot be the duty to respect a person's autonomy, for, even in the view of its advocates, this principle only makes it permissible to grant the patient's wish to be killed, it doesn't make it a duty. And indeed, later decisions explicitly state that the relevant duty is the duty to alleviate the patient's suffering.

The anti-paternalists usually try to square the view of the law with their own view, in the way we already found Kuitert advocating. They say that the question whether a person's suffering is unbearable can only be answered by the person himself. This view seems to me false, ultimately resting on a kind of solipsistic denial of the possibility of access to other minds. It is true that the notion of "unbearable suffering" is subjective in a certain sense: the very same physical condition can be tolerable to one person and intolerable to another, depending on their personalities, personal histories, and basic values. Whether a person's well-being can be exhaustively described in terms of such "subjective" criteria is debatable, but they are relevant on any plausible view.[11] But it doesn't follow that the person himself is always in the best position to assess his condition in terms of even these subjective criteria. This misunderstanding may partially explain the appeal of the anti-paternalist position: people believe that if the patient is not granted full authority, the only alternative is to deny the subjective aspects of well-being.

So the view that a person's suffering is unbearable if he perceives it as unbearable is false. It is not fully shared by the courts either, although there is much confusion about the sense in which suffering is a subjective notion. It is even clearer that on the question whether the patient's suffering is hopeless, the doctor is supposed to form his own judgment. Usually this means that he has to decide whether the patient's physical or psychological state can be improved, or whether further deterioration can at least be stopped by any viable form of treatment. The patient, of course, has the right to reject any treatment the doctor proposes, but as long as a viable alternative exists, the appeal to necessity will then fail as a result. Whether an alternative is viable may to some extent again depend on the perspective of the patient. For example, a patient will be allowed to reject total sedation, the palliative use of high doses of morphine, resulting in a complete loss of consciousness, if it is very important to him to remain "in control." But, again, that the patient's perspective is relevant doesn't imply that his assessment is authoritative. That a request for euthanasia or for assistance in suicide is not always motivated by severe suffering, even when it exists, is proven by the exceptional case in which the patient rejects a viable alternative, because he does not want to surrender his "claim." It is well known that suicides by people who are not suffering from any physical disease may be motivated by strong disappointments or resentments, for abandonment by others, or loss of honor. We cannot be sure *a priori* that patients in the terminal stage of a fatal illness will never be guided by such motives.

THE INFLUENCE OF THE REIGNING DOCTRINE

I have argued that the law and the doctors do not accept the decisive importance of self-determination.[12] That does not mean, however, that the dominant doctrine has no influence on legal decisions or medical behavior at all. Concerning medical behavior we have to rely on anecdotal evidence. An illuminating case can be found on an American video recording, called "An Appointment with Death," dating from the early '90s. It concerns a HIV-infected patient in an early stage of his disease. He has witnessed the struggle of some of his friends on their path downwards, and he decides that he will have none of this. So he asks his doctor to assist his suicide, even if at present he doesn't suffer from any of the accompanying illnesses and handicaps of AIDS. The doctor clearly feels very uncomfortable about this request. He points to the many AIDS patients who succeed in going on for some years and finding some happiness in their lives, and he explains that the law requires unbearable suffering. Then the patient asks "Unbearable, from whose point of view? Whose values are decisive, yours or mine?" The doctor, looking even more unhappy, answers, "yours." And he starts the required consultation procedure. This doctor obviously is making the mistake I discussed. That the values of the patient are decisive doesn't mean that his assessment of his situation in terms of them is final.

How the dominant view influences the position of the Royal Dutch Society, and ultimately even the law, can be illustrated by the discussion about the acceptability of assisting the suicide of psychiatric patients. From 1984 on the courts have rejected making further requirements on the condition of unbearable and hopeless suffering, for instance, that the patient should be in a terminal stage of his illness (which is the case about 90% of the time), or that it should derive from a somatic disease or defect. The Minister of Justice, however, wanted to be absolutely certain about this, and so brought a number of test cases to the courtroom, involving psychiatric patients. As a matter of fact, though most psychiatrists don't rule out assisting suicide completely, it only occurs in some five cases a year, half of which involve patients who are also suffering from a severe physical illness.[13] The Royal Dutch Society therefore asked a committee of experts to prepare a report on the problem.[14] One of the most important points discussed in the report is the question whether a psychiatric patient can be competent in making a life-or-death decision. Isn't there always room for the suspicion that his wish to be dead is directly caused by his illness?, or is it possible that it results from a sober assessment of the condition his illness has brought him into? The committee begins by affirming the reigning doctrine that judgments of competence should solely be based on the decision-making process, not on its outcome. It then gives a list of possible criteria of competence, listed in order of stringency, and it accepts the view that we should require more stringent criteria to be satisfied, as the decision to be assessed is more important.[15] It then seems obvious that we should insist on the most stringent set of criteria in the case of a life-or-death decision. But the committee then observes that it would show a lack of compassion always to insist on this. Consequently, the committee wants to justify the decision to grant the patient his wish on respect for his autonomy, not on compassion, but it lets its assessment whether his decision deserves such respect be influenced by compassion.

The verdicts of the courts show the same pattern. They insist that in the case of a psychiatric patient it should be most carefully established that his death wish isn't directly caused by his illness, but they go on to accept the appeal to necessity in cases in which this isn't clear at all.[16] So it seems that their judgments of competence are motivated, indeed, by compassion. The result is a very unsatisfactory compromise. A patient in a permanent state of severe depression who steadfastly wants to be dead cannot be granted his wish, but a patient who, intermittently between similar periods of deep depression, has some relatively normal moments, will be eligible for assistance, because compassion with his suffering will require us not to heed our doubts concerning his competence.

These examples show that clarity about the ultimately justifying ground is still needed; it will make a difference, both in the hospital and in the courtroom.[17] It is particularly needed for discussing the most difficult class of requests for assisted suicide: those that are motivated by the fear of mental decay, as in the beginning stages of Alzheimer's disease. Neither the Royal Dutch Society nor the courts have clearly made up their minds about these cases. As a matter of fact the discussion about them has started only very recently. Of course, the anti-paternalists see no special problem. But if we reject their position, as I shall argue we should, we seem to be confronted by an unsolvable dilemma.

I will not attempt a full investigation of alleged justifying grounds; this would imply a discussion of the value or perhaps the values, of life, which requires a paper on its own.[18] I will proceed on the assumption that it is possible for life to become a burden, a prison, or even a hell to the person who is living it, and therefore to have negative value on the whole. I will concentrate on two points. First, I will argue that respect for a person's self-determination cannot be a sufficient justifying ground for killing him, because an additional principle which is needed for completing the justification is not valid without restriction. This is the so-called *Volenti* principle. Secondly, I will discuss whether accepting concern for a patient's well-being as a justifying ground implies that unbearable and hopeless suffering is always necessary for granting a patient's wish, and in particular whether it is necessary in the case of the patient with Alzheimer's disease.

IS SO-CALLED INDIRECT PATERNALISM REALLY A FORM OF PATERNALISM?

As I said, appeal to the principle of respect for autonomy will, at most, result in permitting doctors to comply with the unambiguous request of competent patients. But it will only have this result if we accept the principle *Volenti non fit iniuria*: the consenting person cannot be wronged, the fact of a person's consent exculpates you from causing a setback to his interests. Oddly, the fact that this principle is essential to the reigning doctrine has only rarely been observed in discussions of it; advocates hardly ever notice that it is only suicide, not assisting it, which can strictly be a matter of "self-determination."[19]

The *Volenti* principle has always been rejected in traditional medical ethics; as a matter of fact it is rejected in the ethical codes of the classical professions generally. In some countries including, as we saw, the Netherlands, it is now generally accepted that competent patients always have the right to refuse any medical treatment, but that doesn't mean that their consent is also sufficient to start it. On the contrary, this requires an independent (and justifiable) judgment of the doctor that the treatment will be in the best interests of the patient. If I ask my doctor to have my leg amputated, he will feel he has to refuse, unless there is a good medical reason for amputation. The fact, let's say, that I strongly identify with my one-legged grandfather who used to be a street-musician, is not sufficient.

It is, of course, true that doctors do not always live up to this principle. They sometimes give in to patient's pressure, perhaps hoping for a placebo effect, or believing that the patient's well-being is served on the whole if his desires are satisfied. In cosmetic surgery especially, unacceptable risks are sometimes taken by appealing to "psychological needs." These appeals are really forms of the fallacy I discussed of believing that a person's own view of what constitutes his well-being is indisputable. If harms are recognized as such, doctors generally will not feel free to cause them, not even with the patient's consent.

Professional morality on this point is supported by strongly held general moral views which have found legal expression in most, perhaps in all, legal systems. Some rights are held to be inalienable: John Locke classically mentioned the rights to life, to liberty, and to bodily integrity, and this means that if I try to give another person permission to dispose of the goods protected by those rights, I will not succeed. If I make a contract with my enemy, stipulating that we will throw a coin, heads meaning that I get his fortune, tails that he will be allowed to kill me, such a contract is morally and legally void.

Joel Feinberg has argued that, even though some rights are inalienable, that doesn't mean that the goods protected by those rights are inalienable as well.[20] It is true that it is possible to abandon a good without abandoning the *right* to the good, but alienation differs from abandonment, because it involves another person. If I am the owner of a book, I can abandon the book without surrendering any rights of ownership, by throwing the book into the fire, for example. But I cannot abandon the book to your exclusive benefit.

What I actually can do is to release you from some duties which correspond to my right, without surrendering the right itself. This is another and stronger objection to my argument.[21] I can lend the book to you without compromising my ownership, or allow you to enter my bedroom without compromising my right to privacy. Similarly I can request and hence permit my doctor to give me deadly pharmaca without transferring to him my right to life. I don't give him any discretionary power. This is a valid distinction indeed, but in the end it doesn't refute my argument. Consider the right to bodily integrity again. It implies that, even on a valid medical indication, the doctor is not permitted to ampute my leg without my consent. But if there is no such indication, the consent is not sufficient to exonerate the doctor from performing ill-advised treatment. Hence we have to understand the notion of "inalienability" in an extended sense. You cannot give another person the right to maim or to kill you at her own pleasure, but neither can you give her permission to do so at your own direction. (Freedom is an exceptional good, because it doesn't allow for this distinction to begin with.) The Dutch criminal law, as we saw, penalizes killing a person on his own request; it also penalizes robbing a person's freedom, even if he consented to this to begin with.[22] (It does not penalize the consent.) In the notorious Spanner case (concerning sado-masochistic sex) the House of Lords has decided that consent can never be a defense in a case of physical assault, with the only exception of "manly sports." One need not agree with this decision in order to concede that the justifying force of consent is limited.

Even John Stuart Mill argued in *On Liberty* that a person cannot abdicate his own freedom. He has been accused of being a strong paternalist on this account. However, accepting inalienable rights is only so-called indirect paternalism: what is blocked is not the person's own disposing of a good, but the consensual disposing of it by another person. Freedom is again a special case, because I cannot dispose of the good without having you dispose of it, so when your action is blocked, mine is as well. But that does not make blocking your action a form of direct paternalism. Whether indirect paternalism really deserves to be called paternalism at all, I will discuss presently.

Daniel Callahan has argued that the fact that the right to life is inalienable means that euthanasia can never be allowable.[23] That argument cannot be correct, for the right to bodily integrity also being inalienable, it would rule out of court almost all medical activity. The right to bodily integrity is meant to protect an interest, so if my interests on the whole are best served by amputating my leg—for otherwise gangrene will spread through my body—it can, with my consent, be done. The point is only that what is protected is a good, not a freedom.

I have argued that commonly recognized norms of professional and general morality reject the unrestricted *Volenti* principle. This means that the proposal to accept it is a revisionary one; we have to be given reasons for adopting it. The burden of proof is on its advocates.

As I said, restricting the *Volenti* principle is usually called indirect paternalism; it can be thought of as being part of a certain view on the general issue of paternalism, which has been called the balancing view. It is the view that is probably closest to most people's intuitions about this issue, including all those who don't object to being obligated to wear protective helmets and seatbelts. The balancing view holds that the interest in freedom may be one of people's most important interests, but still is only one interest among others, and so occasionally has to be weighed against those others. The weight of the interest in autonomy is relatively slight, when the relevant options which may be open to us aren't really important within our life-plan, like the option not to wear a seatbelt, which will mostly be chosen out of laziness pure and simple, a mild form of weakness of will. When the interest to be weighed against it is improved safety from the risks of death and injury, these may be the weightier ones in the balance. Indirect paternalism seems to be a simple extension of this balancing view: it also weighs the interest in certain forms of freedom against grave harms, which may result from its exercise.

The basic moral objection against the balancing view has been well stated by Joel Feinberg. If people are treated paternalistically, "their grievance is not simply that they have been unnecessarily inconvenienced or 'irked,' but rather they have been violated, invaded, belittled. They have experienced something analogous to the invasion of their property or the violation of their privacy."[24] Someone who interferes with your way of conducting your own life, and does so for your own good, implicitly presupposes a moral asymmetry between him and you: he doesn't treat you as an equal and thereby insults you. So the interest in autonomy is not simply one interest among others, one component of your total well-being to be considered as such. For even before aspects of your well-being are to be taken into account, your standing as a full member of the moral community should be established, and this is at issue in paternalistic acts. For that reason the principle of respect for autonomy has priority on considerations of well-being. It has a deontological appeal.

I am not sure that this objection succeeds in disposing of the balancing view in all its forms, for some forms of paternalism seem more insulting than others, depending again on the importance of the relevant decisions within a person's life-plan. I don't feel insulted by the obligation to wear a seatbelt at all, though I know some people who say they do. My present point, however, is that it is not evident that the objection also applies to indirect paternalism. Let's suppose that all paternalistic interference in the way in which you attempt to execute your decisions is insulting. That doesn't mean that my refusal to help you in any way to execute those decisions is also insulting, not even when it is motivated by the desire not to harm you. Such a refusal only shows concern, not a lack of respect. It is a not a denial of your right to self-determination at all: you are still the master of your own actions, but not of mine. Now, suppose I have decided to assist you, but a third person comes along and prevents me, again from concern for your good. This may be insulting to me, but that is not the question. The question is: is it insulting to you in the way interference is, or not insulting in the way refusal to help is? I submit that it is not insulting, because it again leaves you to be the master of your own actions, but not of mine. So this third person doesn't treat your person as a means only, and not as an end in itself.

It is not difficult to imagine cases in which the action of the third person would be disrespectful indeed. If we make a perfectly valid contract, and I am prevented from performing my part of the agreement by a third person who thinks I am harming you, that is insulting. But that is, I suggest, because the contract actually is a valid one, so you already have a right to expect performance. That right is already part of your moral assets, which is why the action of this third person is analogous to "the invasion of your property or the violation of your privacy." That doesn't rule out certain categories of harmful consequences to invalidate contracts to begin with.

What the example suggests is that the *Volenti* principle is related to the principle of respect for autonomy in an indirect way only. To begin with, its aim is to protect legitimate expectations arising from consenting acts. If a person in good faith performs his part of an agreement, he should not normally be held responsible for any harm befalling his partner to the agreement as a result of that. So the *Volenti* principle does not aim at protecting the autonomy of the consenting party, but rather at shielding the other party from liability.

Only if it is already established on independent grounds that my consent is sufficient for justifying your action, even if the action harms me, is the interference of a third person disrespectful to me. The *Volenti* principle only helps to define the boundaries of the domain of the agent's sovereignty to the extent to which it is valid. So if we hold that it cannot justify killing, maiming, or enslaving people on request, we do not thereby violate those persons' autonomy. We should not only require a clear request in any case in which communication is possible; we have also to require that the interest which is protected by the inalienable right to life doesn't exist any more and is even converted into its opposite.[25]

THE APPEAL TO THE INTEGRITY OF ONE'S LIFE

This brings me to my second question: does this always mean that there should be unbearable and hopeless suffering?[26]

In particular, if a person in the beginning stage of Alzheimer's disease asks the doctor to help him to kill himself, can it ever be acceptable to agree? I observed that this is a case of the most difficult kind. It is so for several reasons. One reason that I will only mention, but not discuss extensively, is the problem whether and why there should be any task for a doctor in such cases, in which the patient mostly is not disabled, either physically or mentally, to act on his own behalf. The reasons why some people argue that there is a task are the following. First, we want to be sure that the death wish is authentic, unambiguous, well-informed, particularly concerning the prognosis and the available options of treatment and care. Secondly, if you want to kill yourself, there are strong reasons to prefer doing so by using pharmaca, which in the Netherlands (and the argument goes: for good reasons) are only available on a doctor's prescription: this is the only way that is almost failure-proof, not risky in the sense of causing severe physical damage if it fails, relatively mild (I stress the "relatively") and least traumatizing to others. I will not really try to evaluate the force of this argument on this occasion, but assume that it succeeds. We then come up to the other reason why the case is so difficult. A person might want to wait for the moment when he actually has lost almost all his mental capacities. For many people this decisive moment has arrived when they are definitely unable to recognize any one of their close relatives and friends. But it is impossible to require a doctor to kill a person who, at that moment, doesn't want to be dead and who is not actually suffering, perhaps even feeling well most of the time, just because this same person —really the same person?—requested this to be done some years before. From the point of view of the present person you cannot say that his life has negative value, even if you cannot say either that he benefits from going on. This means that a person who doesn't want to reach that stage of mental degradation, has to act on his own initiative as long as he still is in a position to make competent decisions. But that may well be at a time that he is still fully capable of appreciating the goods of life. (And cannot be fully sure about the diagnosis.) So even if we can sympathize with his wish in a general way, it always seems either too early or too late to act on it.

It is sometimes suggested that even if a person at that moment is not suffering severely from any other causes, the suffering caused by his fear of his future suffering, or by his aversion of the irreversible loss of his abilities and his personality, may still be unbearable. I suspect that this argument derives most of its apparent force from the mistake, well-known by now, of ascribing final authority to a person's own perception of his condition. But the argument fails anyway. For the person's request in his own sincere view is not motivated by his present suffering at all, but by his expectations for the future. It would show a lack of respect to disregard his own reason, and only consider the effect it has on his state of mind. It would also be unfair, when two people have the same wish for the same reasons, to deny the request of the person who happens to be able to cope with his fear. And in any case, even if the patient's present suffering is unbearable, it is, cynical though it may sound, not hopeless. It will come to an end with the progress of the disease.

If we take the patient's own request seriously, the relevant value that we should consider, is not the prevention of suffering at all, but a value that has been alternatively described as integrity, or authenticity, or the narrative unity of a person's life. What he says is this: I don't want to be remembered by my children or grandchildren as the person I will shortly become, this stage of my life which I am about to enter, cannot be accepted as a significant addition to it at all, if judged by the values that have informed my life as a whole. Is this a justifying ground, which we should, at least sometimes, accept as a valid one? That would mean that we would be allowed to assist a person who wants to end his life—really, unambiguously, steadfastly, wants to end it—if either he is in a state of unbearable and hopeless suffering, or lengthening his life would detract from its overall value, because the additional period would be contrary to the basic character of the life?

Suppose we accept this. What about the AIDS patient I discussed before who believes that the endless struggle with the minor and major pathologies that are characteristic of that illness is something for which he is not made to deal? What about a person who derives the whole meaning of his life from his personal investment in body-building, and doesn't see any point in going on when aging brings the inevitable end of this basic ambition? Either we are back at the anti-paternalistic position, only requiring the patient to argue his decision in terms of the narrative unity of his life, as we require the woman who wants an abortion to argue her decision in terms of need. Or we have to require someone—the doctor?—to evaluate the claims those persons make. I am sure the medical profession will refuse the job. And rightly so. For this is a judgment which no one can be in a position to make with sufficient confidence, neither the person whose life it concerns nor anyone else, before the person's life has actually ended. We cannot at one particular moment construct a life's profile from its history and then require circumstances to allow this life to continue to have the same profile. For, as we tend to forget, perhaps forgivably, our life still is and always will remain a hostage to fortune, as it has been expressed so forcefully in the mediaeval hymn *Media vita in morte sumus*. You can have an accident while driving home tonight. It will always be necessary to cope with unexpected circumstances, and we know that people are often able to do so in unexpected ways. They sometimes succeed in adapting themselves to the most extreme conditions, such as life in a concentration camp, and not only to survive, but even to go through the painful process of integrating such episodes into their lives.

The narrative unity of one's life can only be constructed *ex post facto*, because it cannot be taken to exclude either unexpected adaptations to unexpected circumstances or conversions. For that reason it cannot normally be a justifying ground for assisting suicide. But I believe that we have to allow for one exception to this rule.

This exception concerns the person with Alzheimer's disease. I argued that the appeal to the narrative unity of a person's life normally fails, because the next stage of his life can necessitate us to reconsider our present construction of it, perhaps to reconsider it fundamentally, and we have no reason to privilege our present point of view. But this argument doesn't apply to the Alzheimer's patient. I don't deny that it is possible for some people to find a meaning in this stage of their lives, for instance because they see it is as preordained by God or because they generally don't place much weight to being in control over their life and they simply take it as it comes. But even in their cases the meaning to be found in the life of the future Alzheimer's patient during the final stages of his illness can already be identified from the point of view of the present person. For the Alzheimer's patient himself during those stages it is not possible to connect his life in any meaningful way to his life as a whole. A process of structural disintegration doesn't leave a self that is able to redefine the narrative unity of its life, or even to allow its redefinition by a sympathetic observer. There is still experience, but, as there is no self, there is no unity. To that extent the common saying that people who are afraid of dementia don't know what they are afraid of, is as misconceived as the similar view concerning the fear of death: there is no mysterious form of life there which you might empathetically enter, if only you knew how. So the only contribution which this stage of one's life can make to the meaning of the whole, is already fully defined before the stage is reached. Therefore the patient and his physician are, exceptionally, already in the position to make the *ex post facto* judgment, which I alleged to be the only judgment concerning the narrative unity of a life that could possibly be reliable. A similar point can be made about people in a persistent vegetative state. But I believe that in almost all other cases, circumstances that seem to threaten the integrity of a person's life should rather be seen as challenges, as invitations to redefinition.

This may seem a rather harsh doctrine, for it seems to saddle people with the burden of redefinition, without respect to the weight of the burden. Two years ago we had the famous Chabot case concerning a psychiatrist who assisted a woman to commit suicide who had lost her two sons, the first from suicide after a failing adolescent love affair and the second from cancer. The psychiatrist had tried to convince her to accept a form of therapy aiming at going through a mourning process, but she refused. Her main argument was, in her own words, that she didn't want to become another person than when she was a mother and happy. This is, in effect, an appeal to the narrative identity of her life. As we have seen, the Dutch Supreme Court has ruled that if a patient refuses a possible treatment, her suffering cannot be considered to be hopeless, so it seems that the criterion of unbearable and hopeless suffering is not satisfied. Does it then follow from my argument that we have no alternative but confronting her with a challenge of redefinition? An American psychiatrist discussing her case draws this conclusion. He correctly observes that she, as a result of her childhood experiences and further personal history, had come to find the meaning of her life exclusively in her role as a mother. This leads him to comment: "she needed someone who could tell her in a friendly but resolute way that she had never even started to live her own life and that it still wasn't too late to start doing so."[27] I think this comment overestimates the resources of psychiatry in dealing with personality disorders. It also seems rather cheerful in its assigning of exceptionally heavy burdens. It could be argued, as it was done by Chabot and by the colleagues whom he consulted, with one exception, that the possibility that she really could benefit from treatment was too low to counterbalance such burdens. If that judgment is right, it would be cruel to require her to accept the invitation to redefinition, something analogous to sending a person to a concentration camp. That doesn't mean, however, that we accept her appeal to the narrative unity of her life; we still only rely on the criterion of unbearable and hopeless suffering. But we recognize that what counts as "hopeless" is subject to a proportionality criterion, as it always is in medicine.

Compassion has the last word.

NOTES AND REFERENCES

1. See Margaret Pabst Battin, *The Least Worst Death* (New York: Oxford University Press, 1994), chapt. 6, "A Dozen Caveats Concerning the Discussion of Euthanasia in the Netherlands," pp. 130–144.
2. H.J.J. Leenen, *Rechten van Mensen in de Gezondheidszorg* (Samsom, Alphen aan den Rijn, 1978), cf. the 3rd ed.: *Handboek Gezondheidsrecht deel I* (Samsom/Tjeenk Willink Alphen aan den Rijn, 1994), pp. 259–295. Summaries of verdicts of the Supreme Court discussed below can be found here as well.
3. E.g. H. van der Klippe, "Wilsonbekwaamheid in de psychiatrie: zes benaderingen," *Maandblad voor de Geestelijke Volksgezondheid* 45 (1990), pp. 535–537.
4. H.M. Kuitert, *Een Gewenste Dood: Euthanasie als Moreel en Godsdienstig Probleem* (Baarn: Ten Have, 1981), chapts. 8–10.
5. In the second edition of his book, *Mag er een Eind Komen aan het Bittere Einde?* (Ten Have Baarn, 1993), pp. 64–69, 86, H.M. Kuitert's wording is more cautious.
6. W.C.M. Klijn and W. Nieboer, *Euthanasie en Hulp bij Zelfdoding* (Utrecht: 1984); Th. Beemer, "Tegen een gehalveerde ethiek" in *Euthanasie Wetgeving: Andere Wegen*, . D. van Tol, Ed. (Amsterdam: VU Press,1986), pp. 33–47.
7. In particular C. Spreeuwenberg, *Huisarts en Stervenshulp* (Van Loghum Slaterus Deventer, 1981). Cf. R.J.M. Dillmann, "Euthanasie: de morele legitimatie van de arts," in J. Legemaate & R.J.M. Dillmann, *Levensbeëindigend handelen door een arts: tussen norm en praktijk* (Bohn Stafleu Van Loghum Houten/Diegem: 1998). For a more nuanced position in health law see J.K.M. Gevers, "Euthanasia or Assisted Suicide and the Non-Terminally Ill," in O. Aycke, A. Smook, B. de Vos-Schippers (Eds.), *Right to Self-Determination* (Amsterdam: VU Press, 1990), pp. 67–68.
8. G. van der Wal, P.J. van der Maas, *Euthanasie en Andere Medische Beslissingen rond het Levenseinde* (den Haag: SDU Uitgevers, 1996), pp. 52–53.
9. Robert Pool, *Vragen om te Sterven, Euthanasie in een Nederlands Ziekenhuis* (WYT Uitgeefgroep: Rotterdam, 1996). Comparable data in another anthropological study, focusing more on the role of nurses: Anne-Mei The, "Vanavond om 8 uur...," *Verpleegkundige Dilemma's bij Euthanasie en Andere Beslissingen rond het Levenseinde* (Houten/Diegem: Bohn Stafleu Van Loghum, 1997).
10. H.J.J. Leenen, "Euthanasia in the Netherlands,", in *Medicine, Medical Ethics and the Value of Life*, Peter Byrne, Ed. (Chichester: John Wiley, 1990); J.K.M. Gevers, "What the Law Allows: Legal Aspects of Active Euthanasia on Request in the Netherlands," in R.I. Misbin (Ed.), *Euthanasia: The Good of the Patient, the Good of Society* (Frederick, MD:

University Publishing Group, 1992); Govert den Hartogh, "Recht op Leven. Recht op de Dood: een Conflict van Plichten?," *Trema,* no. 6 (1995), pp. 176–182.
11. Cf. Joseph Raz, *The Morality of Freedom* (Oxford: Oxford University Press, 1986), pp. 289 ff.
12. Last year a bill has been proposed to Parliament, which to a large extent codifies the existing legal situation which so far has relied on judge-made law. At some points, however, the bill makes concessions to what I have called the reigning doctrine. In particular it makes it possible for physicians to act on the fomerly declared will of the patient in cases in which the patient is unable to express a present will anymore, as in PVS or dementia cases.
13. G. van der Wal, P.J. van der Maas, *Euthanasie en Andere Medische Beslissingen rond het Levenseinde* (den Haag: SDU Uitgevers, 1996), pp. 202–217.
14. *Discussienota IV, Hulp bij Zelfdoding bij Psychiatrische Patiënten,* van de Commissie Aanvaardbaarheid Levensbeëindigend Handelen KNMG (1993), pp. 19–21, cf. *Discussienota III, Ernstig Demente Patiënten* (ibid. 1993), pp. 29–31. In the final version of the report, *Medisch Handelen rond het Levenseinde bij Wilsonbekwame Patiënten* (Houten/Diegem: Bohn Stafleu Van Loghum, 1997), p. 161, the appeal to compassion is more direct.
15. A. Buchanan and D.W. Brock, *Deciding for Others* (Cambridge: Cambridge University Press, 1989), pp. 43–47, show that this view itself implies the recognition of autonomy and well-being as independent values.
16. Cf. the first and the third case discussed in: B.E. Chabot, *Sterven op Drift* (Nijmegen: SUN, 1996), chapt. 6, pp. 101–133.
17. A recent study of public opinions about euthanasia and assisted suicide reports that more than 60% of the Dutch population believes that euthanasia can be justified by a person's right to decide on the moment of his own death. See Joop van Holsteyn and Margo Trappenburg, *Het Laatste Oordeel, Meningen over Nieuwe Vormen van Euthanasie* (Ambo Baarn: 1996). But the authors also argue that people's judgments on concrete cases tend to rely to a considerable extent on considerations of compassion, pp. 145–148.
18. Cf. Govert den Hartogh, "The Values of Life," *Bioethics,* Vol. 11 (1997), 43–66
19. Exceptions include G.A. van der Wal, "Bestaat er een recht op sterven?" in G.A. van der Wal (Ed.), *Euthanasie, Knelpunten in een discussie* (Baarn: Ambo, 1987); Helen Keasberry, "Enkele rechtsfilosofische aspecten van euthanasie," in J. Elders a.o., *Euthanasie, recht en ethiek* (Assen/Maastricht: Van Gorcum, 1985).
20. Joel Feinberg, "Voluntary Euthanasia and the Inalienable Right to Life," *Philosophy and Public Affairs* 7 (1978), 93–123.
21. A. Soeteman, "Zelfbeschikking en uitzichtloze noodsituatie," *Filosofie en Praktijk* 8 (1987), pp. 57–74.
22. Wetboek van Strafrecht, Art. 274.
23. Daniel Callahan, *What Kind of Life?* (New York: Simon & Schuster, 1990) pp. 230–231. Cf. E.M.H. Hirsch Ballin, "Over het leven beschikken," *Nederlands Tijdschrift voor Rechtsfilosofie en Rechtstheorie* 13 (1984), pp. 182–187.
24. Joel Feinberg, *Harm to Self* (New York: Oxford University Press, 1986), p. 27
25. There may be some additional reasons why the *Volenti* principle is specially unacceptable in professional ethics.
26. I have profited from discussions of this subject with Henri Wijsbek and Boudewijn Chabot.
27. Herbert Hendin, *De Dood als Verleider* (Haarlem: Gottmer, 1996), p. 63. [Dutch translation of *Seduced by Death* (New York/London: W.W. Norton & Co.].

Jurisprudence in the Age of Biotechnology
An Israeli Case Analysis

DALIA DORNER

Justice, Supreme Court of Israel, Sha'arei Mishpat Street, Kiryat David Ben-Gurion, Jerusalem 91909, Israel

INTRODUCTION

Advances in biotechnology in recent decades have brought the world revolutionary improvements in health care, new cures and treatments for diseases, and great promises for the future. At the same time, these developments have raised both hopes and concerns about the potential uses and abuses of new technology which affect not only the medical field, but also social, political and legal relations as well. For example, we are certainly all aware of the recent public debates concerning biological weapons, genetic cloning, and other forms of eugenics. On the political level, there have been great efforts to draft treaties and agreements regulating the use of biotechnology. Although the legal issues that arise as a result of this recent technology are new, we can mold existing legal principles to solve the dilemmas in accordance with principles of equality and justice.[1]

I would like to share with you one example of how biotechnology has presented the Israeli Supreme Court with such a challenge, and to show how we, as judges, can draw on legal tools to resolve novel issues. The case that I am referring to is *Nachmani v. Nachmani*,[2] decided finally in September 1996, which arose from the medical possibility of childbearing through *in vitro* fertilization.

THE *NACHMANI* CASE

Danny and Ruti Nachmani were married in 1984. Like most married couples, they wished to have children. Unfortunately, Ruti became afflicted with a malignant illness and had to undergo a hysterectomy. Nevertheless, medical technology offered the couple an opportunity to have their own biological children—the removal of Ruti's ova, *in vitro* fertilization, and implantation in a surrogate mother. The couple chose this option, despite the risks associated with the medical procedure.

The medical procedure itself, however, turned out to be the least of their worries. At the time, Israeli national health regulations prohibited implantation of ova in surrogate mothers. The couple tried instead to pursue the processs in the United States, but discovered that they could not afford it, despite their success in raising $30,000.

Ruti and Danny thus appealed to the High Court of Justice, seeking an order allowing the fertilization process at least to take place at an Israeli hospital. After a legal battle that lasted three years, an agreement was reached with the Ministry of Health, granting the couple's request.

Subsequently, for a period of eight months, Ruti underwent difficult medical treatments to remove ova from her body. Eleven ova were then successfully fertilized by Danny's sperm and were frozen for the purpose of future implantation. At the same time, Danny and Ruti signed a financial agreement with an American surrogacy agency and made initial payments to the agency.

However, two months after signing the financial agreement, Danny left Ruti and moved in with another woman. While Ruti refused to divorce her husband, Danny fathered a child with the other woman. Nonetheless, Ruti, who had no other means of bearing children of her own, wanted to continue with the implantation process, but Danny refused to grant his consent.

Ruti turned to the courts seeking possession of the pre-embryos from the hospital in which they were kept. The District Court of Haifa granted her request, and Danny appealed. The Supreme Court, hearing the case as a panel of five, reversed the lower court, denying possession to Ruti.[3] Because of the novelty of the issue, the Supreme Court decided to hear the case again as a panel of eleven justices, an unprecedented event. The Court held, seven to four, in favor of Ruti. I myself joined the majority ruling.[4]

THE LEGAL QUESTION

When reduced to its bare bones, the legal question in this case can be conceptualized as follows: is the right of the husband not to be a parent, which is based on his "ownership" of half of the genetic material of the embryos, dominated by the right of the wife, the provider of the remaining half of the genetic material, to be a parent?

All of the justices, including myself, agreed that there was no statute directly on point. A number of statutes were related, but, for a variety of reasons, did not govern this case.[5] The closest legal analogy perhaps concerns reproductive rights—that is, the respective rights of men and women regarding procreation and termination of pregnancy. Israeli law defines these rights in reference to a specific, identifiable point in time: that of conception. Thus, before conception, consenting adult men and women are equally free to choose to procreate, or to take measures to avoid procreation. After conception, however, the woman alone has the right to choose whether or not to continue the pregnancy, regardless of the wishes of her male partner. This right is subject only to the approval of a statutory committee relating to abortion.[6]

The *in vitro* fertilization process, however, poses a challenge to this doctrine. At what point exactly is the moment of conception? When the ova are removed? When they are fertilized? When they are implanted in the surrogate mother? Or is this even a relevant consideration?

A second attempt to squeeze the *Nachmani* case into an existing legal doctrine is by reference to contract law. The claim could be made that Danny bound himself to the continuation of the implantation process upon signing the agreement with the surrogacy agency. However, public policy considerations dictate that such a contract is unenforceable by courts.[7]

JUDICIAL ANALYSIS—VARIED APPROACHES TO LAW AND JUSTICE

The *Nachmani* decision, because it tests the boundaries of medicine, ethics, and law, was produced by a deeply divided court. Although the Court ruled seven to four in favor of Ruti, each of the eleven justices on the panel wrote a separate opinion explaining his or her reasoning.

The opposing decisions of the minority and majority justices conflict fundamentally on the jurisprudential question of whether law and justice are to be differentiated. Three of the four minority Justices[8] distinguished from the outset between law and justice. They believed that only through adherence to legal principles could a just result be reached. The Justices in the minority shared a reluctance to rely on justice—or according to their rhetoric, a subjective sense of justice—as a basis upon which to exercise judicial discretion. As judges, the minority felt bound to follow the "king's road" of the law before wandering into the uncertain and subjective paths of justice. The legal issue, thus, became whether or not Danny's consent was required for every step of the *in vitro* process, and, if so, whether or not Danny had explicitly or implicitly given such consent.[9]

Using legal principles of contract interpretation, the Justices in the minority concluded that Danny had not consented to the completion of the *in vitro* fertilization process. The Justices looked at the intent of the parties at the time of their original agreement to begin the *in vitro* process, and found that the agreement was based on the marital relationship of Danny and Ruti and was thus dependent on the continuity of that partnership. Given the change in their marital circumstances, the original consent could not control, and it was necessary that new consent be obtained from both sides. The Justices concluded that new consent was clearly lacking on Danny's part. Therefore, in the minority's view, Ruti was left with no legal basis for obtaining possession of the pre-embryos for the purpose of completing the process that the two of them had begun.[10] They emphasized that in finding for Danny their opinions were just, because their opinions were based purely on legal principles.

The Justices in the Majority, including myself, rejected the claim that law and justice are distinct and separable. This concept has been recognized by legal philosophers from time immemorial. In the *Nichomachean Ethics*, Aristotle asserted that a judge's duty is to make justice in the case before him, even if the law does not give him express guidance.[11] The Talmud warns us, "Jerusalem would not have been destroyed had its rulers gone beyond the letter of the law to seek out justice."[12] English law has also made room for principles of justice where the common law alone would lead to unjust results. The English doctrines of equity were developed to facilitate a degree of flexibility in the application of the common law, through consideration of the particular circumstances of the case and the possibility of remedies not available under the law.[13] These doctrines have been accepted in Israeli law as well.[14]

Professor Ronald Dworkin, one of the preeminent legal philosophers of our time, has also endorsed this approach. In his seminal work, *Taking Rights Seriously*, he argues that judges have an obligation to appeal to principles of justice and morality in the course of their reasoning, especially when confronted with "hard cases."[15] Scholars such as Chief Justice Barak, who view the judge's role as involving a wide degree of discretion, assert that judges must refer to the principles and values behind legal norms in balancing conflicting interests.[16] Former Justice Berenson stressed that not only must we appeal to justice in applying the law, but also that law and justice are one; if law is correctly interpreted, "law is law if it is just."[17]

In considering the novel question raised by the *Nachmani* case, we must look to the principles and equities underlying each side's position. In the words of former Israeli Supreme Court Justice Vitcone:

> As is the case in most legal and life problems in general, it is not the choice between good and evil that makes deciding difficult. The difficulty is in determining between differing considerations, that are all good and worthy of attention, but which conflict with each other. We are required to determine their respective merit.[18]

Among the Justices who followed this approach, the reasons and analyses provided were many and varied. However, the different approaches to justice can be placed into three main categories: an absolute approach to justice, justice as that which does the least harm, and justice as a balance of the rights and circumstances of each side.

Two Justices in the Majority followed an absolutist approach. Justice Kedmi advocated upholding the right to be a parent under all circumstances. He based his approach on the principle of creation of life and the inherent connection between each "maker" and his or her "creation." In an analogy to conception as the critical point beyond which the balance of rights shifts, the theory points to the moment of fertilization of the ovum as the moment of creation.[19] Distinct from the conception rule, this theory states that the wish of either the mother or the father to be a parent must always be upheld. Justice Tirkel also took an absolutist approach, finding justice always to be on the side of life. Unlike Justice Kedmi's decision, however, Justice Tirkel did not define the exact point at which life begins. Instead, his theory finds the potential for life that exists in the pre-embryos to be a sufficient reason to prefer whichever side that leads to birth.[20]

An absolute approach can be applied to favor the other side, the person who does not wish to be a parent, as well. This preference is based on the principle that recognizes and protects the autonomy of the individual. To force parenthood on one party would constitute a breach of this fundamental right of autonomy. Therefore, the decision to bring a child into the world is subject to the mutual consent of both partners. To force parenthood on one party would constitute a breach of his fundamental right of autonomy.[21]

The second category of opinions defines justice as the choice that will lead to the relatively least amount of harm. Under this view, Justice Goldberg found that the harm caused to Ruti in effectively denying her the self-realization experienced through parenthood was far greater than the emotional and economic harm done to Danny in imposing a child upon him against his will.[22] Also in this category was a theory of rights that Justice Mazza developed in order to arrive more scientifically at the decision that leads to the least harm. He analyzed Ruti's right to be a parent as a general right of great importance. Danny's right not to be a parent, on the other hand, was merely a specific application of a general right, because he was not demanding never to be a parent, but only not to be a parent to Ruti's child. At the same time, the harm Danny sought to impose on Ruti was a general limitation of her right—that is, because this was Ruti's only opportunity to become a biological mother, his position would effectively negate her right completely. The harm Ruti sought to impose on Danny, however, was only a specific limitation of his right—that is, he was left with the choice not to be a parent under all other circumstances.[23]

The third approach, which was my own and which was endorsed by two of my colleagues,[24] avoids absolute standards in favor of a balance of the respective principles and circumstances underlying each party's claim. There were two sets of competing principles in this case. On one hand are the principles underlying the right to be a parent. Freedom, in the full sense of the word, is not merely negative freedom from control by others, but has positive aspects as well. Freedom includes the ability of a person to direct his own life, to realize his basic needs and wishes, and to choose among a variety of possibilities using personal discretion. In our society, one of the most fundamental and important manifestations of this freedom is parenthood. Parenthood is not only a biological function but an existential one as well, which defines and symbolizes a person's uniqueness. Ruti's desire to have a child stemmed directly from the principles of self-realization underlying her right to parenthood.

The competing principles, of course, are those underlying the right not to be a parent. As we have seen, this right stems from the autonomy and privacy of the individual. Under this principle, the rights of others cannot be realized in such a way as to interfere with one's autonomous decision-making by imposing positive obligations on an unwilling party. We found significant the fact that Danny's argument was not based on his unwillingness to be a parent—he was already enjoying fatherhood of a child that he bore with his new partner. Nor was his claim based on the impossibility or the unwillingness to bear the financial burden of the potential child.

These competing principles cannot be weighed in a vacuum, though. We looked to the circumstances of the case to illuminate the gravity due each principle. As United States Supreme Court Justice Holmes noted, "General propositions do not decide concrete cases. The decision will depend on a judgment or intuition more subtle than any articulate major premise."[25]

In balancing the interests of Ruti against those of Danny, we had to consider the parties' good faith in the exercise of their rights. In the Israeli system, the requirement of good faith in the exercise of rights is a fundamental principle and a source of justice in the framework of the law. Thus, even if Danny had a right not to be a parent, in weighing his claims against those of Ruti, we had to examine whether or not he exercised such rights in good faith.

In the particular circumstances of this case, there were three additional factors that we considered crucial in our pursuit of justice. These factors included (*a*) the point at which Danny sought to discontinue the process; (*b*) the representations, expectations, and actions taken by the parties in reliance on such representations; and (*c*) the alternative possibilities for each party's realizing his or her respective rights. I will discuss these in order.

(*a*) In general, the further a couple is in the process of *in vitro* child bearing, the more weighty is the right of the one who wishes to complete the process. As we have suggested, the right to be a parent and the right not to be a parent arise from the principle that the human being is the master of his or her own body, and that no one can impose on another party a bodily action for the sake of realizing the other party's right. The situation is different in circumstances in which the realization of the right to be a parent is not dependent on the undermining of the other's right over his or her body. This was the situation in the *Nachmani* case. The process was already at an advanced stage and required no additional physical action from either side. Ruti's right to be a parent did not remain in the realm of mere hope but was already well into the process of realization.

(*b*) The principle of estoppel prevents a party who has made certain representations to another party from denying the legal effect of those representations, when the other party has acted in a reasonable manner in reliance on those representations to his or her detriment. As one student of the legal resolution of *in vitro* fertilization disputes has commented:

[T]he doctrine of reliance should be applied to resolve a dispute between gamete providers. The consistent application of a reliance-based theory of contract law to enforce promises to reproduce through IVF will enable IVF participants to assert control over their reproductive choices by enabling them to anticipate their rights and duties, and to know with reasonable certainty that their expectations will be enforced by the courts.[26]

In our case, Ruti had relied to her detriment on Danny's representations that he wanted to have a child with her. She invested considerable time and money and underwent painful medical treatments toward the achievement of this goal. The fertilization of her ova with his sperm effectively prevented her from being able to use these ova with another partner. These are important considerations, but do not solve the case by themselves.

(c) Finally, and significantly, we examined the alternative possibilities that each side has in realizing his or her right. As discussed above, Ruti was left with no physical alternative by which to become a biological mother. Thus, to rule in favor of Danny would leave Ruti with no other possibility of having children of her own. In making our determination, we adopted the view that where the right of one completely destroys the right of the other, it is the latter's right that should be preferred. Thus, because Danny's right to avoid reproduction completely destroys Ruti's right to become a parent, it is Ruti's right that must be preferred.[27]

Such a rationale is not a particularly "feminist" resolution, however. Should the circumstances have been reversed—that is, if Danny had been left with no alternative means of becoming a biological parent and wanted to continue the process against Ruti's will—I would have ruled in his favor. In this case, however, the balance of the rights and privileges involved made it clear to me, and a majority of my colleagues, that Ruti should be allowed to realize her right to be a parent.

THE STATUTORY RESPONSE: THE AGREEMENTS FOR CARRYING FETUSES ACT

Detailed agreements between the involved parties to a surrogacy agreement can help us prevent some of the dilemmas that result from the use of new reproductive technologies. By making plain the intent of the parties, these agreements can aid us, as well, in finding just solutions to future conflicts between the parties. However, prior to working out the intricate details of what a statute regulating surrogacy should look like, a legislature must first decide the basic premise whether surrogacy agreements should be permitted at all.

Arguments for prohibiting surrogacy agreements completely are based on the view that such arrangements threaten notions of bodily integrity and human identity and have great potential to harm surrogate mothers psychologically. Such arrangements, it is argued, devalue human life and exploit class advantages. This is precisely what is claimed to have occurred in the famous New Jersey *Baby M.* case,[28] which involved a custody dispute between the genetic father and mother, who had made a surrogacy agreement. The trial court's reliance on the "best interests of the child" standard in deciding who gets custody of a child pursuant to a surrogacy agreement, it is argued, permitted the trial court to make class-biased and idiosyncratic determinations in ruling against the biological mother and for the biological father.[29] Other than in extreme cases, it is nearly impossible to make such a determination. Implicitly recognizing as much, the New Jersey Supreme Court held that surrogacy contracts are unenforceable as contrary to public policy.[30] Since then, other American states have followed New Jersey's lead and have passed statutes legislating that surrogacy agreements are void and unenforceable.[31]

Those believing that surrogacy agreements should be enforced claim that the approach prohibiting such agreements neglects to account for the diversity of women's interests and the full range of societal values involved. Some women might value the opportunity to help an infertile couple while assisting their own families financially. Infertile couples—who have no other means to conceive a child with genetic ties to at least one parent—benefit significantly from such transactions as well.[32] Furthermore, proponents argue that complete enforcement of surrogacy agreements protects reproductive autonomy and contractual responsibility. Giving full effect to such agreements, it is argued, will discourage women who are ambivalent about the process from participating as gestational mothers, thus minimizing costly disputes.

In Israel, the Knesset decided against banning surrogacy agreements, but rather, to regulate them in an effort to accommodate all the interests implicated. The Israeli Agreements for Carrying Fetuses Act[33] is tailored to avoid problems that result from the status of the parties involved and the resulting child by viewing the issue from a religious—in particular Jewish—perspective. This statute reflects the extent to which such regulation must be drafted so as to meet the needs of the specific community and legal framework in which it operates and also reflects the difficulty of drafting a comprehensive international treaty.[34] Still, national and state regulation may prove extremely valuable in helping parties foresee potential rights and responsibilities.

The Act restricts surrogacy agreements to situations in which a written agreement between the intended parents and gestational mother, supported by medical, psychological, and other expert opinions and counseling, has been approved by an Authorization Committee established by the Act. Included on the Committee, in order to provide a wide spectrum of expert analysis concerning the suitability of the parties to undergo surrogacy, are medical doctors, a clinical psychologist, a social worker, a public representative who is also a lawyer, and a clergy member of the parties' religion. There are certain regulations provided by the Act to avert certain potential complications deemed important by the Legislature. For instance, all parties involved in an agreement must be adult residents of Israel. The surrogate mother must not be married or a relative of either of the prospective parents, unless the Committee is convinced that the prospective parents were unable, through reasonable efforts, to reach an agreement with an unmarried woman. Also, the sperm must be that of the prospective father and the ova not that of the gestational mother. The gestational mother and prospective mother must also be of the same religion, unless, no party to the agreement is Jewish and such a decision is supported by the opinion of the clergy member of the Committee.

In order to approve an agreement of this sort, the Committee must be convinced that the parties to the agreement are acting voluntarily and with a full understanding of the meaning and consequences of the agreement. The agreement may not include any conditions that would deprive or infringe upon rights of the potential child or the parties. However, the Committee may authorize conditions for payment of the gestational mother to cover actual expenses, which include legal-advice expenses, insurance, and compensation for loss of time, income, or capacity to work, and for suffering, as well as any other reasonable reimbursement. In the case of a substantial change in circumstances, facts, or conditions on which such a decision was based, the Committee is authorized to review its authorization decision as long as the fertilized ova are not yet implanted in the gestational mother.

Although this statute did not control in the *Nachmani* case, it is hoped that its emphasis on social and psychological counseling prior to such agreements will enable us to avoid such dilemmas in the future. Unforeseen controversies will inevitably arise, but the approach of the new legislation will enable us to concentrate on human needs and feelings and find solutions that maximize the well-being of all parties.[35]

CONCLUSION

The *Nachmani* case illustrates how the law can respond to new legal dilemmas that result from new technologies. Reproductive advancements are particularly challenging because they involve extremely sensitive ethical and legal conflicts. The *Nachmani* case was, however, just the beginning. I expect that in the coming years we will be faced with many more such cases. Even the *Nachmani* case itself is not fully resolved. If and when the ova are implanted and a child is born, a host of novel issues may be raised concerning, for example, the child's legal identity, the rights and obligations of the father, and succession rights.[36] Thus, the obligation falls on judges to reconsider, reapply, and modify traditional paradigms and principles of justice to take into account new medical and social realities as needed. This is often an exceedingly difficult task, because as Justice Wideyer of the High Court of Australia pointed out: "Law [marches] in medicine but in the rear and limping a little."

NOTES AND REFERENCES

1. See generally E.B. Brody, *Biomedical Technology and Human Rights* (Aldershot, England: Dartmouth Publishing Co. Ltd. 1993).
2. A.H. 2401/95, *Nachmani v. Nachmani*, 50(4) P.D. 661.
3. See C.A. 5587/93, *Nachmani v. Nachmani*, 49(1) P.D. 485.
4. A.H. 2401/95.
5. For example, the National Health Regulations (In Vitro Fertilization), 1987, K.T. 5053 deal with the role of hospitals in the *in vitro* process, but do not explicitly cover the relationship between the male and female partners. The Agreements for Carrying Fetuses Act (Authorization of Agreement and Status of the Newborn), 1996, S.H. 1577, was more directly on point but was passed subsequent to the Nachmanis' actions and was consequently inapplicable.
6. See Penal Law, 1977, secs. 314-16; C.A. 413/80, *Doe v. Doe*, 35(3) P.D. 57, 67.
7. Cf. D. Freedman and N. Cohen, *Contracts,* Vol. A (Jerusalem: Aviram Publishers, 1992), p. 326; A. Bendor, "The Legal Status of Political Agreements," *Mishpat U'Mimshal,* Vol. 3 (1995), pp. 297, 316 [both in Hebrew].
8. Justices Strasberg-Cohen, Or, and Zamir are the three justices to whom I am referring.
9. Opinion of Justice Strasberg-Cohen in A.H. 2401/95. Although all four Justices agreed that the central issue to be decided was whether consent had been given, the Justices came to this conclusion differently. The opinion of Justice Zamir in A.H. 2401/95 found an implicit requirement of consent by examining the statutory framework, namely, the consent requirement for a divorced woman to implant her ova fertilized with her ex-spouse's sperm and the requirement that to preserve frozen pre-embryos beyond five years, both partners must give their consent. In contrast, the

Opinion on Chief Justice Barak in A.H. 2401/95 found its consent requirement by examining the nature of the rights involved; specifically, that the right of parenthood and the right not to be a parent are freedoms that do not create obligations on others.
10. Opinions of Justices Or, Strasberg-Cohen, Barak, and Zamir in A.H. 2401/95.
11. Aristotle, *Etica: Mahadurat Nikomakos* [Ethics: Nichomachean Edition] (Jerusalem: Shoken Publishing, Yosef G. Leibs trans., 1973), p. 134.
12. Babylonian Talmud, *Baba Metziya*, p.30 at col. 2.
13. See, for example, H.G. Hanbury and R.H. Maudsley, *Modern Equity* (13th ed., London: Sweet & Maxwell, 1989), pp. 5–15; G.S. Bower and A.K. Turner, *The Law Relating to Estoppel by Representation* (London: Butterworths 1977), 3rd ed.
14. See opinion of Justice Elon in H.C. 702/81, *Mintzer v. Central Committee of the Israeli Bar Ass'n and Others*, 36(2) P.D. 1, 18.
15. R. Dworkin, *Taking Rights Seriously* (Cambridge, MA.: Harvard University Press, 1979), p. 22.
16. A. Barak, *Interpretation in Law* (Vol. 1: The General Theory, Jerusalem: Nevo Publishing, 1992) p. 301 [Hebrew]. See also D. Lyons, *Moral Aspects of Legal Theory* (Cambridge: Cambridge University Press, 1993), pp. 94–101.
17. T. Berenson, "Words of Justice Berenson on the Day of His Retirement," *Mishpatim*, Vol. 8, (1977), at 3, 5. See also I. Zamir, "In Honor of Justice Tzvi Berenzon," *Mishpat U'Mimshal*, Vol. 2 (1994), pp. 325, 327–330 [both in Hebrew].
18. C.A. 461/62, *Tsim Yachting Co. of Israel v. Mazi'ar*, 17(2) P.D. 1319, 1337.
19. Opinion of Justice Kedmi in A.H. 2401/95. This view was similar to the rationale applied in the U.S. case of *Kass v. Kass*, No. 19658/93, 1995 WL 110368 (N.Y. Sup. Jan. 18, 1995), *rev'd*, 663 N.Y.S.2d, which was later reversed on appeal. Judge Roncallo of New York asserted: "In my opinion there is no legal, ethical or logical reason why an *in vitro* fertilization should give rise to additional rights on the part of the husband. From a propositional standpoint it matters little whether the ovum/sperm union takes place in the private darkness of a fallopian tube or the public glare of a petri dish. Fertilization is fertilization and fertilization of the ovum is the inception of the reproductive process. Biological life exists from that moment forward." 1995 WL 110368, at *3.
20. Opinion of Justice Tirkel in A.H. 2401/95. This approach was endorsed by another U.S. case. In the case of *Davis v. Davis*, 842 S.W.2d 588 (Tenn. 1992), the Supreme Court of Tennessee held that parenthood, as a general rule, cannot be imposed on an unwilling party. However, the Court went on to hold that this rule ought not apply in cases where upholding a party's right not to be a parent would in effect deprive the other party, absolutely and finally, of the right to be a parent. In the words of Judge Daughtrey: "Ordinarily, the party wishing to avoid procreation should prevail, assuming that the other party has a reasonable possibility of achieving parenthood by means other than the use of the pre-embryos in question. If no other reasonable alternative exists, then the argument in favor of using the pre-embryos to achieve pregnancy should be considered.... [T]he rule does not contemplate the creation of an automatic veto... 842 S.W.2d at 604.
21. Chief Justice Barak took an absolutist approach, but one not dependent on principles of autonomy; rather, the Chief Justice defined justice as always being in favor of equality. Thus, he reasoned, what is crucial is that both potential mother and father have equal powers with regard to the pre-embryos. Since, according to him, the consent of both sides was a legal requirement at each stage, each has equal power to cancel the process by not granting his or her consent. This remains true, regardless of any specific facts or circumstances of either potential parent. See Opinion of Chief Justice Barak in A.H. 2401/95.
22. Opinion of Justice Goldberg in A.H. 2401/95.
23. Opinion of Justice Mazza in A.H. 2401/95.
24. Opinions of Justices Tal and Bach in A.H. 2401/95. Several scholars also endorsed this approach. See A. Marmor, "The Frozen Embryos of the Nachmani Case—A Reply to Chaim Gas," *Tel Aviv University L.R.*, Vol. 20 (1995), at 443; D. Barak-Erez, "Symmetry and Neutrality: Reflections on the Nachmani Case," *Tel Aviv University. L.R.*,

Vol. 20 (1996), at 197; S. Davidow-Motola, "A Feminist Decision? The *Nachmani* Case from Another Perspective," *Tel Aviv University L.R.*, Vol. 20 (1996), at 221.
25. *Lochner v. New York*, 198 U.S. 45, 76 (1905) (Holmes, J., dissenting).
26. Comment, "Disputes Over Frozen Embryos: Who Wins, Who Loses, and How Do We Decide," *Creighton L.R.*, Vol. 24 (1991), pp. 1299, 1302–1303. See also note, "The Davis Dilemma: How to Prevent Battles Over Frozen Preembryos," *Case Western Reserve L.R.*, Vol. 41 (1991), pp. 543, 547.
27. Interestingly, two years following the decision in this case, a molecular biologist and lawyer team reached the same conclusion as I did in this case based on similar reasoning. L.M. Silver and S.R. Silver, "Confused Heritage and the Absurdity of Genetic 'Ownership,'" *Harvard J. of Law & Technology*, Vol. 11 (1998), at 593. See also J.A. Robertson, "Prior Agreements for Disposition of Frozen Embryos," *Ohio State L.J.*, Vol. 51 (1990), at 407, 420 ("If the right to reproduce and the right to avoid reproduction are in conflict, favoring reproduction is not unreasonable when there is no alternative way for one party to reproduce.")
28. *In the Matter of Baby "M"*, 525 A.2d 1128 (N.J. Super. Ct. Ch. Div., 1987)
29. N. Taub and L.M. Rarles, "In the Matter of Baby M," *Women's Rights L. Reporter.*, Vol. 14 (1992), at 243, 249, n.45. For instance, the trial court, in ruling against the biological mother in the custody battle, emphasized that she would be a less fit parent because, among other reasons, she dropped out of high school in tenth grade and she and her husband had declared bankruptcy in the past, whereas the biological father and his wife were financially stable and both of them possessed doctoral degrees. *In the Matter of Baby "M"*, 525 A.2d at 1167–70.
30. *In the Matter of Baby "M"*, 537 A.2d 1227 (N.J. 1988).
31. See, for example, Ariz. Rev. Stat. Ann. §25–218(A) (West 1991); D.C. Code Ann. § 16-401 (1993); Ind. Code Ann. §§31–20–1–1, 31–20–1–2 (Michie 1997); Mich. Comp. Laws Ann. §722.855 (West 1993); N.D. Cent. Code §14–18–05 (1991); Utah Code Ann. §76–7–204 (1995); Va. Code Ann. § 64.1–7.1 (Michie 1993).
32. D.L. Rhode, *Justice and Gender* (Cambridge, Mass: Harvard University Press, 1989), p. 224–25.
33. The Agreements for Carrying Fetuses Act (Authorization of Agreement and Status of the Newborn), 1996, S.H. 1577.
34. For example, an official West German Commission has considered a total ban on surrogacy except between relatives. The European Commission has recommended that a contract should not be enforceable against a surrogate mother who changes her mind at any point during the pregnancy or after delivery. E.B. Brody, *Biomedical Technology and Human Rights* (Aldershot, England: Dartmouth Publishing Co. Ltd., 1993), p. 90.
35. Such a solution is advocated in the context of human rights and biomedical technology so as to focus on human needs and feelings rather than on legal-judicial issues. E.B. Brody, *Biomedical Technology and Human Rights* (Aldershot, England: Dartmouth Publishing Co. Ltd. 1993), p. 65.
36. For a discussion of these issues, see J. Gunning and V. English, *Human In Vitro Fertilization* (Aldershot, England: Dartmouth Publishing Co. Ltd., 1994); G. Douglas, *Law, Fertility and Reproduction* (London: Sweet & Maxwell, 1991); A. Liu, *Artificial Reproduction and Reproductive Rights* (Aldershot, England: Dartmouth Publishing Co. Ltd., 1997).

Reproductive Liberty and the Right to Clone Human Beings

JOHN A. ROBERTSON

School of Law, University of Texas at Austin, 727 E. 26th Street, Austin, Texas 78705, USA

INTRODUCTION

The birth of Dolly, the sheep cloned from the mammary cells of an adult ewe, is a turning point in ethical and social debates over the use of assisted reproductive technologies. Prior to Dolly, two sets of issues dominated ethical discussion. One set focused on the creation, storage, and discard of human embryos, and the impact of those practices on respect for human life. A second set of issues concerned the family and kinship effects of recombining genetic, gestational, and social aspects of parenthood, as occurred in gamete donation and surrogacy.

The birth of Dolly—and thus the prospect of human cloning—raises a third set of issues that will attract the ethical spotlight for some years to come. Having not yet fully resolved embryo and kinship issues, we must now come to terms with the growing ability to choose, manipulate, or engineer the genome of offspring. That we would eventually have to face selection issues was, of course, expected; the suddenness with which cloning arrived was not. The resulting dilemmas are among the most difficult issues posed by technological control over birth and conception.

The prospect of human cloning presents in stark form the question of the extent to which techniques to select, manipulate, and engineer the genes of offspring should be developed and used. Cloning is only the first of several selection techniques that will be available in the relatively near future. Germline gene therapy, which has a clear therapeutic intent and the benefit of fixing a genetic problem in subsequent offspring, may soon be available. In its wake will come nonmedical genetic enhancement, and even cases of genetic diminishment, as portrayed in the film *Bladerunner* and suggested by the efforts of deaf parents to have a deaf child. Many other situations of genetic alteration will also arise to test the limits of parental manipulation of offspring characteristics.

Note that the main technical barriers to achieving such control lie in the realm of genetics and not in the limitations of reproductive manipulation itself. The ability to micromanipulate eggs and embryos, as evident in intracytoplasmic sperm injection (ICSI), assisted hatching, cytoplasmic transfers, and embryo biopsy, show that the mechanical ability to handle eggs and embryos to the extent needed for genetic manipulation exists in, or could easily be acquired by, many IVF clinics and laboratories both in the United States and the developed world. The main difficulties lie in the realm of genetic knowledge and technique. We are still ignorant of the mechanisms and processes by which complex behavioral and phenotypic traits are produced genetically. In addition, we are only beginning to develop safe and effective vectors for inserting genes in humans. Little genetic work with human embryos has yet occurred, and it will be some time before the techniques of inserting and deleting genes will be available. Although somatic cell nuclear transplant may ultimately prove less attractive and less threatening than other forms of genetic manipulation, its operation at the level of the entire genome rather than individual genes makes it much more available for future use.[1]

The ability in the near future to engage in somatic cell nuclear transfer cloning, and the ability thereafter to manipulate or select other offspring characteristics, presents a complicated set of ethical dilemmas. People have always engaged in certain kinds of genetic selection, as in the choice of a marriage or reproductive partner, carrier screening, and the extensive screening of pregnancies, often followed by abortion, that now are a routine part of obstetrics and gynecology in developed countries. In addition, parents have done many things after birth that also improve or affect the characteristics of offspring, through education, training, medications, and cosmetic surgery. We have generally regarded such practices as part of parental freedom or liberty. If we take reproductive freedom seriously, how can we deny parents the ability to select and choose offspring characteristics prior to birth through the use of prenatal and preconception selection and manipulation techniques? Yet if we recognize a right of genetic selection as part of procreative liberty, do we not risk commodifying offspring and creating other harms?

I would like to sharpen this dilemma by presenting more precisely the argument for genetic selection as part of one's procreative liberty.[2] I will argue that a robust right to choose and select offspring characteristics follows from prevailing conceptions of reproductive and parental freedom. Given the strong commitment to reproductive freedom that exists in ethical, legal, and social practice, a presumptive right to use somatic cell nuclear transfer human cloning in certain circumstances should follow. Yet that prospect—at least initially—seems unpalatable. Reconciling these two positions is a major challenge for future uses of assisted reproductive and genetic selection technology.

GENETIC SELECTION AS PART OF PROCREATIVE LIBERTY

The most powerful argument for a rights claim to use prebirth methods of selecting offspring characteristics derives from an individual's liberty to make decisions concerning reproduction. Although one can also make an argument based on family autonomy in rearing children, the main support for a right to engage in prebirth selection rests on the close connection between the expected characteristics of offspring, and the decision whether or not to reproduce.

Procreative liberty—the freedom to have or not have offspring—has a firm moral basis in the importance that reproductive decisions have for individuals. Such decisions are among the most important that an individual will make in her lifetime. Having or not having offspring will determine central aspects of her personal identity and definition of self. It will also determine the physical, social, and psychological responsibilities that she will have—or not have—toward others. Because reproductive events have such personal significance and impact, the decision whether or not to reproduce should clearly be within an individual's personal discretion.

In the United States, for example, procreative liberty also has a firm legal basis, even though this has not always been explicitly articulated. Reproductive decisions receive legal protection against both private and public interference. Private interference with decisions to reproduce is a civil wrong, recognized as the torts of wrongful pregnancy and wrongful birth.[3] In addition, the United States Supreme Court has recognized a constitutional right to avoid reproduction, both before and after conception, in *Grisworld v. Connecticut*,[4] *Eisenstadt v. Baird*,[5] *Roe v. Wade*,[6] and *Casey v. Planned Parenthood*,[7] albeit with some limitations.

The Supreme Court has also recognized the right to have offspring without undue state interference, though mainly in dicta,[8] because few cases of direct interference have reached the Court. In *Skinner v. Oklahoma*, the Court, in striking down a compulsory sterilization law on equal protection grounds, stated that reproduction "is one of the basic civil rights of man."[9] This holding and later dicta[10] strongly suggest that courts would apply strict scrutiny and invalidate state interference with coital reproduction by married, and possibly unmarried, persons unless the state could show compelling justification for the restriction. If the Constitution protects coital reproduction from state interference, it should also protect infertility treatments because such treatments are essential to allowing coitally infertile individuals to reproduce. Although there is some uncertainty about whether the Constitution would protect an infertile couple's use of donor gametes and surrogates, there are strong grounds for concluding that it would protect the use of noncoital techniques involving the couple's own gametes to the same extent as their efforts to reproduce coitally.[11]

If the moral and legal right to choose whether or not to reproduce is a fundamental right, then a large measure of prebirth control over offspring traits and characteristics should follow. If reproductive decisions are fundamental, then access to information material to the decision to reproduce should be equally fundamental.[12] If a person would choose not to reproduce if she knew that the child would have a disability or some other undesired characteristic, then she should be entitled to have that information and to act on it. Her right to avoid reproduction for any *reason* would entitle her to avoid reproduction for a particular *reason*. Similarly, her right to have offspring generally should entitle her to have offspring only if she thinks that offspring will have particular characteristics.

Such protected status of prebirth selection follows from the fact that individuals seek to reproduce or to avoid reproduction precisely because of the types of experiences, situations, and responsibilities that reproduction or its absence will entail. A person who chooses to reproduce chooses to accept the experiences and responsibilities entailed in reproduction and child-rearing, unknown and vague as they may be at the time of choice. If the package of burdens and responsibilities differs markedly from one that she would find acceptable, then that person might choose not to reproduce. Thus, denying a person information about the package of burdens, benefits, and rearing responsibilities that will ensue, or denying her the ability to avoid or engage in reproduction based on that information, could affect her decision whether to reproduce at all and thus interfere with her procreative liberty.

The right to information and actions that enable one to avoid offspring with certain characteristics, or to reproduce only if offspring have certain other characteristics, may be articulated as a prebirth right to select or control offspring characteristics. If a couple would not reproduce if a child had gene A, but would if it had gene B, procreative liberty should protect their decision not to reproduce in the first case and to reproduce in the second. Denying them information about A or B, or denying them the ability to make reproductive choices based on that information, would interfere with their procreative liberty.

Procreative liberty, however, is a presumptive, not an absolute, right. If reproductive decisions are fundamental rights, then attempts to restrict them should be strictly scrutinized by the courts or others who are committed to protecting fundamental rights.[13] If cognizable in a judicial action, courts should presumptively protect actions involving procreative liberty against state interference until the point at which the reproductive choice in question harms or intrudes upon the tangible interests of others. The reasons for seeking to restrict information relevant to the decision to reproduce, or for prohibiting reproductive decisions based on such information, will determine whether interference with procreative liberty is justified. A court deciding such a case, as well as policymakers or professionals confronting those circumstances, would have to analyze the interests served by the interference, and the harms and sufferings it tries to prevents. This inquiry inevitably involves a form of balancing, but a balancing that, because of the importance of procreative liberty, should be weighted heavily in favor of procreative choice. Only when those seeking to limit procreative choice could show that unrestricted choice would cause compelling, tangible harm to others should interference with procreative choice be permitted. If the harms and concerns are of lesser weight (for example, if they conflict with particular notions of what is natural or desirable in reproduction or if they present the potential to indirectly harm as a class, women or persons with disabilities), private or public interference with a couple's efforts to use genetic selection or other techniques presumptively protected as part of procreative liberty should not be permitted. In that case, however, a range of policy options short of interference or prohibition, such as denial of subsidies, establishment of professional standards for providing or withholding the service, and provision of education and counseling, would have to fill the regulatory gap.

The ultimate scope of the liberty prior to birth to select or control offspring characteristics thus depends on two inquiries. The first is whether the characteristic in question is one that is central or material to a reproductive decision—whether the characteristic determines whether reproduction will occur. If so, the law should give this choice the same respect and weight it gives to other decisions about whether or not to reproduce. If not, if the characteristic is only a preference as to offspring characteristics but not one that determines whether reproduction will occur, then choice over it may not be part of procreative liberty and may not deserve the respect accorded procreative choices generally.

The second inquiry is into the nature, severity, and probability of the harms of untoward effects that allegedly flow from prebirth selection efforts. Alleged harms include destruction of embryos and fetuses, harm to offspring, confusing kinship relations, instrumentalizing or commodifying human life and children, discrimination on the basis of gender and disability, and facilitating coercive forms of eugenics. Courts and policymakers, as well as ethicists and others concerned with the use of a selection technology, will have to analyze and assess alleged harms carefully to see whether they rise to the compelling level that justifies interference with procreative choice.

WHEN DOES A PROCREATIVE INTEREST IN GENETIC SELECTION EXIST?

If the criterion for determining whether a prebirth selection decision falls within procreative liberty is the effect on or materiality of the information or trait to reproductive decisions, then many forms of genetic selection and manipulation should qualify. A variety of prebirth selection activities have become part of routine medical and obstetrical practice precisely because they are so clearly material to reproductive choice. Medical specialists routinely screen Ashkenazi Jews, African-Americans, siblings of persons with cystic fibrosis, and other groups to determine their status as carriers of genetic diseases.[14] Individuals then use the information from these tests to make decisions about marriage, conception, prenatal diagnosis, and abortion, and thus whether to forego reproduction or to go forward with it. Many women over thirty-five have amniocentesis or chorionic villus sampling to screen for Down's syndrome. It is estimated that doctors now screen more than 75% of United States pregnancies for neural tube defects. Although not everyone is willing to undergo carrier and prenatal tests and then make reproductive decisions based on the results, enough people do so that there can be little doubt that information derived from these tests is determinative of their decision to reproduce.

The growing knowledge of the human genome will increase the number of diseases, and eventually other traits, that prospective parents can discover at both carrier and prenatal stages, and thus avoid by selection decisions prior to birth. Although many of these diseases will be worse or comparable in severity to those presently screened and selected, many others will be less severe. In addition, screening will detect susceptibility genes that simply create a higher than normal risk that the disease will occur. In these cases, the materiality of the information to individual decisions to reproduce will vary, with some, but perhaps fewer, people willing to undergo screening or to avoid births under those circumstances. In some instances individuals many have idiosyncratic preferences to avoid certain characteristics.

Individuals will also vary in their demand for or acceptance of positive means of selection, such as cloning, germline gene therapy, nonmedical enhancement, and intentional diminishment of offspring. Most people will have little need to consider using such procedures, for standard coital and noncoital means of conception will better serve their needs. But some individuals whose reproductive needs cannot be met in more traditional ways may find it desirable or advantageous to use certain forms of positive selection.[15] For some subset of them, the opportunity to engage in positive forms of selection, say reproductive cloning, will determine whether or not they form a biologically related family.

A crucial issue is how to measure the materiality of a particular genetic trait to a decision whether or not to reproduce. A purely subjective standard would allow anyone to select on the basis of any trait, as long as they asserted either that they would not reproduce if the child had trait or gene A or that they would reproduce only if it had trait or gene B. This standard would place no limits on what is understood as reproductive freedom as long as the person creditably asserts that the trait or procedure is a *sina qua non* for their reproduction. An objective standard, however, would require that a reasonable person find that the trait, and hence the means to acquire or avoid it, is determinative of her reproductive choice. But reproductive decisions are highly personal, and as such, are often arbitrary and subjective, not easily judged by a reasonable-person standard. Some mix of objective and subjective factors no doubt will emerge to negotiate these differences, as it has for informed consent, self-defense, and many other legal doctrines.[16] At the outer limits, questions of the materiality of prebirth selection practices to reproductive decisions will ultimately require judgments that are constitutive of why reproductive freedom receives heightened protection.

The stage at which individuals engage in prebirth selection and the methods they use may also affect assessments of the importance of the reproductive interest in genetic selection. This cuts both ways. The fact that a person is willing to undergo significant bodily intrusion, such as undergoing a cycle of *in vitro* fertilization or having an abortion in order to avoid the birth or offspring with particular characteristics, arguably shows the material importance of that trait to reproductive choice. At the same time, the fact that someone is willing to go to what others would deem extreme lengths to avoid or to have a child with a particular characteristic may indicate that selection on that basis is such a radically subjective position that it cannot be an important reproductive interest.

The objective materiality of some traits to reproductive decisions will attenuate as we move from genes for severe genetic disease and susceptibility traits to genes for gender and hair and eye color, and from negative methods of selection, such as carrier screening and prenatal diagnosis, to positive methods such as nontherapeutic enhancement, cloning, and intentional diminishment. Individuals may still claim that having or not having a child with the gene or trait in question is central to their decision and thus should presumptively receive protection, but at some point the divergence from what most people view as central to reproductive meaning will diminish the perceived importance of the reproductive interest at stake, and suggest that selection on that basis should not be part of procreative liberty.[17] Unless courts then protect that instance of selection under the rubric of some other right, the state would only need to show a rational basis for restriction.

Drawing the line between protected and unprotected traits and methods is likely to be difficult. Decisions to avoid the birth of offspring with severe disabilities appear clearly connected to reproductive choice, and thus are presumptively protected. In contrast, prebirth selection efforts that focus on trivial genetic traits, nonmedical enhancement, cloning, or intentional diminishment initially seem more questionable as exercises of procreative liberty. A person may attach a subjective importance to control over a particular factor. However, if that factor is too attenuated or deviant from common understandings or reproductive meaning, courts and other decisionmakers may not find it material to reproductive choice, despite the subjective claim, because it is judged to be beyondprevailing understandings of practices that give reproduction meaning. As noted, the judgments made in such cases will ultimately constitute that which is considered distinctively and centrally reproductive.

As particular issues of genetic selection arise, the problem in each instance will be to determine how centrally or trivially connected to decisions to reproduce the selection activity is, while recognizing that there may be wide subjective variation in the willingness of people to make reproductive choices on the basis of that characteristic. If prebirth control over whether offspring have these traits falls within the sphere of procreative liberty, government may restrict selection on that basis only when such control threatens tangible harm to others. Conversely, if the selection activity is not protected, government must show only a rational basis for limiting those selection decisions.

APPLICATION TO HUMAN CLONING

I want to suggest briefly how this analysis of procreative liberty might apply to human cloning.[18] Under this standard there may well be instances where a married couple, intent on having and rearing biologically related offspring, might use somatic cell nuclear transfer cloning as the best solution to their desire to have and rear offspring. Three plausible cases for using nuclear transfer cloning to achieve reproductive goals are easily imagined. One would be where a couple is infertile because of male infertility attributed to, say, severe oligospermia or azoospermia, so that not even ICSI (intracytoplasmic sperm injection) is possible. A variation on this need would be where the couple are carriers for a genetic disease and choose to use the DNA of one of them instead of adopting or seeking a gamete donor.[19] In either case, rather than resort to commercial or anonymous sperm banks, with whom they will have no genetic connection, they decide to use the DNA of one of them for reproductive cloning. This will assure the genetic kinship link, and enable the source's genes to create a later bond. Unless they can use this source of DNA, they creditably assert that they will not have children at all.

A second case would be where a couple that lacks gametic function in both partners, but the wife is still capable of gestating, decide to seek embryo donation. However, rather than utilize the leftover frozen embryos of other couples, or have new embryos created with donor sperm and donor egg, they decide to use the DNA of one of them or a third party to form the embryo, which they then place in the woman for gestation. Again, unless they can use this source of DNA, they convincingly assert that they will not have children at all.

A third case would arise when the couple has an existing child who might need future organs or tissue to treat a life-threatening disease. Because of the shortage of suitable donors, the couple decides to have another child who could serve as a tissue donor, if the need arose. However, since only children who are a close genetic match would be effective donors, they decide to use DNA from an existing child (it could be the potential recipient or another child who is a suitable match, but who cannot, for other reasons, be a donor). As in the other cases, unless they could select this DNA, they would not have another child at all. Obviously, to be acceptable, the later retrieval of organs or tissue would have to respect the rights and interests of the donor, for example, and not occur without that child's actual or substituted consent.

None of these cases is preposterous nor, on their face, illegitimate. The use of donor sperm is now widely accepted, as is the right of the couple to have some say in the choice of donor. Indeed, commerical sperm banks in the United States distribute brochures with the height, weight, hair and eye color, ethnic origin, education, and hobbies of donors listed. Embryo donation occurs on a much more limited scale, and so a practice of actual selection of embryos does not now exist, as it does with sperm donation. Yet there is no reason why couples desiring an embryo donation would not want some degree of choice over the embryos that they receive. Finally, starting with the Ayala case in California in 1992, more than 50 cases of parents having children by coital means to serve as tissue or organ donors have been reported.[20] The use of nuclear cell transfer cloningwould enable that goal to be achieved more precisely and effectively.

Finding that certain family-centered uses of reproductive cloning fall within the scope of procreative liberty does not, of course, end the inquiry. We must then ask whether such uses pose such grave harm to others that they can be justifiably restricted. With cloning, there is a need to examine more thoroughly the harms that are said to flow from its use. In the United States, the National Bioethics Advisory Commission cited threats to physical safety, individuality, autonomy, instrumentalization, and eugenics as grounds for a five-year criminal ban on nuclear cell transfer.[21] The Council of Europe has cited threats to the "dignity and identity of all human beings" in adopting a ban on human cloning in its Convention for the Protection of Human Rights and Dignity with Regard to the Application of Biology and Medicine.[22]

Upon closer analysis, however, it appears that few of the alleged harms of cloning rise to the level of gravity and certainty needed to justify infringement of procreative or other basic liberties. Illustrative is the claim of a threat to individuality of the resulting child—the fear that he will be too identified with the DNA source to live his own life in freedom and dignity. But there are many reasons to think that this claim does not hold for the plausible uses of human cloning described above. The clone is clearly a separate and different individual with a separate identity, despite genomic similarity. In addition, genotype is not identical with phenotype, and there is no reason to expect total identity between the first- and later-born identical twin. The clone will have been gestated and reared at a different time than the clone source, and thus be more different from the clone source than identical twins are, which already is considerable. In the most plausible cloning situations, the couple choosing a source of DNA, while assigning it certain meaning or expectations, will also have interests in viewing the child as an individual in his own right, albeit one with a chosen genome.[23] In any event, whatever psychological problems presented, they would hardly constitute the wrongful life or severe compromise of welfare that would make it a harm or wrong to the child to be born in that way. Nor is the clone source's identity or dignity compromised in a significant way.[24]

Obviously much more needs to be said about the various harms of human cloning, and other selection techniques.[25] I hope that I have indicated sufficiently that claims of harm must be more carefully scrutinized than has been the case to date in the cloning debate. Given the variations in how people assign meaning to procreation, and the recognition that reproductive choices are largely reserved to individual choice, no particular view of how reproduction should occur can be imposed, if a practice otherwise implicates the key values and interests involved in reproduction. Only tangible harm to others justifies banning or greatly restricting a practice when that practice involves an exercise in fundamental liberty such as the right to reproduce. Whether human cloning poses such harm (or is even a fundamental liberty) remains to be seen. Yet a reasonable argument exists that reproductive cloning, while presenting novel variations on kinship relations, causes no more harm than the many forms of assisted reproduction and genetic selection now in use, and therefore should be treated similarly as a constitutionally protected way of forming a family.

IMPLICATIONS FOR FUTURE DEBATE

The above analysis has shown that if we take reproductive liberty seriously, as our moral, legal, and social traditions do, then a large measure of presumptive freedom to choose offspring characteristics should follow, subject to restriction or regulation to avert serious harm. If that proposition is correct, then a wide variety of genetic-selection practices, including reproductive cloning by somatic cell nuclear transfer, should also be presumptively protected. The most plausible uses of reproductive cloning are so similar to practices that enable couples or individuals to have healthy, biologically related offspring to rear that it will be difficult to deny cloning similar protected status.

An important implication of this position is that reproductive cloning should not be barred or prohibited in all circumstances—only when sufficient harm can be shown to justify the infringement of basic liberty. Although an official United States Commission, the Council of Europe, the UNESCO Bioethics Committee, and many other countries have called for a ban on human cloning, they have not presented convincing reasons for doing so. They have neglected to analyze the reproductive interests that are implicated and have rarely gone beyond slogans and generalities in identifying harm. Indeed, if a ban on cloning is justified, then a ban on many other forms of assisted reproduction and genetic selection should be as well, yet few persons are prepared to go that far. A much fuller debate and more thorough analysis of the competing interests is needed before we can determine the most desirable public policies for reproductive cloning and genetic selection generally.

A second implication is that not all attempts to clone, or to choose or select offspring characteristics, will fall within the protective canopy of procreative liberty. An important set of future issues will concern whether all uses of cloning and other selection techniques are centrally located within procreative liberty at all. Indeed, one can imagine some uses of cloning that would not deserve that protection (e.g., an entrepreneur who purchases DNA from film and sports stars, buys eggs from young women, and then hires surrogates to gestate them, with the resulting children then provided, in exchange for the expenses of production, to couples seeking children for adoption). Whether future interventions, such as non-medical genetic enhancement or intentional diminishment of offspring, will or will not be seen as part of legitimate procreative liberty, will require a much more precise and thorough analysis of procreative liberty than society has yet confronted.

A third implication of presumptive protection for cloning and genetic selection is that much closer attention must be paid to the alleged harms of these practices. It will not suffice to assert arguments of the form that "If X is done, Y *could occur.*" [26] Not only will it be necessary to establish that Y is truly harmful, but also that the probability that X will produce Y is very high indeed. Speculation about untoward effects, which have not been shown to be highly likely to occur, will not justify intrusions on fundamental liberties. They are, however, an adequate basis for action or interference if no fundamental liberty is at stake. Future work will be needed to analyze the meaning of harm, and the kinds and likelihood of harm that might legitimately justify restrictions on procreative liberty. Shibboleths about protecting human identity and dignity, and preventing the commodification or instrumentalization of children who have no other way to be born but with the technique at issue, may be much less adequate as a basis for restricting procreative choice than previously thought.

Finally, attention to rights-based arguments for reproductive cloning and other forms of genetic selection leads us to an awareness of the constitutive nature of many of the ethical, legal, and social policy choices presented. The meaning of procreative liberty, though determined in part by analogy to existing instantiations of that liberty, is not deducible in the abstract from a set of logical premises. Rather, its meaning is created and constituted by the choices that individuals and societies make in confronting the very questions of procreative liberty presented. Similarity to existing reproductive norms and practices will play a major role in that assessment, but ultimately the choice is one for individuals and societies to make anew as they confront these issues.

NOTES AND REFERENCES

1. Cloning by nuclear transfer repeats the entire nuclear genome of an individual, and does not manipulate or alter particular genes as other forms of genetic alteration might.
2. For a greatly amplified account of this argument, and its application to several different kinds of genetic selection, see John A. Robertson, "Genetic Selection of Offspring Characteristics," *Boston University Law Review,* Vol. 76 (1996), pp. 421–482.
3. *Smith v. Cote,* 513 A.2d 341 (N.H. 1986) (allowing a mother's action for wrongful birth against a physician who failed to advise her of the risk of birth defects in a fetus exposed to rubella); *Nelson v. Krusen,* 678 S.W.2d 918 (Tex. 1984) (upholding a wrongful birth suit against a physician who negligently advised a woman that she was not a carrier of a genetic disease).
4. 381 U.S. 479, 503 (1965) (striking down a Connecticut law prohibiting the use of contraceptives).
5. 405 U.S. 438, 454-55 (1972) (striking down a Massachusetts statute prohibiting unmarried persons from obtaining contraceptives).
6. 410 U.S. 113, 164-65 (1973) (upholding a woman's unqualified right to an abortion during the first trimester of her pregnancy, and permitting only reasonable state restrictions subsequent to that time and prior to viability).
7. 505 U.S. 83, 878-79 (1992) (affirming *Roe v. Wade,* but permitting state regulation of abortion so long as it does not constitute an undue burden upon a woman).
8. *Meyer v. Nebraska,* 262 U.S.390, 399 (1923) (noting that constitutional liberty includes the right of an individual "to marry, establish a home and bring up children").
9. 316 U.S. 535 (1942).
10. *Cleveland Bd. of Educ. v. LaFleur,* 414 U.S. 632, 639-40 (1973) (commenting that "freedom of personal choice in matters of marriage and family life is one of the liberties protected by the Due Process Clause of the Fourteenth Amendment); *Stanley v. Illinois,* 405, U.S. 645, 651 (1972) ("The rights to conceive and to raise one's children have been deemed 'essential,' 'basic civil right of man,' and 'rights far more...precious than property rights.'" [internal citations omitted]); *Eisenstadt v. Baird,* 405 U.S. 438, 453 (1972) (contending that "[i]f the right of privacy means anything, it is the right of the individual, married or single, to be free from unwarranted governmental intrusion into matters so fundamentally affecting a person as the decision whether to bear or beget a child").
11. For a fuller discussion of collaborative reproduction, see John A. Robertson, *Children of Choice: Freedom and the New Reproductive Technologies* (Princeton, NJ: Princeton University Press, 1994), pp. 119–145.
12. The right to have and act on information about the expected characteristics, like other reproductive rights, is a negative right against state or third-party interference. It is a right to have and use that information if one has the means to obtain it and then act on it, and not a right to have such services funded, unless one is operating in a health care or social welfare system in which infertility or other health services are substantially funded.
13. The comments that follow are based on the structure of fundamental rights in the United States, and may not be applicable in all jurisdictions.
14. See John F. Meany *et al.,* "Providers as Consumers of Prenatal Genetic Testing Services: What Do the National Data Tell Us?," *Fetal Diagnosis & Therapy,* Vol. 8 (Spring Suppl. 1993) (noting that 60% to 70% of all pregnancies in the United States are now screened in one form or another).

15. As the Supreme Court notes in *Casey*, an undue burden is determined, not by how many people are affected by a restriction, but by how substantially those affected are burdened in their ability to exercise the right. 505 U.S. 83 (1992).
16. For example, *Canterbury v. Spence*, 464 F.2d 772, 791 (D.C. Cir.), cert. denied, 409 U.S. 1064 (1972) (holding, in a landmark case on the right of a patient to receive information material to medical decision-making, that doctors disclose information that "a prudent person in the patient's position" would find material to a decision to consent to medical care); see also *Tex. Penal Code Ann.* §932.2(2) (West 1994) (stating that a person is justified in using deadly force in self-defense "if a reasonable person in the actor's situation would not have retreated").
17. See *Canterbury*, 464 F.2d at 791 (concluding that the test for the materiality of information to a patient's decision should be part objective and part subjective).
18. A more complete analysis of human cloning as an aspect of procreative liberty is found in John A. Robertson, "Liberty, Identity, and Human Cloning," *Texas Law Review*, Vol. 76 (1998); John A. Robertson, "Two Models of Human Cloning," *Hofstra Law Review* 27, pp. 604–638 (1999).
19. The resulting child would be a carrier of the trait but not himself have the disease, because mating of two carriers is necessary to produce a child with the disease.
20. See Robertson, *Children of Choice*, at 214–217, note 11 *supra*.
21. National Bioethics Advisory Commission, *Cloning Human Beings: Report and Recommendations of the National Bioethics Advisory Commission* (Rockville, Maryland, June 1997).
22. Council of Europe: Draft Additional Protocol To The Convention On Human Rights and Biomedicine On The Prohibition of Cloning Human Beings With Explanatory Report and Parliamentary Assembly Opinion (Adopted September 22, 1997), XXXVI International Legal Materials 1515 (1997).
23. Even though the chosen genome will not automatically determine all the child's characteristics or prevent the child from being an individual in his own right, it will undoubtedly have some effect. In any event, the desire to resort to cloning to found a family may reflect a desire for genetic kinship or the assurance of healthy offspring, rather than replication of the characteristics of another person as such.
24. A strong case for requiring the clone source's consent to use of her DNA can be made, even when no bodily invasion of the source has occurred.
25. The alleged harms from human cloning are analyzed in Robertson, "Liberty, Identity, and Human Cloning," note 18 *supra*.
26. The National Bioethics Advisory Commission report on human cloning is vulnerable to this criticism. See John A. Robertson, "Wrongful Life, Federalism, and Procreative Liberty: A Critique of the NBAC Cloning Report," *Jurimetrics*, Vol. 38, pp. 69–82 (1997).

Clones, Genes, and Reproductive Autonomy
The Ethics of Human Cloning

JOHN HARRIS

The Center for Social Ethics and Policy, The University of Manchester, Oxford Road, Manchester M13 9PL, England, U.K.

INTRODUCTION

The recent announcement of a birth in the press has caused a sensation probably unparalleled for two millennia and has highlighted the impact of the genetic revolution on our lives and personal choices. More importantly perhaps, it raises questions about the legitimacy of the sorts of control individuals and society purport to exercise over something which, while it must sound portentous, is nothing less than human destiny. This birth, that of "Dolly" the cloned sheep, is also illustrative of the responsibilities of science and scientists to the communities in which they live and in which they serve, and of the public anxiety that sensational scientific achievements sometimes provoke.

NUCLEAR SUBSTITUTION: THE BIRTH OF DOLLY

Dolly's birth[1] was reported in *Nature* on February 27, 1997.[2] The event caused an international sensation: President Clinton of the United States called for an investigation into the ethics of such procedures and announced a moratorium on public spending on human cloning; the British Nobel Prize winner, Joseph Rotblat, described it as science out of control, creating "a means of mass destruction"[3]; and the German newspaper *Die Welt*, evoking the Third Reich, commented: "The cloning of human beings would fit precisely into Adolph Hitler's worldview."[4]

More sober commentators were similarly panicked into instant reaction. Dr. Hiroshi Nakajima, Director General of the World Health Organization said: "WHO considers the use of cloning for the replication of human individuals to be ethically unacceptable as it would violate some of the basic principles which govern medically assisted procreation. These include respect for the dignity of the human being and protection of the security of human genetic material."[5] WHO followed up the line taken by Nakajima with a resolution of the *Fiftieth World Health Assembly,* which saw fit to affirm "that the use of cloning for the replication of human individuals is ethically unacceptable and contrary to human integrity and morality."[6] Federico Mayor of UNESCO, equally quick off the mark, commented: "Human beings must not be cloned under any circumstances. Moreover, UNESCO's International Bioethics Committee (IBC), which has been reflecting on the ethics of scientific progress, has maintained that the human genome must be preserved as [the] common heritage of humanity."[7]

The European Parliament rushed through a resolution on cloning, the preamble of which asserted (Paragraph B):

> [T]he cloning of human beings..., cannot under any circumstances be justified or tolerated by any society, because it is a serious violation of fundamental human rights and is contrary to the principle of equality of human beings as it permits a eugenic and racist selection of the human race, it offends against human dignity and it requires experimentation on humans...

It then went on to claim that (Clause 1)

> ...each individual has a right to his or her own genetic identity and that human cloning is, and must continue to be, prohibited.[8]

These statements are, perhaps unsurprisingly, thin on argument and rationale; they appear to have been plucked from the air to justify an instant reaction. There are vague references to "human rights" or "basic principles," with little or no attempt to explain what these principles are, or to indicate how they might apply to cloning. The WHO statement, for example, refers to the basic principles that govern human reproduction and singles out "respect for the dignity of the human being" and "protection of the security of genetic material." How, we are entitled to ask, is the security of genetic material compromised? Is it less secure when inserted with precision by scientists, or when spread around with the characteristic negligence of the average human male?[9]

The UNESCO approach to cloning is scarcely more coherent than that of the WHO: how does cloning affect "the preservation of the human genome as common heritage of humanity"? Cloning cannot be said to have an impact on the variability of the human genome; it merely repeats one infinitely small part of it, a part that is repeated at a natural rate of about 3.5 per thousand births.[10]

GENETIC VARIABILITY

So many of the fears expressed about cloning, and indeed about genetic engineering more generally, invoke the idea of the effect on the gene pool or upon genetic variability or assert the sanctity of the human genome as a common resource or heritage. It is very difficult to understand what is allegedly at stake here. The issue of genetic variation need not detain us long. The numbers of twins produced by cloning will always be so small compared to the human gene pool in totality, such that the effect on the variation of the human gene pool will be vanishingly small. We can say with confidence that the human genome and the human population were not threatened at the start of the present millennium in the year 1000 AD, and yet the world population was then perhaps 1% of what it is today. Natural species are usually said to be endangered when the population falls to about one thousand breeding individuals; by these standards fears for humankind and its genome may be said to have been somewhat exaggerated.[11]

The resolution of the European Parliament goes into slightly more detail; having repeated the now mandatory waft in the direction of fundamental human rights and human dignity, it actually produces an argument. It suggests that cloning violates the principal of equality, "as it permits a eugenic and racist selection of the human race." Well, so does prenatal and pre-implantation screening, not to mention egg donation, sperm donation, surrogacy, abortion and human preference in choice of sexual partner. The fact that a technique could be abused does not constitute an argument against the technique, unless there is no prospect of preventing the abuse or wrongful use. To ban cloning on the grounds that it might be used for racist purposes is tantamount to saying that sexual intercourse should be prohibited because it permits the possibility of rape.

The second principle appealed to by the European Parliament states that "each individual has a right to his or her own genetic identity." Leaving aside the inevitable contribution of mitochondrial DNA,[12] we have seen that, as in the case of natural identical twins, genetic identity is not an essential component of personal identity,[13] nor is it necessary for "individuality." Moreover, unless genetic identity is required either for personal identity, or for individuality, it is not clear why there should be a right to such a thing. But if there is, what are we to do about the rights of identical twins?

Suppose there came into being a life-threatening (or even disabling) condition that affected pregnant women and that there was an effective treatment, the only side effect of which was that it caused the embryo to divide, resulting in twins. Would the existence of the supposed right conjured up by the European Parliament mean that the therapy should be outlawed? Suppose that an effective vaccine for HIV was developed which had the effect of doubling the natural twining rate; would this be a violation of fundamental human rights? Are we to foreclose the possible benefits to be derived from human cloning on so flimsy a basis? We should recall that the natural occurrence of monozygotic (identical) twins is one in 270 pregnancies. This means that in the United Kingdom, with a population of about 58 million, more than 200 thousand such pregnancies have occurred. How are we to regard human rights violations on such a grand scale?

HUMAN DIGNITY

Typical of appeals to human dignity was that contained in the World Health Organization statement on cloning issued on March 11, 1997:

> [The] WHO considers the use of cloning for the replication of human individuals to be ethically unacceptable as it would violate some of the basic principles which govern medically assisted procreation. These include respect for the dignity of the human being...

Appeals to human dignity, are of course universally attractive; they are also comprehensively vague. A first question to ask when the idea of human dignity is invoked is: whose dignity is attacked and how? If it is the duplication of a large part of the human genome that is supposed to constitute the attack on human dignity, or where the issue of "genetic identity" is invoked, we might legitimately ask whether and how the dignity of a natural twin is threatened by the existence of her sister and what follows as to the permissibility of natural monozygotic twinning? However, the notion of human dignity is often linked to Kantian ethics and it is this link I wish to examine more closely here.

A typical example, and one that attempts to provide some basis for objections to cloning based on human dignity, was Axel Kahn's invocation of this principle in his commentary on cloning in *Nature*. Kahn, a distinguished molecular biologist, helped draft the French National Ethics Committee's report on cloning. In *Nature* Kahn states[14]:

> The creation of human clones solely for spare cell lines would, from a philosophical point of view, be in obvious contradiction to the principle expressed by Emmanuel Kant: that of human dignity. This principle demands that an individual—and I would extend this to read human life—should never be thought of as a means, but always also as an end. Creating human life for the sole purpose of preparing therapeutic material would clearly not be for the dignity of the life created.

The Kantian principle, invoked without any qualification or gloss, is seldom helpful in medical or bioscience contexts.[15] As formulated by Kahn, for example, it would surely outlaw blood transfusions. The beneficiary of blood donation, neither knowing of, nor usually caring about, the anonymous donor uses the blood (and its donor) exclusively as a means to her own ends. The recipient of blood donations does not usually know of or even care about the identity of the blood donor. The donor figures in the life of the recipient of blood exclusively as a means. The blood in the bottle has after all less identity, and is less connected with the individual from which it emanated, than the chicken "nuggets" on the supermarket shelf. An abortion performed exclusively to save the life of the mother would also, presumably, be outlawed by this principle.

INSTRUMENTALIZATION

This idea of using individuals as a means to the purposes of others is sometimes termed "instrumentalization," particularly in the European context. The "Opinion of the group of advisers on the ethical implications of biotechnology to the European Commission,"[16] for example, in its statement on "ethical aspects of cloning techniques," uses this idea repeatedly. For example, referring to reproductive human cloning (paragraph 2.6) it states: "Considerations of instrumentalization and eugenics render any such acts ethically unacceptable."

Applying this idea coherently or consistently is not easy! If someone wants to have children in order to continue his or her genetic line does that person act instrumentally? Where, as is standard practice in IVF, spare embryos are created, are these embryos created instrumentally?

Kahn responded in the journal *Nature* to these objections.[17] He reminds us, rightly, that Kant's famous principle states: "respect for human dignity requires that an individual is *never* used...*exclusively* as a means" and suggests that I have ignored the crucial use of the term "exclusively." I did not of course, and I am happy with Kahn's reformulation of the principle. It is not that Kant's principle does not have powerful intuitive force, but that it is so vague and so open to selective interpretation and its scope for application is consequently so limited, that its utility as one of the "fundamental principles of modern bioethical thought," as Kahn describes it, is virtually zero.

Kahn himself rightly points out that debates concerning the moral status of the human embryo are debates about whether embryos fall within the *scope* of Kant's or indeed any other moral principles concerning persons; so the principle itself is not illuminating in this context. Applied to the creation of individuals, which are, or will become autonomous, it has limited application. True the Kantian principle rules out slavery, but so do a range of other principles based on autonomy and rights. If you are interested in the ethics of creating people, then, so long as existence is in the created individual's own best interests, and the individual will have the capacity for autonomy like any other, then the motives for which the individual was created are either morally irrelevant or subordinate to other moral considerations. So that even where, for example, a child is engendered exclusively to provide "a son and heir" (as so often occurs in so many cultures), it is unclear how or whether Kant's principle applies. Either other motives are also attributed to the parent to square parental purposes with Kant, or the child's eventual autonomy, and its clear and substantial interest in or benefit from existence, take precedence over the comparatively trivial issue of parental motives. Either way the "fundamental principle of modern bioethical thought" is unhelpful.

It is therefore strange that Kahn and others invoke it with such dramatic assurance or how anyone could think that it applies to the ethics of human cloning. It comes down to this: either the ethics of human cloning turn on the creation or use of human embryos, in which case as Kahn himself says "in reality the debate is about the status of the human embryo" and Kant's principle must wait upon the outcome of that debate. Or, it is about the ethics of producing clones that will become autonomous human persons. In this latter case, as David Shapiro also comments,[18] the ethics of their creation are, from a Kantian perspective, not dissimilar to other forms of assisted reproduction, or, as I have suggested, to the ethics of the conduct of parents concerned exclusively with producing an heir, or preserving their genes or, as is sometimes alleged, making themselves eligible for public housing. Debates about whether these are *exclusive* intentions can never be definitively resolved.

Kahn then produces a bizarre twist to the argument from autonomy. Kahn defines autonomy as "the indeterminability of the individual with respect to external human will" and identifies it as one of the components of human dignity. This is of course hopeless as a definition of autonomy: those in a persistent vegetative state (PVS), and indeed all newborns, would on such a view have to count as autonomous! However Kahn then asserts: "The birth of an infant by asexual reproduction would lead to a new category of people whose bodily form and genetic make-up would be exactly as decided by other humans. This would lead to the establishment of an entirely new type of relationship between the "created" and the "creator" which has obvious implications for human dignity. Kahn is, I'm afraid, wrong on both counts. As Robert Winston has noted: "[E]ven if straight cloning techniques were used, the mother would contribute important constituents—her mitochondrial genes, intrauterine influences and subsequent nurture."[19] These, together with the other influences, would prevent exact determination of bodily form and genetic identity. For example, differences in environment, age, and number of years between clone and cloned would all come into play.

Lenin's embalmed body lies in its mausoleum in Moscow. Presumably a cell of this body could be de-nucleated and Lenin's genome cloned. Could such a process make Lenin immortal and allow us to create someone whose bodily form and genetic makeup, not to mention his character and individuality, would be "exactly as decided by other human beings"? I hope the answer is obvious. Vladimir Ilyich Ulyanov was born on April 10, 1870 in the town of Simbirsk on the Volga. It is this person who became and who is known to most of us as V.I. Lenin. Even with this man's genome preserved intact we will never see Lenin again. So many of the things that made Vladimir Ilyich what he was cannot be reproduced even if his genome can. We cannot recreate pre-Revolutionary Russia. We cannot simulate Lenin's environment and education. We cannot recreate his parents to bring him up and influence his development as profoundly as they undoubtedly did. We cannot make the thought of Karl Marx seem as hopeful as it must then have done. We cannot, in short, do anything but reproduce his genome and that could never be nearly enough. It may be that "manners maketh man," but genes most certainly do not.

Autonomy, as we know from monozygotic twins, is unaffected by close similarity of bodily form and matching genome. The "indeterminability of the individual with respect to external human will" will remain unaffected by cloning. Where then are the obvious implications for human dignity?

When Kahn asks: "Is Harris announcing the emergence of a revisionist tendency in bioethical thinking?" the answer must be, rather I am pleading for the emergence of "bioethical *thinking*" as opposed to the empty rhetoric of invoking resonant principles with no conceivable or coherent application to the problem at hand.

Clearly the birth of Dolly and the possibility of human equivalents has left many people feeling not a little uneasy, if not positively queasy at the prospect. It is perhaps salutary to remember that there is no necessary connection between phenomena, attitudes, or actions that make us uneasy, or even those that disgust us, and those phenomena, attitudes, and actions that there are good reasons for judging unethical. Nor does it follow that those things we are confident *are* unethical must be prohibited by legislation or controlled by regulation. These are separate steps, which require separate arguments.

PROCREATIVE AUTONOMY

We have examined the arguments for and against permitting the cloning of human individuals. At the heart of these questions is the issue of whether or not people have rights to control their reproductive destiny and, so far as they can do so without violating the rights of others or threatening society, to choose their own procreative path. We have seen that it has been claimed that cloning violates principles of human dignity. We will conclude by briefly examining an approach that suggests that *failing* to permit cloning might violate principles of dignity.

The American philosopher and legal theorist, Ronald Dworkin, has outlined the arguments for a right to what he calls "procreative autonomy" and has defined this right as "a right to control their own role in procreation unless the state has a compelling reason for denying them that control."[20] Arguably, freedom to clone one's own genes might also be defended as a dimension of procreative autonomy because so many people and agencies have been attracted by the idea of the special nature of genes and have linked the procreative imperative to the genetic imperative.

> The right of procreative autonomy follows from any competent interpretation of the due process clause and of the Supreme Court's past decisions applying it... . The First Amendment prohibits government from establishing any religion, and it guarantees all citizens free exercise of their own religion. The Fourteenth Amendment, which incorporates the First Amendment, imposes the same prohibition and same responsibility on states. These provisions also guarantee the right of procreative autonomy.[21]

The point is that the sorts of freedoms that freedom of religion guarantees, freedom to choose one's own way of life and live according to one's most deeply held beliefs, are also at the heart of procreative choices. And Dworkin concludes:

> ...that no one may be prevented from influencing the shared moral environment, through his own private choices, tastes, opinions, and example, just because these tastes or opinions disgust those who have the power to shut him up or lock him up.[22]

Thus it may be that we should be prepared to accept both some degree of offence and some social disadvantages as a price we should be willing to pay in order to protect freedom of choice in matters of procreation and perhaps this applies to cloning as much as to more straightforward or usual procreative preferences.[23]

The nub of the argument is complex and abstract but it is worth stating at some length. I cannot improve upon Dworkin's formulation of it.

> The right of procreative autonomy has an important place...in Western political culture more generally. The most important feature of that culture is a belief [in] individual human dignity: that people have the moral right—and the moral responsibility—to confront the most fundamental questions about the meaning and value of their own lives for themselves, answering to their own consciences and convictions....The principle of procreative autonomy, in a broad sense, is embedded in any genuinely democratic culture.[24]

The rationale that animated the principle of procreative autonomy was made the subject of a submission to the United States Court of Appeals by Ronald Dworkin and a group of other prominent philosophers. Their submission was in a case concerning voluntary euthanasia and it is interesting because it cites a number of United States Supreme Court decisions and their rationales:

> Certain decisions are momentous in their impact on the character of a person's life decisions about religious faith, political and moral allegiance, marriage, procreation and death, for example. Such deeply personal decisions reflect controversial questions about how and why human life has value. In a free society, individuals must be allowed to make those decisions for themselves, out of their own faith, conscience and convictions. This Court has insisted, in a variety of contexts and circumstances, that this great freedom is among those protected by the Due Process Clause as essential to a community of "ordered liberty." *Palko v. Connecticut*, 302 U.S. 319, 325 (1937).

> In its recent decision in *Planned Parenthood v. Casey*, 505 U.S. 833, 851 (1992), the Court offered a paradigmatic statement of that principle: ...matters involving the most intimate and personal choices a person may make in a lifetime, choices central to a person's dignity and autonomy are central to the liberty protected by the Fourteenth Amendment.

> As the Court explained in *West Virginia State Board of Education v. Barnette*, 319 U.S. 624, 642 (1943): If there is any fixed star in our constitutional constellation, it is that no official can prescribe what shall be orthodox in politics, nationalism, religion, or other matters of opinion or force citizens to confess by word or act their faith therein.

> Interpreting the religion clauses of the First Amendment, this Court has explained that "the victory for freedom of thought recorded in our Bill of Rights recognizes that in the domain of conscience there is a moral power higher than the State." *Girouard v. United States*, 328 U.S. 61, 68 (1946).

> And, in a number of Due Process cases, this Court has protected this conception of autonomy by carving out a sphere of personal family life that is immune from government intrusion. See e.g., *Cleveland Bd. of Educ. v. LeFleur*, 414 U.S. 632, 639 (1974) ("This Court has long recognized that freedom of personal choice in matters of marriage and family life is one of the liberties protected by the Due Process Clause of the Fourteenth Amendment."); *Eisenstadt v. Baird*, 405 U.S. 438, 453 (1973) (recognizing right "to be free from unwarranted governmental intrusion into matters so fundamentally affecting a person as the decision to bear and beget a child");

> *Skinner v. Oklahoma,* 316 U.S. 535, 541 (1942) (holding unconstitutional a state statute requiring the sterilization of individuals convicted of three offenses, in large part because the state's actions unwarrantedly intruded on marriage and procreation, "one of the basic civil rights of man");
>
> *Loving v. Virginia,* 388 U.S. 1, 12 (1967) (striking down the criminal prohibition of interracial marriages as an infringement of the right to marry and holding that "the freedom to marry has long been recognized as one of the vital personal rights essential to the orderly pursuit of happiness by free men").[25]
>
> These decisions recognize as constitutionally immune from state intrusion that realm in which individuals make "intimate and personal" decisions that define the very character of their lives.

In so far as decisions to reproduce in particular ways or even using particular technologies constitute decisions concerning central issues of value, then arguably the freedom to make them is guaranteed by the constitution (written or not) of any democratic society, unless the state has a compelling reason for denying them that control. To establish such a compelling reason the state (or indeed a federation or union of states, like the European Union for example) would have to show that more was at stake than the fact that a majority found the ideas disturbing or even disgusting.

As yet, in the case of human cloning, such compelling reasons have not been produced. Suggestions have been made, but have not been sustained, that human dignity may be compromised by the techniques of cloning. Dworkin's arguments suggest that human dignity and indeed democratic constitutions may be compromised by attempts to limit procreative autonomy, at least where greater values cannot be shown to be thereby threatened. This paper has argued that no remotely plausible arguments exist as to how human cloning might pose significant dangers or threats or that it may compromise important human values. It has shown that there is a *prima facie* case for regarding human cloning as a dimension of procreative autonomy that should not be lightly restricted.

NOTES AND REFERENCES

1. Some of the material in this paper was presented to the UNDP/WHO/World Bank Special Programme of Research, Development and Research Training in Human Reproduction Review Group Meeting, Geneva (25 April 1997) and to a hearing on cloning held by the European Parliament in Brussels (7 May 1997). I am grateful to participants at these events for many stimulating insights. I must also thank Justine Burley, Christopher Graham and Pedro Lowenstein for many constructive comments. The issues raised by cloning were discussed in a special issue of the *Kennedy Institute of Ethics Journal,* Vol. 4, No. 3 (September 1994) and in my *Wonderwoman and Superman: The Ethics of Human Biotechnology* (Oxford: Oxford University Press, 1992), especially Chapter 1. Versions of the ideas expressed here have appeared in my "Goodbye Dolly: The Ethics of Human Cloning," *The Journal of Medical Ethics,* Vol. 23, No. 6, 353–361, and in my "Cloning and Human Dignity," *Cambridge Quarterly of Healthcare Ethics,* Vol. 7 (1998), pp. 163–167. Readers will note that this is a modified and abbreviated version of my "Clones, Genes and Human Rights," which appeared in Justine Burley (Ed.), *The Genetic Revolution and Human Rights* (Oxford: Oxford University Press, 1998), pp. 61–95. My participation in the meeting that gave rise to this volume was made possible by a generous grant by The British Council.
2. Wilmut *et al.* "Viable Offspring Derived from Fetal and Adult Mammalian Cells," *Nature* (27 February 1997).
3. *The Guardian* (26 February 1997).

4. Reported in *The Guardian* (28 February 1997).
5. WHO Press Release (WHO/20 11 March 1997).
6. WHO document (WHA50.37 14 May 1997), despite the findings of a Meeting of the Scientific and Ethical Review Group (see note 1), which recommended that "the next step should be a thorough exploration and fuller discussion of the [issues]."
7. UNESCO Press Release No. 97-29.
8. The European Parliament, Resolution on Cloning, Motion dated 11 March 1997. Passed 13 March 1997.
9. Perhaps the sin of Onan was to compromise the security of his genetic material?
10. It is unlikely that "artificial" cloning would ever approach such a rate on a global scale and we could, of course, use regulative mechanisms to prevent this without banning the process entirely. I take this figure of the rate of natural twinning from Keith L Moore and T.V.N. Persaud, *The Developing Human* (Philadelphia: W.B. Saunders, 1993), 5th ed. The rate mentioned is 1 per 270 pregnancies.
11. Of course if *all* people were compulsorily sterilized and reproduced only by cloning, genetic variation would become fixed at current levels. This would halt the evolutionary process. How bad or good *this* would be could only be known if the course of future evolution and its effects could be accurately predicted.
12. Mitochondrial DNA individualizes the genotype even of clones to some extent.
13. Although, of course, there would be implications for criminal justice since clones could not be differentiated by so called "genetic fingerprinting" techniques
14. Axel Kahn "Clone Mammals...Clone Man," *Nature*, Vol. 386 (13 March 1997), p. 119.
15. See my "Is Cloning an Attack on Human Dignity," *Nature*, Vol. 387, 754 (19 June 1997).
16. *Opinion of the Group of Advisers on the Ethical Implications of Biotechnology to the European Commission* No 9 (28 May 1997). Rapporteur: Dr. Anne McClaren.
17. Axel Kahn, *Nature*, Vol. 388, 320 (24 July 1997).
18. *Nature,* Vol. 388, 511 (7 August 1997).
19. Robert Winston, *British Medical Journal,* Vol. 314 (1997), pp. 913–914.
20. Ronald Dworkin *Life's Dominion* (London: Harper & Collins, 1993), p. 148.
21. Ronald Dworkin, *Life's Dominion,* p. 160.
22. Ronald Dworkin *Freedom's Law* (Oxford: Oxford University Press, 1996), pp. 237–238.
23. Ronald Dworkin has produced an elegant account of the way the price we should be willing to pay for freedom might or might not be traded off against the costs. See his *Taking Rights Seriously* (London: Duckworth, 1977), chapt. 10 and his *A Matter of Principle* (Cambridge, MA: Harvard University Press, 1985), chapt. 17.
24. Ronald Dworkin, *Life's Dominion,* pp. 166-167.
25. *State of Washington et al. Petitioners, v Harold Glucksberg et al., Respondents; Dennis C. Vacco, Attorney General of New York, et al., Petitioners, v. Timothy E. Quill, et al.,* Respondents. Nos. 5-1858, 96-110 (10 December 1996). Brief for Ronald Dworkin, Thomas Nagel, Robert Nozick, John Rawls, Thomas Scanlon and Judith Jarvis Thomson as *amici curiae* in support of respondents.

Genetic Research
Conversation across Cultures

JOAN McIVER GIBSON

Director, Health Sciences Ethics Program, #368 Nursing/Pharmacy Building, University of New Mexico, Albuquerque, New Mexico 87131, USA

INTRODUCTION

Pneumatic tubes might be effective vehicles for mechanically transporting written messages from sender to receiver. They are, however, woefully inadequate metaphors for communication and understanding. Nevertheless the belief persists that good communication requires detailed, content-driven packaging, that a linear, one-directional conduit is up to the task, and that the receiver merely needs to be willingly open and able to receive the pre-packaged message. Nowhere is the pneumatic tube approach to communication and understanding more set than in the theory and practice of informed consent. And nowhere does communication fail more thoroughly than with informed consent.

This paper will focus on communication and understanding within the context of medical treatment and research, specifically informed consent for genetic research across diverse populations. In the United States we voice concern about the effect of others' culture and ethnicity on *their* attitudes toward research. Such reflection, however, reveals more about communication generally, about ways to create shared understanding that cut across populations, and about the inadequacy of our word-heavy manner of creating and expressing meaning within our own groups, where we assume there are few if any cultural influences, let alone barriers. Several years ago a Navajo woman remarked to me, as we were discussing cross-cultural issues in advance directives: "Too many words. You white people think that if you use enough words you'll understand what is happening. Have you ever tried listening to silence?"

INFORMED CONSENT, AUTONOMY, AND MONOLOGUE

The report of the U.S. President's Advisory Committee on Human Radiation Experiments[1] urges researchers and the public alike to remain vigilant in insisting that valid and effective informed consent be obtained. How best to do this remains unaddressed. The current enthusiasm for research, especially genetic research on populations and culturally or ethnically homogeneous groups, affords us the opportunity to revisit the philosophy and practice of informed consent in light of contemporary communication theory. This is not, in my opinion, an exercise only for historians, philosophers, and lawyers. Interested individuals generally, as well as population groups as a whole (i.e., potential subjects) will certainly become more involved in the identification, design, and conduct of research protocols involving human subjects. Their power to sanction such research—as well as their willingness to do so—will likewise grow. I submit that there exists a social franchise that scientists and medical researchers must maintain: they need the public's trust and understanding for their research to proceed. Without these, continuing research is jeopardized, as demonstrated by public reaction to recent disclosures about cloning, banking of DNA, and cell line research.

Americans of Anglo-Saxon and Western European heritage worship at the altar of autonomy. For us, rights and duties repose in individuals, and we are forever struggling to understand and establish connections and relationships with other rights-bearing individuals. Such individualism drives our approach to communication, and informed consent, in its philosophical, legal, clinical, and research manifestations, provides us a paradigm, if not a caricature, of how meaning is created and expressed—though not necessarily shared—through soliloquy and monologue. In a soliloquy the speaker reveals her/his *own* thoughts and concerns. A monologue is a protracted speech by only one person. Informed consent as it has evolved in the United States discourages genuine conversation and dialogue, especially in health care and research settings. Its increasingly legal and formal functions focus mainly on content and the written word, rather than on shared understanding. I suspect this is the case for reasons more fundamental and troublesome than simply the hurried pace of the health care environment, or even the fear of liability. Informed consent as it is commonly administered, at least in the United States, rests on a uniquely a-contextual, monologic approach to the creation and communication of meaning that continues to dominate the philosophical, legal and scientific literature.

As others look to adopt our informed consent procedures for permission to treat or to enroll research subjects, I invite them to pause and reflect on how it is we really do create and share meaning. In America we have much to learn from others, both within and outside our borders, where individuals acquire rights, duties, and identity from their community (not vice versa), where genuine dialogue is a fixture of professional, social, and public discourse, and where listening is more than waiting to talk. Medical ethics in the 21st century, especially in the United States, will pay more attention to the role of family, community, and society in matters of medicine, research and policy. How to bind individuals and diverse groups in community is the work of the 21st century. We have a ways to go.

The influence of individualism on the evolution of informed consent in medicine and research is strong. The term "self-determination" appeared in the early part of the 20th century to describe the duty to obtain a patient's consent.[2] The Nuremberg Code begins: "The voluntary consent of the human subject is absolutely essential."[3] "Informed consent" as a term first appeared in 1957; the first serious discussion around it occurred in 1972, and in 1982 the U.S. President's Commission for the Study of Ethical Problems in Medicine and Biomedical and Behavioral Research, "…held that informed consent is ultimately based on the principle that competent persons are entitled to make their own decisions from their own values and goals, but that the context of informed consent and any claim of 'valid consent' must derive from active, shared decision making. The principle of self-determination was described as the 'bedrock of the commission's viewpoint.'"[5]

In Israel, the recently developed **Patients' Rights Act of 1996** mirrors this commitment to self-determination. The Act begins with: "This Act aims to establish the rights of every person who requests medical care or who is in receipt of medical care, and to protect his dignity and privacy."[6] As in the United States, dignity, privacy and respect for persons are paramount. What begs for attention is how to promote "active, shared decision making."

Informed consent in scientific and medical communication has focused more on formal ethical and legal requirements and less on the way in which people actually communicate, that, is, create, express, and share meaning. Procedure has trumped process. Despite the best efforts of Institutional Review Boards, it is questionable whether informed consent is really, commonly accomplished. G. Kent, in "Shared understandings for informed consent: the relevance of psychological research on the provision of information"[7] observes that information rarely is provided in a way that subjects can understand, that the language used to describe risks and benefits is almost always ambiguous, and that there is a real need for those who understand the concepts and content to work with those who understand psychology and process.

METAPHORS AND DIALOGUE

Let us return to the pneumatic tube metaphor, or, as Lakoff and Johnson in *Metaphors We Live By*[8] characterize the language we use to explain language, the "conduit metaphor," where ideas (or meanings) are objects, linguistic expressions are containers, and communication is sending. "The speaker puts ideas (objects) into words (containers) and sends them (along a conduit) to a hearer who takes the idea/objects out of the word/containers."[9] Implicit in the conduit metaphor are the assumptions that words and sentences have meanings in themselves, independent of any context or speaker, and that meanings have existence independent of people and contexts.[10] This certainly captures a common assumption we hold while attempting to design the perfect consent form. If only we might package the meaning of the research (the *researcher's* meaning, of course), and format it according to the template of risks and benefits—leaving nothing out—then the conditions for effective communication are largely met.

Lakoff and Johnson suggest an alternate account of effective communication, what they refer to as the "experientialist myth"—an explanation which I argue comports more closely with how we actually construct and convey meaning. "Within the experientialist myth, understanding emerges from interaction, from constant negotiation with the environment and other people."[11] A physician colleague once explained: "I tell my patients and their families that understanding is created and decisions made in the spaces between us." In reality there is no self-executing consent form to explain either medical treatment or a research protocol. Context and the "situatedness" of all the involved parties requires designing and implementing a process that goes beyond the content and form of the consent.

Conversations across cultures likewise call for negotiation. Lakoff and Johnson continue:

> To negotiate meaning with someone, you have to become aware of and respect both the differences in your backgrounds and when these differences are important.... Metaphorical imagination is a crucial skill in creating rapport and in communicating the nature of unshared experience.... Problems of mutual understanding are not exotic; they arise in all extended conversations where understanding is important.... When the chips are down, meaning is negotiated: you slowly figure out what you have in common, what it is safe to talk about, how you can communicate unshared experience or

create a shared vision. With enough flexibility in bending your world view and with luck and skill and charity, you may achieve some mutual understanding." [12]

Applying contemporary narrative theory to informed consent[13] yields yet another perspective on communication between physician and patient, between researcher and subject, where monologue is the typical pattern of speech. M. Bakhtim describes the effects of strict monologism as follows: "Ultimately, *monologism* denies that there exists outside of it another consciousness, with the same rights, and capable of responding on an equal footing, another equal *I(Thou)*. For a monologic outlook (in its extreme or pure form), the 'other' remains entirely and only an *object* of consciousness. No response capable of altering everything in the world of my consciousness is expected of this other. The monologue is accomplished and deaf to the other's response; it does not await it and it does not grant it any *decisive* force. Monologue makes do without the other; that is why to some extent it objectifies all reality. Monologue pretends to be the *last word*."[14] This otherwise literary description aptly captures the dilemma for the researcher, who has been trained to think objectively and yet needs to communicate with potential subjects in a way that is clearly *intersubjective*. Subjects rarely are given the opportunity to both "tell their story" and be heard, thus making and reflecting back their own sense of the information communicated. Even when subjects do respond, their narratives are routinely cut short and interpreted by the listener's (i.e., the researcher or the researcher's deputy) own historical stance. And there is no interpretation without blind spots. This is the challenge for informed consent: is there a spot or place within the subject's text from which scientists and researchers regularly avert their gaze? I submit that there is, and it is not a uniquely cross-cultural phenomenon.

Regardless of culture, status or profession, research has *meaning* for both the researcher and subject alike, and the meaning of the research (especially genetic research) provokes an emotional response to the perceived value of such research. Ideas that matter give rise to feelings. Martha Nussbaum observes: "Our cognitive activity...centrally involves emotional response. We discover what we think about these events partly by noticing how we feel.... Emotional response can sometimes not be just a *means* to practical knowledge, but a constituent part of the best sort of recognition of one's practical situation." [15] We place great emphasis on packaging and sending the meaning of the research from the perspective of the researcher. Seldom if ever does the meaning for the subject play a role in the design of either the research project or the consent process.

Our recent work on advance directives within and across cultures, where we examine how best to clarify for ourselves and others what matters to us with respect to medical treatment, reveals the primacy of context and dialogue in creating and communicating meaning and value. A principlist approach to clinical decision making, where moral principles are considered to be self-evident and self-executing in specific situations, ignores other determinative factors. Roles, relationships and process matter and literally constitute *de novo* situation-specific values. Each of us inhabits multiple roles which organize and weight our values differently in different situations. In any given situation, the connection between the involved persons, as well as power differences, play a part in organizing values. And process, the manner and company in which we reflect, talk, and approach decision making, affects the outcome, as well as whose voice and values are heard, and whose are not.

Clearly there is a general failure to align the informed consent process with what we know about how people actually communicate and share information; there is failure across the board to consult with subjects—especially with diverse populations—who serve as collective subjects, about *their* views of a successful consent process; rarely do we use such information, when we have it, in designing and tailoring informed consent forms and processes to the population at hand; and we have only begun to inquire of different groups and communities what values are important to them with respect to the content and prospects of genetic research.

WHAT WE HAVE LEARNED

In New Mexico we have begun to talk with individuals and their communities about informed consent and genetic research. The following questions have been suggested as ways to help create a better understanding of what matters to potential subjects as well as to researchers. What we do with the answers remains to be seen.

1. What are the features of an effective informed consent for different individuals and groups? To what extent have potential subjects and/or their communities been involved in designing the consent forms and process? Is consent for a given group best accomplished through negotiation or full participation? How are levels of trust established/diminished?

2. How effective are existing models of consent? Consider the following excerpts from the Department of Energy/National Center for Human Genomic Research (DOE/NCGHR), which strongly encourages researchers to use similar, if not the same language and format when seeking consent for cell line research and DNA banking. Currently the Navajo Nation is radically revising this consent. What values are communicated in the following form? Which ones that might matter are omitted?

CONSENT FOR USE OF [TISSUE] SAMPLES TO MAKE A CELL LINE AND A DNA LIBRARY FOR THE HUMAN GENOME PROJECT

This research is part of the Human Genome Project, the principal goal of which is to map and sequence all of the genes contained in human DNA. You are being asked to provide samples of ____ [tissue] to create a "cell line" and a "library" of DNA to be used in research as part of the Human Genome Project. This form describes the research that will be done and what providing samples would mean, so that you can decide whether or not you want to donate samples. The choice is completely up to you.

What we will do with your [tissue] samples, what they will be used for, and who will use them. We will divide your sample into two parts. We will take cells from one part of your sample and treat them so that they become a permanent "line," which means that they can be grown in the laboratory whenever they are needed. [**N.B.:** In case of sperm donors, thislanguage will obviously need to be changed to indicate that a blood sample will also be taken in order to construct a cell line.] Creating a cell line will allow us to have a source of your DNA to use for research in the future, without having to come back to you to ask for another [tissue] sample.

From the other part of your [tissue] sample, we will isolate the DNA and prepare it for "cloning," which means making multiple copies of it. To do this, we will cut the DNA up into pieces. These pieces will then be joined with a "vector," which is a kind of DNA that allows your DNA to be grown in a [host] and to make millions of copies, or clones, of each piece. The collection of all of the cloned pieces of your DNA is known as a "clone library." The library we make will consist of a complete collection of all your genetic material.

Clone libraries, like the one we will make from your [tissue] are very useful for genetic research. At present, clone libraries are used for two purposes. One is to map genes, which means finding out on which chromosome, and where on that chromosome, an individual gene is located. The second is to determine the sequence of the bases in those genes, which means finding out how the DNA sentences (genes) are spelled; this process is called DNA sequencing. In the future, the clone libraries may be used for other types of research.

Because of its usefulness, the clone library we plan to construct from your DNA will be shared with researchers around the world for gene mapping and DNA sequencing research. Some of these researchers work in universities and research institutions; others work in commercial organizations. The results of the mapping and sequencing of genes carried out by the Human Genome Project will be put in databases that are available to the public. Other results, particularly those obtained by researchers from commercial organizations, may not be made public but may make important contributions to the development of useful medicines, diagnostic tests, and other products that will be available to the public. It is also possible that some companies may restrict the use of the information they obtain to those who pay a licensing or royalty fee....

Risks of allowing your [tissue] to be used to create a cell line and a DNA library. [The risks of providing blood samples are those associated with drawing blood, namely, pain or bruising at the site as well as a very small possibility of infection.] The actual process of providing sperm poses no health risks.] There are, however, some other risks of providing [tissue] for this project that you should know about that could occur in the unlikely event that your identity were to become known.

Although every effort will be made to ensure that this does not happen, someone may find out that you are donating [tissue] for this project. There has been public interest in whose DNA is being sequenced in the Human Genome Project. If someone found out that you are one of the DNA donors, representatives of the media or other people might want to interview you or represent you. Some people are opposed to this type of research and may criticize you for your participation. These responses could be embarrassing or annoying to you.

Other things could happen if someone found out which DNA sequences were obtained from your DNA, particularly if one or more of the sequences showed a mutation or change in the DNA that caused or predisposed you to have a particular disease. If your particular DNA sequence were to become known: You could be distressed if you found out about a risk of illness that you had not known about before; you might have a harder time than you otherwise would have had in getting or keeping a job or health insurance if you were found to have a disease-causing or disease-promoting mutation. Some laws have already been enacted, and others are being considered, that attempt to protect people from such job and insurance discrimination. You should know, however, that the laws that are currently in place do not provide people with complete protection from being discriminated against on the basis of their genetic information.

There may be other risks that we do not yet know about. This makes it hard to say for sure whether any new risks may arise in the future.

Optional: [Payment for your donation. You will be paid $_____ when you provide a [tissue] sample for your time and inconvenience. To help protect your confidentiality, you will not get checks directly from the [investigator's institution]; rather, [consent/contact person] will pay you out of a separate fund.]

Compensation for your contribution and for any injuries that may result from your participation. If you suffer from unwanted media attention, emotional distress, or discrimination in the unlikely event that your identity or genetic makeup became known in the absence of negligence or malfeasance, you will not be compensated (by [the investigator], by the [investigator's home institution], by the [Department of Energy/National Center for Human Genome Research], or by any other person or entity that is using or storing the DNA for sequencing the human genome.)

Below is a replica of the consent form:

I AGREE TO THE USE OF DNA OBTAINED FROM MY [TISSUE] TO CREATE A CLONE LIBRARY TO BE DISTRIBUTED FOR RESEARCH. THIS CONSENT APPLIES ONLY TO THE SAMPLES I PROVIDE NOW.

I HAVE READ THIS FORM AND UNDERSTAND THE POSSIBLE CONSEQUENCES FOR ME AND MY FAMILY OF ALLOWING MY DNA TO BE USED IN THIS WAY. I UNDERSTAND THAT, WHILE I AM FREE TO DECIDE IN THE FUTURE THAT I NO LONGER WANT MY DNA TO BE USED, THERE ARE SIGNIFICANT LIMITATIONS ON MY ABILITY TO PREVENT FUTURE USE.

I HAVE HAD MY CONCERNS AND QUESTIONS ADDRESSED AND KNOW THAT I CAN ASK MORE QUESTIONS IF THEY COME UP. I HAVE BEEN GIVEN A COPY OF THIS FORM FOR MY FUTURE REFERENCE.

_____ [*signature*]

_____[*witness*]

_____ [*date*]

****

There are further questions that need to be considered:

3. What are the values (interests, hopes, fears) associated with genetic research—from the viewpoint of the subjects? the community? the researchers? What are the foreseeable effects on individuals? families? populations?

4. What are the issues of privacy and confidentiality around future uses of tissue? How do people's self-concepts of body and identity affect their willingness to participate in such research?

5. What are the issues surrounding population-based research as distinct from individual studies and how well do subjects (individuals as well as communities) understand the difference?

6. What is the relationship between religious beliefs and the meaning of genetic research in the eyes of the participants? The sacredness of body tissue is an important issue for many.

7. What should the role of individuals and their communities be in the initial protocol design and plans for implementation?   William L. Freeman, M.D., M.P.H., Chair of the Indian Health Service IRB, writes, "Research is a valued activity that should be nurtured, and ... research is dependent upon the good will of the society that funds it and the communities and volunteer participants with whom it takes place. Research is not an autonomous activity by autonomous researchers, but is an activity interdependent with community-partners and individual volunteer-partners."[16]

Genetic research enjoys perhaps the highest profile of any research currently being conducted, and its reach into and across population groups is expanding. Human genetic research is the study of genetic factors (and the interaction of such factors with the environment), responsible for human traits, both normal and abnormal, including the identification of all genes composing the human genome, the gene functions, and the characterization of normal and disease conditions in individuals, families, and populations.[17] Of international and cross-cultural importance is the Human Genome Diversity Project (HGD). In the Introduction to the North American Regional Committee/Human Genome Diversity Project's "Model Ethical Protocol for Collecting DNA Samples,"[18] the HGD is introduced as an

> ...international effort to collect, preserve, analyze, and make genetic and ethnographic information from all people around the world. The project expects that its work will lead to advances in understanding the biological development and the history of our species and, ultimately, in understanding the treating many diseases with genetic components. The Project will collect DNA samples and ethnographic information from communities throughout the world, thus correcting the current bias in research in human genetics toward people of European descent. The Project expects that the samples will be preserved in repositories where they will be available to all qualified researchers.[20]

In my home state of New Mexico, Navajo and northern New Mexico Hispanic communities are populations of real interest to the HGD project. Research has shown[19] that Amerindians and Hispanics share a common historical, cultural, and genetic background. The historical/genetic relationship between Hispanics and Amerindians regionally provides a very powerful scientific tool, and also means that findings in one group can also be usefully applied to related populations. As we trace the roots of various population groups, shared features rather than differences may turn out to be the more striking motif. We have not, however, adequately involved these groups in the design of either the research or the consent protocols.

Canada has recognized that research with indigenous or native groups must consider the present and future effects of research on the group as a whole. The Tri-Council's Code of Conduct for Research Involving Humans contains the following articles:

— 13.5 The researcher must seek to protect the members of the collectivity, and the collectivity itself from harm. Where this is not possible, the researcher must clearly inform the collectivity of the harms involved.

— 13.6 When undertaking research with a family, community or other collectivity, the researcher may not begin until permission has been obtained from the appropriate authorities for that collectivity. Furthermore, obtaining group *and* individual consent before beginning any research involving a collectivity, or its members, must be regarded as a minimum requirement. Permission from the community as well as effects of research on the group as a whole are key considerations when designing and carrying out such research.

Equally important is the *meaning* of such research to the subjects themselves. For many groups, the specimens used to collect DNA such as hair, blood, mucus, and other tissues are considered to be sacred and remain so even after collection. It is important that subjects who hold such beliefs be involved in approving research protocols. Freeman offers the following table to illustrate the continuum of passivity to active involvement of subjects with respect to research.[20] It challenges researchers who profess commitment to "shared decision making."

> Six conceptual levels of the researcher–community relationship are arranged along a continuum, from the researcher using a group and its people that are passive, to full partnership involving the group and the researcher, to the group itself initiating part of the research.
>
> 'Bleed and run,' 'safari,' or 'helicopter' research—the researchers drop into the group, do the research or obtain the specimens, and then leave with the tissues and data for good. The group and its members are passive.[20]
>
> The researcher comes back, to report the research results to the group, which still remains relatively passive when it receives the report.
>
> The group negotiates with the researchers so that they arrange for more services as a *quid pro quo* for doing the research in or with the group.
>
> The researchers increase the competence and capacity of the group's or of some of its members, i.e., improves the capabilities of the group to deliver services or do research. The group exercises that expanded competence and capacity.
>
> The group and researchers are partners in the design, execution, analysis, and reporting of the research. (The group's resources and ideas often make the research succeed.) The group and its members are quite active and pro-active.
>
> The group determines its research priorities and initiates the research. It calls in researchers as needed to be partners/consultants in the design, execution, analysis, and reporting of the research. The research is the group's.

CONCLUSION

While basic scientists as well as medical researchers may share a similar level of understanding and enthusiasm for genetic research, the same cannot be said for many groups and individuals around the world. In the United States where our worship of autonomy and individual rights is legendary, we have high hopes for informed consent as the mechanism-of-choice to insure that potential subjects participate in shared decision making. Generally we fail. We do not understand the intrinsically dialogic nature of communication. We train our professionals to speak in monologue, thereby foreclosing on any possibility that there is a conscious "other," who must be heard, who is a constitutive participant in any consent process, and whose values and context inevitably shape the exchange as much as those of the researcher. We have begun to explore the power and utility of narrative in clinical encounters. I propose we extend this to informed consent in research arenas. We fail to appreciate the contextual nature of the decision-making environment, especially for individuals and cultures where community identity, not the individual, comes first.

Genetic research, such as stem cell line research and the creation of DNA libraries, will require much greater support from the public than currently exists. We must mount an educational effort that listens as much as it speaks, that fosters collaboration across cultures, among nations, with indigenous populations, among scientists, and that regularly tests the strength of research's social franchise with the general public and with the research subjects themselves.

NOTES AND REFERENCES

1. "Executive Summary and Guide to Final Report," *The Final Report of the Advisory Committee on Human Radiation Experiments* (1995).
2. *Schloendorff v. New York Hospital* (1914).
3. Germany (Territory Under Allied Occupation, 1945–1955: US. Zone) Military Tribunals. 1947. "Permissible Medical Experiments," in *Trials of War Criminals Before the Nuremberg Tribunals Under Control Law,* No. 10, pp. 81–84.
4. T. Beauchamp and R. Faden, "History of Informed Consent," in Warren Thomas Reich (Ed.), *Encyclopedia of Bioethics,* Vol. 3 (New York: Simon and Schuster Macmillan, 1995), p. 1232.
5. Beauchamp and Faden, "History of Informed Consent," p. 1237.
6. *Patients' Rights Act, 1996.* Passed by the Knesset on 1 May 1996
7. G. Kent, "Shared Understandings for Informed Consent: The Relevance of Psychological Research on the Provision of Information," *Social Science Medicine,* Vol. 43, No. 10 (1996), pp. 1517–1523.
8. G. Lakoff and M. Johnson, *Metaphors We Live By* (Chicago: University of Chicago Press, 1980), pp. 10–11.
9. Lakoff and Johnson, *Metaphors We Live By,* p. 10.
10. Lakoff and Johnson, *Metaphors We Live By,* p. 11.
11. Lakoff and Johnson, *Metaphors We Live By,* p. 230.
12. Lakoff and Johnson, *Metaphors We Live By,* pp. 231–232.
13. This material is adapted from a scholar of narrative theory, David Morris, Ph.D., and is drawn from material he prepared for a seminar he conducted in Spring 1997, at the University of New Mexico School of Medicine. The seminar title was: "Listening at the End of Life: Narrative Competencies and the Dying Patient."
14. M. Bakhtim, *Problems of Dostoevsky's Poetics,* Caryl Emerson (Ed. and Trans.) (Minneapolis: University of Minnesota Press, 1984), p. 318.
15. M. Nussbaum, *The Fragility of Goodness: Luck and Ethics in Greek Tragedy and Philosophy* (Cambridge: Cambridge University Press, 1986), pp. 15–16.
16. William L. Freeman, *The Role of Community in Research with Stored Tissue Samples,* Unpublished paper, 1997. Dr. Freeman is the Chair of the Indian Health Service IRB.
17. Canadian Tri-Council's "Code of Conduct for Research Involving Humans," electronic version (http://www.ethics.ubc.ca/code/sec-05.html, Section 15).

18. Model Ethical Protocol for Collecting DNA Samples. North American Regional Committee/Human Genome Diversity Project, September 1, 1995. Permission received from Jean Doble, Morrison Institute for Population and Resource Studies, to cite this draft protocol as published on the web. (http://www.leland.stanford.edu/grop/morrinst/Protocol.html).
19. R.C. Williams, W.C. Knowler, D.J. Pettit, *et al.* "The Magnitude and Origin of European-American Admixture in the Gila River Indian Community of Arizona: A Union of Genetics and Demography," *American Journal of Human Genetics*, Vol. 51 (1992), pp. 101–110.
20. Freeman, *The Role of Community in Research with Stored Tissue Samples, op. cit.*, p. 8.

Organ Transplantation without Brain Death

ROBERT D. TRUOG

*Children's Hospital, Farely 517, 300 Longwood Avenue,
Boston, Massachusetts 02115, USA*

INTRODUCTION

More than thirty years ago, an *ad hoc* committee at Harvard Medical School promulgated criteria for the transplantation of vital organs from one person to another.[1] Although the Harvard Committee described the necessary condition of the donor as a state of "irreversible coma," in the years that followed this condition came to be known as "brain death." The Harvard Committee was explicit in noting that one of the important purposes of its document was to enable the nascent field of organ transplantation. Although there are many who remain skeptical about the success of organ transplantation, I will assume for the purposes of this paper that development of the ability to transplant vital organs like hearts, livers, and kidneys has been an unqualified success, saving the lives of thousands of people who would otherwise have suffered a premature death, and in most cases providing these individuals with a fully satisfactory quality of life. My purpose is therefore not to raise objections to the process of organ transplantation *per se*, but rather to question the justifications that underlie the removal of vital organs from one person for purposes of transplantation into another.

HISTORICAL ASPECTS

Any discussion of brain death must begin by addressing the more fundamental philosophical questions of: "What is death?" and "How do we diagnosis it?" Logic would indicate that the criteria for the diagnosis should follow from an understanding of the definition, but historically the reverse has been true. Indeed, until the last few decades, there was no doubt about the appearance of death: cold, blue, and stiff. The debates were about how to make the diagnosis without error. Historian Martin Pernick has written a fascinating account of this topic.[2] According to him, one of the most commonly used safeguards to assure the certainty of the diagnosis of death was the imposition of a waiting period between the diagnosis of death and the burial of the person. An early description of this practice came from an ancient Jewish sect that observed bodies for three days before burying them. Napoleon also required a 24-hour delay between the diagnosis of death and burial in his empire. At the turn of the century, mortuaries were constructed in Europe with the explicit purpose of providing a place to observe the newly-presumed-dead bodies. They were built so that a centrally stationed guard could observe several of the guests at a time. The guards made regular rounds to check the guests for any signs of life, and the latest in resuscitation devices were always available. Indeed, these mortuaries could be seen as the predecessors of modern day intensive care units!

Others emphasized the lack of circulation as an indictor of death. For example, in 1846 a Frenchman won a prize from the Paris Academy of Sciences for his claim that two to three minutes of careful auscultation of the heart provided an unfailing sign of death. In 1930 an American physiologist recommended the routine slashing of the wrists to demonstrate the absence of pulse. A less mutilating but more creative technique involved intravenous injection of the drug fluorescin—if the eyeballs failed to turn green, there was a demonstrated lack of circulation.

Still others focused upon the lack of respiration, determined by, for example, holding a feather, candle, or mirror to the mouth, or by submerging the body in a tub of water and looking for bubbles. Finally, some were interested in neurological function, showing that the patient failed to respond to smelling salts or to having a trumpet blown into the ear.

Given the variety of approaches, it should not be surprising that *batteries* of tests were proposed. For example, in 1904 a bill was placed before the Massachusetts General Court that would have fined doctors who diagnosed death prior to documenting eleven specific and separate signs. This emphasis upon using batteries of tests persists in our current approach to the diagnosis of brain death.

Despite all of the interest in clarification of the diagnosis of death, it was not until after the development of mechanical ventilation that there was serious discussion about the definition of death. Although the phenomenon of decapitation has been known ever since man first butchered a chicken, it did not substantially challenge the common understandings of death, since decapitation is uniformly followed by the quick cessation of pulse and respiration. With the development of mechanical ventilation in the 1950s, however, a new condition emerged that was the physiological equivalent of anatomic decapitation. This was described by French neurophysiologists in 1959 as *coma depasse* (literally, beyond coma). With mechanical ventilation, for the first time it was possible to separate the cessation of neurological function from the cessation of pulse and respiration.

This phenomenon was of only theoretical interest, however, until 1967, when the first heart was transplanted in a patient in Cape Town. Literally overnight, the question of whether a person without neurological function was still "alive" acquired enormous practical significance. The following year, the Harvard Committee published its criteria, as noted above. In 1970, Kansas became the first state in America to adopt a neurological standard for death into law. The 1970s were awkward from a legal perspective, since some states had brain death legislation and others did not, and it was thereby possible to be alive in one state and dead in another. In 1981, a President's Commission was appointed to suggest legislation that could be adopted uniformly by all of the states.[3] The Commission developed a duel approach to the definition of death known as the Uniform Determination of Death Act (UDDA), which has subsequently been adopted (in some cases with slight variation) by most of the States. It says:

"An individual who has sustained either:

(1) irreversible cessation of circulatory and respiratory functions, or

(2) irreversible cessation of all functions of the entire brain, including the brain stem, is dead.

A determination of death must be made in accordance with accepted medical standards."

Only two States have significant exceptions to the UDDA. In response to the Orthodox Jewish community, New Jersey has written a religious exemption into its law.[4] New York has a weaker exemption, requiring only "reasonable accommodation" to religious beliefs.

The President's Commission left the actual tests to be used for the diagnosis of brain death to be determined by "accepted medical standards." A panel of medical consultants to the Commission built upon the work of the Harvard Committee to propose tests that were designed to demonstrate the "irreversible cessation of all functions of the entire brain."[5]

From a conceptual perspective, the central nervous system is divisible into three parts: the cerebrum, the brainstem, and the spinal cord. The "cessation" of function of the cerebrum is indicated by unreceptivity and unresponsivity (i.e., coma). The cessation of brainstem function is diagnosed by the absence of all brainstem reflexes, including respiratory drive. The absence of respiratory drive must be very carefully documented through the performance of the apnea test, following a strict protocol. With regard to the spinal cord, the Harvard Committee indicated that cessation of function of the spinal cord should be demonstrated through the loss of all tendon reflexes. For unclear reasons, the President's Commission dropped this requirement, permitting the diagnosis of brain death even in the absence of spinal cord death. This has given rise to the interesting neurological phenomenon known as the "Lazarus sign," where stimulation of the spinal cord neurons (such as often occurs from either hypoxia or ischemia during the apnea test) leads to massive reflex activity that manifests as the patient sitting up in bed![6] While this response does not preclude the diagnosis of brain death, it has been cited as a reason not to have the family present at the bedside during the apnea test, since the "lifelike" activity can be difficult to explain to medically unsophisticated laypersons.

In addition to showing that all brain functions have ceased, it is also necessary to show that this cessation is irreversible. First and foremost, the cause of the findings must be known, and the cause must be sufficient to explain the findings. In other words, one should not diagnose brain death in a patient where the cause and extent of the brain injury is not clearly known. Along this line of reasoning, it is important to rule out drug intoxication, especially with sedatives or neuromuscular blocking agents (which create a pharmacological paralysis). In addition, the patient must not be hypothermic or in shock, since these can themselves depress brain function. Finally, one should perform two complete examinations over at least a 6–24-hour period, to demonstrate that the findings persist over time.[7]

CRITIQUE OF THE CONCEPT

Although the diagnosis of brain death is among the most straightforward in the practice of medicine, there is evidence that clinicians are frequently confused by the concept. For example, one study of physicians and nurses who were frequently involved with questions of brain death and organ donation found that only 35% were able to correctly identify the legal and medical criteria for determining death. Most of the respondents used inconsistent concepts of death, and most did not believe that the brain dead patients were "really" dead, but nevertheless felt comfortable with the process of organ procurement, on the basis of the fact that the patients were permanently unconscious and/or imminently dying.[8] Rather than conclude that these clinicians were either unsophisticated or poorly trained, an editorial that accompanied this article expressed the view that this confusion about the concept was actually *appropriate*, given the inherent inconsistencies within the concept itself.[9] In this next section of the paper, these inconsistencies will be explored in some detail.[10]

The key question in trying to make sense out of the concept of brain death centers around interpretation of the phrase "the irreversible cessation of all functions of the entire brain." This phrase can be interpreted in at least three ways, but unfortunately none of them turns out to be entirely satisfactory.

The first interpretation takes the phrase to mean exactly what it says: that *all* brain functions must have ceased. This understanding is severely flawed, however, since there are multiple lines of evidence indicating residual brain function in many (if not most) patients diagnosed as brain dead. For example, studies have demonstrated that a substantial minority of brain-dead patients do not have diabetes insipidus.[11] In other words, these patients retain the integrated secretion of antidiuretic hormone from the posterior pituitary. Not only does this represent brain function, but it represents a fairly sophisticated brain function in terms of the brain's role in maintaining the body's homeostasis. With regard to diagnosing brain death, the emphasis placed upon the absence of pupillary constriction (a neurological reflex with little physiologic significance) is in striking contrast to the lack of any testing at all for diabetes insipidus (a neurological function with enormous physiologic significance).

In addition, studies have demonstrated that patients diagnosed as brain dead may retain physiologic responsiveness to pain. In one series, for example, brain-dead patients had significant elevations of both heart rate and blood pressure at the time of surgical incision for organ procurement.[12] Although it may be possible for some of this reflex activity to originate at the level of the spinal cord, most likely this response does represent some degree of brainstem functioning.

The issue of temperature regulation presents a catch-22. On one hand, patients cannot be diagnosed as brain dead if they are hypothermic. On the other hand, temperature regulation is itself a brain function. So one of the requirements for making the diagnosis of death (absence of hypothermia) actually precludes the diagnosis (since absence of hypothermia implies brain function).

Finally, there is the ever-controversial question of the electroencephalogram (EEG). Many patients diagnosed as brain dead have electrical activity on their EEG (20% in one large series).[13] The relevant question is whether or not this electrical activity represents true "function" or whether it represents the uncoordinated firing of isolated neurons. While the answer to this question is theoretically unknowable at this time, it is interesting to note that in at least some cases, the activity seen is similar to the activity seen in dreamlike states.[14]

Taken together, there is significant evidence that many patients currently diagnosed as brain dead do not satisfy a literal interpretation of the requirement for "the irreversible cessation of all functions of the entire brain."

The second possible interpretation of the phrase, "the irreversible cessation of all functions of the entire brain," focuses not upon all functions, but only upon those functions that are *significant*, in the sense that they support the integration of the "organism as a whole." This is the interpretation favored by James Bernat and other supporters of the current standard.[15] In this context, the loss of integration of the organism as a whole is manifested by the inevitable development of a cardiac arrest within a short period of time, regardless of the intensity of support provided. During the 1960s and 1970s, this was one of the cornerstones for justifying the emerging concept of brain death—patients who met the clinical criteria for brain death would almost invariably suffer a cardiac arrest within 7 to 14 days of the diagnosis, even when receiving the best intensive care of the time.

While compelling in many ways, this second interpretation of the concept of brain death is also seriously flawed, both conceptually and empirically. First, at an empirical level, the diagnosis of brain death is no longer predictive of a cardiac arrest. Over the past thirty years, intensive care has improved dramatically, and the modern ICU is able to artificially replace most of the functions of the brainstem. Hormonal deficiencies and imbalances that once led to the loss of integration of the organism as a whole can now be easily managed. This is illustrated by those tragic cases in which a pregnant woman becomes brain dead and an effort is made to support her somatic existence until the fetus can reach a viable gestation. These efforts have been successful for up to a couple of months, and there is no reason to believe that they could not succeed almost indefinitely.[16] In other words, one of the most important empirical foundations for the concept of brain death is no longer true.

Second, and perhaps more damning, is the logical confusion inherent in this line of reasoning. To say that the diagnosis of brain death is equivalent to death because the patient will soon experience a cardiac arrest confuses a *prognosis* with a *diagnosis*. Certainly it would be accurate to say that these patients are dying, but this does not imply that they are *already* dead.[17] This error in reasoning becomes even more clear if we consider a patient in the terminal phases of advanced malignancy, when one could say with virtual certainty that the patient will have a cardiac arrest within the next 7 to 14 days. Again, while it would be perfectly correct to claim that this person is dying, it would be terribly mistaken to claim that this person is already dead.

The third possible way of interpreting the phrase "the irreversible cessation of all functions of the entire brain," is perhaps the most philosophically compelling, but fails because of its practical implications. Like the second interpretation discussed above, this also assumes that the only functions that matter are *significant* functions, but understands "significant" as referring to those brain functions that support consciousness. This is also known as the "higher-brain" definition of death, since it focuses exclusively upon the functions of the cerebral hemispheres. This formulation is intuitively compelling to both philosophers and laypeople, because it accords with the common belief that our personhood is inseparable from our consciousness, and the correlate belief that loss of consciousness corresponds to loss of personhood.[18] Despite this intuitive appeal, however, this third interpretation is also problematic. The difficulty concerns those patients who are permanently unconscious but who retain enough brainstem function to breathe without mechanical assistance. These are patients who have been diagnosed as being in the permanent vegetative state, as well as newborns with anencephaly. The difficulty is that by defining these patients as dead, we should be logically and emotionally comfortable with the notion of either cremating them or burying them. Yet most people would find it unthinkable to consider burial or cremation for a breathing person, no matter how convinced one was at an intellectual level that the person was "dead." Of course, some have argued that the way to deal with this is to administer a "lethal injection" to stop the breathing before cremation or burial, on the grounds that this injection would not be killing (since the patient is already considered dead), but would be done for purely aesthetic reasons. Even with these intellectual gymnastics, however, the hurdles that this approach would have to overcome seem insurmountable from the perspectives of social acceptance and public policy.

RECONSIDERING BRAIN DEATH

Having reviewed three possible interpretations of the phrase, "the irreversible cessation of all functions of the entire brain," and having found all of them to have serious empirical, logical, or practical problems, it makes sense to pause and ask the prior question, "Why was the concept of brain death developed in the first place?" To answer this question, it is instructive to return to the work of the Harvard Committee from 1968. Review of the Committee's paper indicates four questions that the Committee was trying to address with this new notion:
  (1) When should life support be withdrawn for the benefit of the patient?
  (2) When should life support be withdrawn for the benefit of society?
  (3) When is a patient ready to be cremated or buried?
  (4) When is it permissible to remove organs from a patient for transplantation?

In 1968, the first question was very important because removal of a ventilator from a living patient was legally viewed as a homicide. In 1999, however, the situation is entirely different. In most ICUs, more than half of those patients who die do so after some form of life-sustaining therapy is discontinued. The relevant question before removal of a ventilator is not, "Is the patient dead?," but rather, "Do the burdens of mechanical ventilation exceed the benefits?" The notion of using brain death to address the question of when to withdraw life support for the benefit of the patient, so central to the reasoning of the Harvard Committee in 1968, has therefore become virtually irrelevant over the last three decades.

In contrast, the second question about the allocation of scarce resources is perhaps even more important now than it was in 1968. Yet the problem is not whether our ICUs are going to be overrun by brain-dead patients on ventilators occupying ICU beds that are needed by others. In 1998, the question is whether we can continue to provide expensive treatments with marginal benefits to individuals at the extremes of their lifespan or with profoundly diminished capacities. These are difficult questions, but they cannot be solved by the concept of brain death.

The third question differs from the first two in that it is essentially noncontroversial. We have always buried or cremated our loved ones after they have ceased to have pulse and respiration. Even when a person is diagnosed as dead by neurological criteria, the ventilator is removed and the clinicians wait until the patient is pulseless and without breath before removing the body to the morgue. Again, the concept of brain death is irrelevant to this question of the Harvard Committee.

Finally, we are left the question of when it is permissible to remove vital organs from one patient for transplantation into another. And from this discussion, it should be clear that the sole reason for maintaining the concept of brain death is to identify a category of persons from whom this is possible. No wonder clinicians are confused by a category of death that is important, not for making the diagnosis of death *per se*, but solely to facilitate the procurement of organs for transplantation. At the very least, this type of convoluted reasoning should prompt us to re-evaluate whether the linkage between brain death and organ transplantation still makes sense, or whether there might be better ways to address the need for transplantable organs.

AN ALTERNATIVE PROPOSAL

For reasons that are not entirely clear, organ transplantation developed under an inchoate standard that has since been labeled as the "dead-donor rule." In other words, from the beginning there was the implicit belief that vital organs could only come from patients who had been declared dead. As a result, the concept of brain death was invented, specifically to create a category of patients who could supply transplantable organs. Given the importance of the transplantation enterprise, the problems and inconsistencies in the concept of brain death have been largely overlooked (or perhaps, intentionally ignored) so as not to threaten the necessary supply of organs.

Again, the purpose of this manuscript is not to question the value of organ transplantation, but instead to critically examine the justifications that underlie the procurement of the transplantable organs, and to offer an alternative.

As a segue to considering alternatives to the "dead-donor rule," it is instructive to examine the ethical principles that underlie the practice of *living related* organ transplantation. In this process, a relative of the potential recipient agrees to donate a non-vital body part, such as a single kidney, a lobe of the liver, or a lobe of the lung. In addition, this process also differs from "cadaveric" transplantation in that the potential benefits to the recipient must be balanced against the possible risks to the donor. In this setting, the relevant questions are:

(1) Does the prospective donor give his permission or consent for the donation?; and,
(2) What is the chance that the prospective donor will be harmed by the donation?

It is critical to understand that the consent of the prospective donor is necessary but not sufficient in this situation. For example, if a parent wants to donate a kidney to a child, the parent must undergo an extensive pre-donation evaluation. If, for example, it turns out that the parent has an unusual vascular supply to the kidneys such that the parent would be at a somewhat greater risk for developing renal insufficiency later in life, then most transplantation centers would refuse to do the transplant from that parent. The criteria for donation are so stringent, in fact, that the long-term renal function of donors who are surviving with only one kidney is collectively better than for the general population with two kidneys.

In other words, the guiding principles behind living related organ transplantation are those of consent and nonmaleficence. The interesting question is whether these same principles can be applied "across the board" for all transplants, even those involving a vital donation like the heart, both lungs, or the entire liver. When considering the transplantation of a vital organ, could we shift the central question from "Is the donor dead?" to "Do we have the donor's permission, and/or would donation significantly harm the donor?"

The recent debate in Japan over the concept of brain death is instructive in this regard.[22] Out of a desire (and pressure?) to facilitate the availability of organs, the Japanese parliament felt compelled to create a category of patients from whom the procurement of vital organs would be permissible. They were reluctant, however, to adopt the notion of brain death as equivalent to the death of the individual. The compromise they reached in June 1997 was essentially in accord with the alternative approach outlined above: Without uniformly recognizing brain death as "death," patients who have given prior permission could become organ donors if they meet certain clinical criteria (i.e., "brain death" criteria). A plausible way of interpreting the Japanese "solution" is that Japan will now allow living patients who have both given their permission and who are "beyond the possibility of being harmed" (i.e., neurological function at or below the level diagnosed by the "brain death exam") to be organ donors.

Other proposals have also been consistent with this approach. In 1994 the Council on Ethical and Judicial Affairs of the American Medical Association adopted a resolution stating that "It is ethically permissible to consider the anencephalic as a potential organ donor, although still alive under the current definition of death," if, among other requirements, the diagnosis is certain and the parents give their permission."[19] Again, the operative principles behind this resolution are those of consent and nonmaleficence, with the implicit assumption that anencephalic newborns, who are unconscious and who never have the possibility of becoming conscious, are beyond the possibility of being harmed. (Of note, this resolution was later retracted following objections from the general membership).

A practice that is currently enjoying a surge of popularity is the procurement of transplantable organs from so-called "non-heart-beating organ donors."[20] Using this strategy, patients who are not "brain dead" but who are dependent upon a life-sustaining treatment like mechanical ventilation or vasoactive agents may be considered for donation upon either their request or that of their family. They are then taken to the operating room, where they are prepped and draped for surgery. They are given anticoagulants and vasodilators to help preserve their organs after the loss of circulation occurs. The life-sustaining treatment is then removed, and they are observed for the development of cardiac arrest. If this occurs, after two minutes of pulselessness they are declared dead, the transplant team enters, and the organs are expeditiously removed.

The purported advantages of this approach are that it does not violate the "dead-donor rule." Nevertheless, many commentators have regarded the protocol as a rather bizarre way of orchestrating the withdrawal of life-support so as to "make the person dead" in a particular way to facilitate the procurement of organs.[21] It is the perceived need to satisfy the dead-donor rule that makes the protocol seem bizarre. Yet again, however, the operative principles seem to be those of consent and nonmaleficence. Once one has permission and has determined that the patient is "beyond the possibility of being harmed," the withdrawal of life support proceeds with the clear purpose of obtaining the organs for transplantation. The questions that beg for answers in this case are "What purpose is served by waiting for this somewhat contrived diagnosis of death? Wouldn't the purposes of the procedure be more transparent, and wouldn't the actions appear more honest, if the organs were simply removed from the patient under general anesthesia, without predicating the procurement upon the diagnosis of death?"

Of course, adoption of this fundamental shift in the justifications for procuring vital organs would have substantial ramifications. First, patients would not be declared dead prior to organ removal, and would therefore be "killed" by the process of organ donation. Clearly, this would require a shift in the legal framework so that the activity of the transplantation physicians would not be construed as homicide. This situation is in many ways similar to the current debate over euthanasia and assisted suicide, where the participation of the physician in the death of the patient must be interpreted in a way that recognizes the cause of death as the underlying disease, rather than either the administration of lethal drugs or the removal of vital organs.

Even so, the question of whether the medical profession should take such an active role in a process that results in the death of the patient is one that must be taken seriously. If one takes the view that the concept of brain death has just been used as a "cover" to permit the procurement of transplantable organs, then one advantage of this alternative strategy is that it forces us to address the issue head-on. Even so, the involvement of physicians at the end of life is already so intimate that this greater degree of involvement could be seen as only an incremental step rather than as a fundamental shift.

Consider, for example, the following thought experiment. In Scenario A, a patient with irreversible neurologic, cardiac, and respiratory failure is supported with extracorporeal life support (ECLS). When the clinicians and family agree that the patient is not going to survive, ECLS is removed, and the patient is allowed to die. In Scenario B, a patient with irreversible neurologic failure (but not "brain dead") is taken to operating room, placed on ECLS, and his heart and lungs are removed for transplantation. ECLS is then discontinued, and the patient is allowed to die. The situation in Scenario A is commonplace, and is not regarded as "killing" by the clinicians. Scenario B is materially the same, yet raises the question of killing. Why the difference?

A final objection to the alternative proposal is that it merely replaces one "gray area" with another. Instead of struggling over the question of "What is death?,"s we are forced to struggle with the questions of "What is harm, and what is sufficient harm that it should preclude the possibility of donation?" Should we say that only persons who fulfill "brain death" criteria are sufficiently beyond the possibility of harm to justify allowing them to be organ donors? This would change the justification for our current practice, but would not change the practice itself. Or should we say that all patients who have permanently lost consciousness are sufficiently beyond the possibility of harm to justify allowing them to be donors? This would allow for the possibility of adopting proposals like that of the AMA regarding anencephalic newborns. Or should we say that even individuals who are not permanently unconscious but who are imminently dying should be allowed to be organ donors? This would allow for patients that are currently being entered into non-heart-beating-organ-donor protocols to be organ donors without first undergoing an orchestrated death.

Each of these is a difficult question. But unlike the debate over brain death, where the very nature of the question (What is death?) obscures our ability to see the real issue ("When is it permissible to procure transplantable organ?"), the alternative proposal forces us to tackle the issues directly. Certainly the changes proposed here will not occur in the next year or even the next decade. Nevertheless, it is difficult to imagine that the flawed concept of brain death can weather the scrutiny of time indefinitely. Alternatives will need to be considered, and ultimately, one will prevail as a better approach. As historian Martin Pernick has noted: "Death is not simply a timeless and permanently definable term. Its meaning has changed over time, in response to changing technology, social structure, and values. The history of past changes should lead us to expect future changes, any of which might invalidate both the specific tests and the basic definition that we adopt for today's use."[22]

NOTES AND REFERENCES

1. Report of the Ad Hoc Committee of the Harvard Medical School to Examine the Definition of Brain Death, "A Definition of Irreversible Coma," *Journal of the American Medical Association*, Vol. 205 (August 1968), pp. 337–340.
2. Martin S. Pernick, "Back from the Grave: Recurring Controversies over Defining and Diagnosing Death in History," in R.M. Zaner (Ed.), *Death: Beyond Whole-Brain Criteria* (Boston: Kluwer Academic Publishers, 1988), pp. 17–74.
3. President's Commission for the Study of Ethical Problems in Medicine and Biomedical and Behavioral Research, Defining Death: A Report on the Medical, Legal, and Ethical Issues in the Determination of Death (Washington, DC: Government Printing Office, 1981).
4. R. S. Olick, "Brain Death, Religious Freedom, and Public Policy: New Jersey's Landmark Legislative Initiative," *Kennedy Institute of Ethics Journal*, Vol. 1 (1991), pp. 275–288.
5. "Guidelines for the Determination of Death," *Journal of the American Medical Association*, Vol. 246 (1981), pp. 2184–2186.
6. Allan H. Ropper, "Unusual Spontaneous Movements in Brain-Dead Patients," *Neurology*, Vol. 34 (1984), pp. 1089–1092.
7. Quality Standards Subcommittee of AAN, "Practice Parameters for Determining Brain Death in Adults (Summary Statement)," *Neurology*, Vol. 45 (1995), pp. 1012–1014.
8. Stuart J. Youngner, C. Seth Landefeld, Claudia J. Coulton, Barbara W. Juknialis, and Mark Leary, "Brain Death' and Organ Retrieval. A Cross-Sectional Survey of Knowledge and Concepts Among Health Professionals," *Journal of the American Medical Association*, Vol. 261, No. 15 (Apr. 1989), pp. 2205–2210.
9. Daniel Wikler and Alan J. Weisbard, "Appropriate Confusion over 'Brain Death'," *Journal of the American Medical Association*, Vol. 261, No. 15 (April 1989), p. 2246.
10. Robert D. Truog, "Is It Time to Abandon Brain Death?," *Hastings Center Report*, Vol. 27, No. 1 (Jan.-Feb. 1997), pp. 29–37.
11. H. Schrader, K. Krogness, A. Aakvaag, O. Sortland, and K. Purvis, "Changes of Pituitary Hormones in Brain Death," *Acta Neurochirurgica*, Vol. 52 (1980), pp. 239–248.
12. Randal C. Wetzel, Nancy Setzer, Judith L. Stiff, and Mark C. Rogers, "Hemodynamic Responses in Brain Dead Organ Donor Patients," *Anesthesia and Analgesia*, Vol. 64 (1985), pp. 125–128.
13. Madeleine M. Grigg, Michael A. Kelly, Gastone G. Celesia, Mona W. Ghobrial, and Emanuel R. Ross, "Electroencephalographic Activity After Brain Death," *Archives of Neurology*, Vol. 44 (September 1987), pp. 948–954.
14. E. Rodin, S. Tahir, D. Austin and L. Andaya, "Brainstem Death," *Clinical Electroencephalography*, Vol. 16 (1985), pp. 63–71.
15. James L. Bernat, Charles M. Culver, and Bernard Gert, "On the Definition and Criterion of Death," *Annals of Internal Medicine*, Vol. 94 (1981), pp. 389–394.
16. David R. Field, Elena A. Gates, Robert K. Creasy, Albert R. Jonsen, and Russell K. Laros, Jr., "Maternal Brain Death During Pregnancy. Medical and Ethical Issues," *Journal of the American Medical Association*, Vol. 260, No. 6 (August 1988), pp. 816–822.
17. Michael Green and Daniel Wikler, "Brain Death and Personal Identity," *Philosophy and Public Affairs*, Vol. 9, No. 2 (1980), pp. 105–133.
18. Robert David Truog and James Courtney Fackler, "Rethinking Brain Death," Critical Care Medicine, Vol. 20, No.12 (December 1992), pp. 1705–1713; Karen Grandstand Gervais, *Redefining Death* (New Haven: Yale University Press, 1986); Robert M. Veatch, "The Impending Collapse of the Whole-Brain Definition of Death," *Hastings Center Report*, Vol. 4 (1993), pp. 18–24.

19. Robert M. Arnold and Stuart J. Youngner, "The Dead Donor Rule: Should We Stretch It, Bend It, or Abandon It?," *Kennedy Institute of Ethics Journal*, Vol. 3 (1993), pp. 263–278.
20. "University of Pittsburgh Medical Center Policy and Procedure Manual: Management of Terminally Ill Patients Who May Become Organ Donors After Death," *Kennedy Institute of Ethics Journal*, Vol. 3 (1993), A1–A15; Robert M. Arnold and Stuart J. Youngner, "Back to the Future: Obtaining Organs from Non-Heart-Beating Cadavers," *Kennedy Institute of Ethics Journal*, Vol. 3 (1993), pp. 103–111; "Guidelines are urged in using organs of heart-dead patients," *New York Times* (21 December 1997).
21. Joanne Lynn, "Are the Patients Who Become Organ Donors Under the Pittsburgh Protocol for 'Non-Heart-Beating donors' Really Dead?," *Kennedy Institute of Ethics Journal,* Vol. 3 (1993), pp. 167–178; J. Weisbard, "A Polemic on Principles: Reflections on the Pittsburgh Protocol," *Kennedy Institute of Ethics Journal*, Vol. 3 (1993), pp. 217–230.
22. Lock, M. "The problem of brain death: Japanese disputes about bodies and modernity," *The Definition of Death: Contemporary Controversies*. S.J. Youngner, R.M. Arnold, and R. Schapiro (Eds.) (Baltimore, MD: The Johns Hopkins University Press, 2000), pp. 239–256.

Genetic Testing, Organ Transplantation, and an End to Nondirective Counseling

DENI ELLIOTT

Director, Practical Ethics Center, The University of Montana, Missoula, Montana 59812, USA

INTRODUCTION

The late twentieth century saw the development of a range of medical miracles, genetic diagnostics and organ transplantation among them. Organ transplantation is heralded as standard or hopeful therapy for a variety of end-stage, life-threatening, or debilitating diseases, including genetic maladies. Here I argue that rather than looking to organ transplantation as a cure for genetic malady, we ought instead to work toward preventing genetic disease through preconceptual and prenatal testing. I argue that health care providers and people who plan to procreate have a moral responsibility to prevent genetic disease where they can. One result of my argument is that the oxymoronic term "nondirective counseling" be replaced with an explicit standard-of-care perspective that moves genetic screening into mainstream medical practice.

I will start with a look at the intersection of genetics and organ transplantation.

GENETICS AND ORGAN TRANSPLANTATION

One of the many common-sense notions that we are proving through the Human Genome Project is that none of us is perfect. It is estimated that "every individual carries a "genetic load" of about 20 genes which are not functioning optimally and which can potentially produce medical or developmental complications. However, —and as a matter of luck, time or outbreeding—most of us are blissfully unaware of the deleterious genes that we carry."[1] It is a matter of luck in that we may inadvertently avoid environmental factors that would trigger the expression of genetic problems, a matter of time in that we may not be aware of late-onset disorders that we carry, and a matter of outbreeding in that "everyone carries four to six genes that are harmless when inherited from one parent but can be deadly when inherited from both."[2] The more genetically similar the partners, the more likely it is that they will both be carriers of the recessive gene that results in a 1-4 chance that each child born will express the genetic disorder. Diseases of this type include Tay-Sachs, cystic fibrosis, sickle cell anemia, Goucher's disease, and Canavan's disease.

Whether through genetic disease, or gestational assault of one sort or another, "about 3% of newborns have anomalies or malformations at birth."[3] "Established genetic disorders now account for almost 50 percent of all childhood deaths in the United States. They also account for as much as 25 percent of all hospital admissions for children."[4]

Transplantation is an expensive treatment of choice for some genetic diseases, specifically for children, who constitute the overwhelming class of transplant recipients for genetic disease. Genetic disease is second only to biliary atresia as the cause of pediatric liver failure.[5] Of all the pediatric transplants, an estimated 35% are provided for genetic illnesses.[6]

These transplants are performed to bring about one of the following results: replacement of an organ that did not develop or is irreparably damaged, providing a site for processing or detoxifying bodily substances, or to manufacture a congenitally absent substance or cell type. [7]

However, transplantation does not always offer a cure. In some cases, transplantation restores a damaged organ, but does not resolve the underlying genetic disease. For example, some children with cystic fibrosis suffer liver failure. Liver transplant restores normal liver function, but cannot change the progress of the fundamental disease. In fact, the immunosuppresents required to prevent rejection may make the lung disease worse.[8]

In other cases, transplantation may bring about a delayed or partial cure for genetic disease. An example of this is Hurler's syndrome. This is an early-childhood-onset disease resulting in growth failure, skeletal deformity and progressive mental deterioration leading to death between 7 and 10 years of age. Bone marrow transplant can stop the progression of the disease. At the time of diagnosis, most children will have some loss of function and will continue to lose function for 4-12 months after bone marrow transplant.[9]

Even in cases in which transplantation provides a cure for the manifestations of the disease and something like a normal, albeit complicated or compromised lifespan, transplantation does not address the underlying genetic cause or the likelihood of the disease's being passed on to yet another generation by the affected individual or to another child through repeated pregnancy. The fact that one child is treated for genetic disease, either through transplant or other means, does not imply that parents understand how to prevent further problems.

Indeed, there is indication that treating physicians may not be educating affected persons or parents of affected children as to the genetic cause for the illness. A study in France of patients with Alport's syndrome regarding knowledge and attitudes toward prenatal testing showed that only 59% of the interviewees knew that gender was the determinant in the progression of the disease; knowledge of the mode of inheritance of the disease was adequate in only 25% of those interviewed.[10] Alport's syndrome results in renal failure and the need for kidney transplant in affected males and has a varying degree of severity in affected females from renal failure to healthy carrier.

Even the possibility of partial cure may not be available to some children because of the shortage of organs. Among transplant candidates younger than 2 years of age, 30% to 50% die before an organ becomes available.[11] In the U.S., "between 1980 and early 1990, 169 infants under 1 year of age underwent heart transplantation. During the same interval, however, approximately 80–100 other infants were registered with organ procurement agencies but died while awaiting donor hearts."[12] Another way to look at this collection of statistics is that if the pediatric transplant candidates who are there for genetic disease were not competing for organs, which constitutes an estimated 35% of the whole, the supply of pediatric organs would come close to matching demand.

My suggestion is not that we deny transplantation to existing victims of serious genetic disease, but that as we move into the twenty-first century, we—policymakers, health care practitioners, and scholars working in the realm of genetics— make a concerted effort to promote prevention as the treatment of choice for serious genetic disease.

PREVENTING GENETIC DISEASE

Preventing detectable genetic disease is not unlike many of life's choices. But before the lay population can be expected to integrate the new tools of genetic screening and diagnostics into their decision-making, those working in the field need to dodge labels like "eugenics," need to accept that selective abortion is not conceptually different from elective abortion, and need to put to rest the myth of nondirective counseling. That is what I hope to do here.

First, let me discuss how and why I think that genetic screening and diagnosis can be easily adopted into individual and community life. Then I will talk about the timing of genetic screening and how "selective" abortion creates a false distinction with "elective" abortion. Finally, I will end with an argument for explicitly directive genetic counseling.

Prevention of genetic disease should become as commonplace as other attempts to prevent fetal injury. The idea that health-care providers and intended parents have obligations to a potential baby is not a new idea. Couples are encouraged to refrain from having children until they can provide a healthful environment for them. Pregnant women are expected to provide as good nutrition to their developing fetus as they are able; they are expected to refrain from exposure to substances that may damage the developing fetus.

What is new is a new collection of new screening and diagnostic tools. With our present state of prenatal diagnosis, knowledge and technology, it is possible to detect, *in utero*, 200 to 300 of the 5,000 hereditary diseases or malformations known to date. The daily discoveries of anomalous genes and genetic combinations through the Human Genome Project guarantees that the number of anomalies we can detect will certainly increase.

But new knowledge brings about new responsibilities. Specifically, if policymakers, health-care providers, and individuals intending to procreate know that certain diseases can be avoided, then they have the moral responsibility to avoid creating children with preventable disease.

Because of the universal, minimalist moral dictate *do not cause unjustified harm,* individuals ought not knowingly produce children with serious genetic disease. In addition to this causal responsibility, those intended to procreate have a role-related responsibility as well. If pregnant women have a responsibility not to cause potential prenatal injury, then it is consistent to argue that they ought not cause avoidable genetic injury as well. New technology does not simply expand reproductive choice; it also expands reproductive responsibility.

Some individuals, communities and nations are already moving in this direction. Individuals who know themselves to be at risk for various genetic disorders are seeking genetic counseling. The Former Soviet Union had a program in place to provide prenatal diagnosis and abortion of affected fetuses for Hurler's and other lysosomal storage diseases. In 1993, cost-benefit analysts in Israel explored the possibility of a nation-wide screening program for cystic fibrosis among the Ashkenazi population. The analysis regarding screening for the five mutations that result in 97% of all CF cases suggest that a voluntary screening program would detect 94% of the Ashkenazi couples with a 1-4 risk for an affected child, and predicted that 92% of persons who voluntarily participated in a CF screening program would be willing to abort if found to be carrying an affected fetus.[14] According to those authors, "Perhaps the major benefit of publicly funded screening is that it provides an option for all individuals to voluntary choose whether or not to be screened, thereby helping persons make more informed reproductive decisions."[15]

A *de facto* national screening program is in place in the United States for prenatal detection of neural tube defect and Down's syndrome. It is the standard of care in the U.S. for every pregnant woman receiving prenatal care to be offered a triple screen —a maternal blood test that analyzes the possibility that the fetus is at increased risk for a neural tube defect or Down's syndrome. Diagnosis of Down's syndrome in the U.S. through amniocentesis carries more than a 90% abortion rate and diagnosis of neural tube defect carries a 75% abortion rate.[16]

One highly successful, if highly controversial, global screening program that takes place preconceptually rather than prenatally is Dor Yeshorim. Dor Yeshorim was begun in 1983 by Rabbi Josef Ekstein, of Brooklyn, New York, after facing the tragedy of having four of his ten children die from Tay-Sachs disease. The idea for the screening was simple. Orthodox boys and girls of marriageable age would have their blood drawn and tested for Tay-Sachs. As being identified as a Tay-Sachs carrier was stigmatizing, the results of the test would be held in confidence. Before a couple began dating seriously or before the matchmaker suggested a pairing, the couple or the matchmaker would contact the Dor Yeshorim hotline, give the number codes of the couple and be told if they were "compatible" or not. Only if both young people were carriers of the Tay-Sachs gene would the couple be notified that they were incompatible. The program has expanded to include testing centers in Israel, Europe, and Canada in addition to the U.S. and now tests for cystic fibrosis, Canavan's disease, Fanconi's anemia, and Gaucher's disease as well. As of November 1997, the test results for more than 80,000 people are now in the computer bank; Dor Yeshorim provides about 8,000 genetic assessments each year. More than 180 prospective couples have been found to be carriers for the same disease and have been given this information. Follow-up genetic counseling for incompatibility is provided as part of the program. Selection of a different, genetically compatible mate might be the decision of choice in traditional communities, but need not be the choice for all individuals.

SELECTIVE ABORTION AND GENETIC TESTING

What about the couple who are both carriers for cystic fibrosis or Tay-Sachs disease and who wish to have an unaffected child? Prenatal genetic testing and the option of selective abortion make these pregnancies possible. While it should be within the couple's choice to abort for fetal anomaly (where culturally acceptable), it is not appropriate to differentiate selective abortion from elective abortion. While I argue this point elsewhere,[17] I will mention two problems with the purported distinction. First the distinction inappropriately creates normative distinctions between women seeking abortion. Abortions performed in the best interest of the fetus are seen as altruistic; those performed regardless of fetal characteristic may be seen as self-centered, not as morally worthy. Yet, if one examines groups of women who abort for fetal characteristic and those that abort for other reasons, the differences blur and disappear. One woman may choose to abort a fetus regardless of characteristics because she believes that she simply can't handle parenthood right now; another woman in identical circumstances may choose to carry the pregnancy to term. One woman may choose to abort a fetus with particular characteristics because she believes that she cannot handle parenting a child with those particular problems; another may make the opposite choice. All selective abortions are elective in that say more about the characteristics of the intended parents than they say about characteristics of the developing fetus. Even in cases of prenatally diagnosed Tay-Sachs disease or anencephaly, the decision of whether to abort or not reflects the worldview of the couples, not the seriousness of the fetal condition.

One unfortunate difference between policies governing selective abortion and elective abortion in the United States is that of availability. Elective abortion is theoretically available up to the point of fetal viability, usually interpreted as 24 weeks from last menstrual period (LMP). Selective abortion can be performed in some states up to actual delivery. Except in the cases of certain fetal or maternal demise, allowing abortion of viable fetuses with anomalies does creates a subclass of the disabled. According to one writer, "States protect fetuses by prohibiting abortions at a time when it is believed that the fetus should be given human consideration. Yet, if "human" consideration and/or legal status is given to a fetus with a defect at a much later date than it is given to a fetus without defects, it is more than a contradiction in terms—not a mere dichotomy of view, but clearly established disparate treatment."[18]

TIMING OF GENETIC TESTING

While selective abortion ought be a legitimate response to genetic disease, at least as long as other sorts of elective abortion are morally permissible, people generally would like to know their genetic risks before conceiving.

For example, Ginsberg *et al.* found that, "98% of Caucasian women in the USA, with similar carrier frequency rates [for cystic fibrosis] to Ashkenazi Jews, said screening should be offered before pregnancy, whereas only 69% said they would accept carrier screening during pregnancy."[19]

In the study of patients with Alport's syndrome, a majority were interested in prenatal testing to determine whether they were carrying an affected fetus, but only two-thirds of them would use selective abortion. This finding is consistent with other studies that found a difference between interest in prenatal testing and the decision to terminate a pregnancy. In a U.S. study of adult onset polycystic kidney disease, slightly more than half of affected or at-risk individuals would use prenatal testing to identify affected fetuses; less than 10% of them, however, would not terminate a fetus with adult polycystic disease, although they claimed that they would terminate the pregnancy for other problems.[20] Consistently respondents report an unwillingness to abort for conditions with which they are familiar. That is, someone who grew up with deaf parents is less likely to abort for congenital deafness.

THE END OF NONDIRECTIVE GENETIC COUNSELING

If we are to assist those making genetic choices, a program of testing potential carriers before they choose to initiate a pregnancy is indicated. The watchword of genetic counseling as been that it is "nondirective." I call "nondirective counseling" an oxymoron because "counseling" implies giving advice or guidance while the word "nondirective" implies an *unwillingness* to supply this advice or guidance.

By whatever name, genetic counseling is and has been value-laden since its inception. Some of the values expressed by the practice of genetic counseling include the belief that the couple may *choose* whether to carry an affected fetus to term or whether to procreate; the counseling indicates a valuing of knowledge about one's self and one's intended offspring. As some counselors will not approve testing if they believe that the couple's reasons for terminating a pregnancy would be trivial (such as fetal sex, the lack of a certain condition or characteristic, or the inability to provide donor bone marrow to an afflicted sibling), normative judgments are clearly in place in the profession. A survey of doctors in France and Canada disclosed admitted judgments about the moral permissibility of bringing to term fetuses with serious genetic disease. Of those surveyed, "a little more than 15 percent of Canadian physicians considered it socially irresponsible to deliberately bring to birth a genetically handicapped child at a time when intrauterine diagnosis and abortion are possible." However, "28 percent of physicians in Quebec and 37 percent in France shared this position."[21]

According to Bouchard, these physicians "think it is impossible to maintain an objective approach to genetic counseling while at the same time wanting to prevent anomalies."[22]

The relationship between medical practitioners and patients has evolved to include the patient as decision-maker, but, generally speaking, medical counseling is far from nondirective. "Physicians, nurses, and psychologists in many areas of clinical practice and public health adhere to professional norms that go beyond value neutrality—they are zealous advocates of the value of health and prevention of disease and disability."[23]

Counselors, doctors, and others in a position to educate intended parents, ought to work explicitly to prevent disease and that includes explicit counseling for prevention. That is their job. These advisors cannot force people to prevent the birth of children with genetic disease any more than medical advisors can prevent people from smoking, drinking, or failing to exercise, but they can assist in creating a culture in which it is acceptable to be tested, to have genetic information about oneself, and to avoid causing genetic injury where possible.

QUESTIONS REMAIN, BUT NOT ALL ARE COMPELLING

Many questions remain regarding the ethics of preventing genetic disease, but I will end by addressing one that I find less than compelling. That is the question of what might have been.

It is interesting that some express concern about what might happen by the elimination of some genetic disorders, but not the elimination of disease caused by virus. It is interesting that some wonder what the world might miss through the avoided conception or birth of some individuals with some genetic diseases without considering this question in the larger context of existing children who are lost to the world because of starvation, neglect, or abuse. The consequences of a "designer" gene pool are not conceptually different from the consequences of other forms of disease prevention.

In a review of 41 articles published between 1966 and 1993 that considered cost-benefits of prenatal testing and selective abortion, the reviewer criticized the articles in that they "generally do not include a discussion of the potential life that is aborted."[24] Another writer says, "Society will not likely lose any scientists, doctors, lawyers, or presidents as a result of genetic testing revealing Down's syndrome.... Is intellectual potential our measuring stick?"[25]

Glover's point that intellectual capacity serves as one of the measures of normalcy is certainly a comment about the state of society at the turn of the century. There are many other aspects of society that make it difficult for some women in some circumstances to have their babies, regardless of fetal characteristics. These comments about society, however, do not imply that it is therefore morally prohibited for individual women to choose abortion in response to their recognized inability to care for the resultant child.

It is true that we never will know what we as individuals or the world as a whole is missing because of the decision to avoid conception or to abort a particular fetus. This is as true, and trivial, as the statement that we will never know what we are missing by having chosen one mate over another. In neither case, do we have a moral responsibility to find out.

NOTES AND REFERENCES

1. R. Anderson and B. Schaefer, "Genetic Counseling Considerations in Pediatric Organ Transplantation," in C. Greiner and D. Elliott, *Transplantation: Parts and Parity* (Hanover, New Hampshire: Institute for the Study of Applied and Professional Ethics, Dartmouth College, 1995), p. 18.
2. G. Cowley, "Made to Order Babies," *Newsweek* (Winter/Spring 1990), p. 94
3. L. Bouchard, M. Renaud, O. Kremp, and L. Dalliare, "Selective Abortion: A New Moral Order? Consensus and Debate in the Medical Community," *International Journal of Health Services*, Vol. 25, No. 1 (1995), pp. 65–84 at 67.
4. A. Caplan, *If I Were A Rich Man Could I Buy A Pancreas?* (Bloomington: Indiana University Press, 1992), at 121.
5. Bazil Zitelli, Carolton Gartner, Jeffrey Malatack, Andrew Urbach and Karen Zamberlan, "Liver Transplantation in Children: A Pediatrician's Perspective," *Pediatric Annals*, Vol. 20, No. 12/December (1991), pp. 691–698, at 692; Sunita Stewart, David Waller, Betsy Kennard, Margaret Benswer and Walter Andrews, "Mental and Motor Development Social Competence, and Growth One Year after Successful Pediatric Liver Transplantation," *The Journal of Pediatrics* (1989), pp. 574–581, at 575.
6. Carl Greiner and Deni Elliott, *Transplantation: Parts and Parity* (Hanover, New Hampshire: Institute for the Study of Applied and Professional Ethics, Dartmouth College, 1995), p. 5.
7. R. Anderson and B. Schaefer, "Genetic Counseling Considerations in Pediatric Organ Transplantation," p. 1.

8. Anderson, *op. cit.*, p. 4.
9. Anderson, *op. cit.*, p. 5.
10. M. Levy, Y. Pirson, B. Boudailliez, H. Nivet, N. Rance, A. Moynot, M. Broyer and J.P. Grunfeld, "Evaluation in Patients with Alport Syndrome of Knowledge of the Disease and Attitudes Toward Prenatal Diagnosis," *Clinical Nephrology*, Vol. 42, No. 4 (1994), pp. 211–220 at 211.
11. Committee on Bioethics, "Infants with Anencephaly as Organ Sources: Ethical Considerations." *Pediatrics*, Vol. 89, No. 6 (1992), pp. 1116–1119, at 1116.
12. S. Ashwal, A. Caplan, W. Cheatham, R. Evans, J. Peabody, "Social and Ethical Controversies in Pediatric Heart Transplant," *Journal of Heart and Lung Transplantation*, Vol. 10 (1991), pp. 860–876, at 860.
13. X.D. Krasnopolskaya, T.V. Mirenburg, and V.S. Akhunov, "Postnatal and Prenatal Diagnosis of Lysosomal Storage Diseases in the Former Soviet Union," *Wiener Klinische Wochenschrift*, 109/3 (1997), pp. 74–80, at 74.
14. G. Ginsberg, Hannah Blau, E. Kerem, C. Springer, Bat-Seba Kerem, E. Akstein, A. Greemberg, A. Kolumbos, D. Abeliovich, E. Gazit, and J. Yahav, "Cost Benefit Analysis of Program a Screening National for Cystic Fibrosis in an Israeli Population," *Health Economics*, Vol. 3 (1994), pp. 5–23, esp. 5–8.
15. G. Ginsberg *et al.*, *op. cit.*, p. 17.
16. N. Glover, and S. Glover, "Ethical and Legal Issues Regarding Selective Abortion of Fetuses with Down Syndrome," Mental Retardation, Vol. 34, No. 4 (1996), pp. 207–214, at 210.
17. D. Elliott, "The Myth of Selective Abortion," Under consideration by *Science and Engineering Ethics Journal*. Presented at the Association for Practical and Professional Ethics Annual Meeting, February 26--9, Dallas, Texas (1998).
18. Glover and Glover, *op. cit.*, p. 210.
19. Ginsberg *et al.*, *op. cit.*, p. 17.
20. M. Levy *et al.*, *op. cit.*, pp. 218-219.
21. Bouchard *et al.*, *op. cit.*, p. 73.
22. Bouchard *et al.*, p. 77.
23. Caplan, *op. cit.*, p. 133.
24. T. Ganaits, "Justifying Prenatal Screening and Genetic Amniocentesis Programs by Cost-Effectiveness Analysis: A Re-evaluation," *Medical Decision-Making*, Vol. 16, No.1 (1996), pp. 45–50, at 46.
25. N. Glover, and S. Glover, "Ethical and Legal Issues Regarding Selective Abortion of Fetuses with Down Syndrome," *Mental Retardation*, Vol. 34, No. 4 (1996), pp. 207–214, 210.

Notes on Contributors

TOM L. BEAUCHAMP is Professor of Philosophy and Senior Research Scholar, Kennedy Institute of Ethics, Georgetown University, Washington, D.C. He holds a Ph.D. in philosophy from the Johns Hopkins University. He served as the staff philosopher of the National Commission for the Protection of Human Subjects of Biomedical and Behavioral Research (NIH), where he wrote the bulk of a research ethics monograph published as *The Belmont Report*. Thereafter he served a three-year term as a member of the Committee on Laboratory Animals of the National Academy of the Sciences, National Research Council (1986-1989). Dr. Beauchamp has authored several books, including *Principles of Biomedical Ethics* (Oxford, 1994, fourth edition, co-author: James F. Childress) and *A History and Theory of Informed Consent* (Oxford, 1985, co-author: Ruth Faden). His research interests include the history of modern philosophy.

RON BERGHMANS is a psychologist and bioethicist working at the Institute for Bioethics in Maastricht. He is affiliated with the Department of Health Ethics and Philosophy of the University of Maastricht. He wrote a Ph.D. thesis on paternalism and coercive treatment in psychiatry, and was a member of the former Dutch National Committee on the Ethics of Medical Research. His major publications are in the fields of ethics in mental health care and in the care for patients suffering from Alzheimer's disease. He is a member of the Health Council of the Netherlands Committee on Dementia.

RAPHAEL COHEN-ALMAGOR is the Fulbright-Yitzhak Rabin Scholar for 1999-2000, and Visiting Professor at UCLA School of Law. He received a B.A. in Political Science, Sociology, and Anthropology from Tel Aviv University (1985); an M.A. in Political Science from Tel Aviv University (1987); and a D.Phil. in Politics, St. Catherine's College, Oxford University (1991). He then lectured and conducted research at the Hebrew University Law Faculty, and at the department of Political Science, Bar-Ilan University. Currently he is a Senior Lecturer at the Department of Communication, University of Haifa. He was a Research Fellow and the Director of The Bioethics Think-tank at the Van Leer Jerusalem Institute (1995–1998), and is a member of the Israel Press Council. Dr. Cohen-Almagor has published essays in the fields of medical and media ethics, political science, philosophy, law, sociology, and history in English, French, Spanish and Hebrew. He is the author of *The Boundaries of Liberty and Tolerance* (Gainesville: University Press of Florida, 1994) and *Speech, Media and Ethics* (London: Macmillan, 2000) and editor of *Basic Issues in Israeli Democracy* [in Hebrew] (Sifriat Poalim: Tel Aviv, 1999), *Liberal Democracy and the Limits of Tolerance: Essays in Honor and Memory of Yitzhak Rabin* (Ann Arbor: University of Michigan Press, 2000) and *Challenges to Democracy: Essays in Honour and Memory of Isiah Berlin* (London: Ashgate, 2000). Dr. Cohen-Almagor is now completing a book entitled *The Right to Die in Dignity: An Argument in Ethics, Medicine, and Law*.

REBECCA J. COOK, A.B. (Barnard) 1970, M.A. (Tufts) 1972, M.P.A. (Harvard) 1973, J.D. (Georgetown) 1982, LL.M. (Columbia) 1988, J.S.D. (Columbia) 1994,

Fellow, Royal Society of Canada, was called to the Bar of Washington, D.C. in 1983. She is a Professor in the Faculty of Law, the Faculty of Medicine, and the Joint Centre for Bioethics at the University of Toronto. She specializes in the international protection of human rights and in health law and ethics, and is Founding Director of the International Human Rights Programme at the law school. She has taught at the School of Public Health at Columbia University and continues to teach there as an adjunct lecturer. She is ethical and legal issues coeditor of *the International Journal of Gynecology and Obstetrics*, and serves on the editorial advisory board of several journals including *Family Planning Perspectives, Human Rights Quarterly* and the *Third World Legal Studies Journal*. She is an occasional adviser to the Commonwealth Medical Association, the Ford Foundation, Profamilia Legal Services for Women, and the World Health Organization. Her publications include more than one hundred books, articles, and reports in the areas of international human rights, the law relating to women's health and feminist ethics. She is the author of *Women's Health and Human Rights* (Geneva: World Health Organization, 1994), the editor of *Human Rights of Women: National and International Perspectives* (Philadelphia: University of Pennsylvania Press, 1994), and co-author of *Considerations for Formulating Reproductive Health Laws* (Geneva: World Health Organization, 1998).

BERNARD M. DICKENS, LL.B. 1961, LL.M. 1965, Ph.D. (Law-Criminology) 1971, LL.D. (Medical Jurisprudence) 1978 (London), Fellow, Royal Society of Canada, called to the English Bar in 1963 and the Ontario Bar in 1977, is a Professor in the Faculty of Law, the Faculty of Medicine, and the Joint Centre for Bioethics, University of Toronto. Professor Dickens specializes in Law and Medicine, and is legal articles editor of the *Journal of Law, Medicine and Ethics*, co-editor of Ethics and Law of the *International Journal of Gynecology and Obstetrics*, serves as a member of the editorial boards of several journals including the *American Journal of Law and Medicine,* and has been involved in a wide variety of organizations in the field of medical jurisprudence. He was Project Director to the Ontario Law Reform Commission's Project on Human Artificial Reproduction and Related Matters, and has been a consultant on several projects of the World Health Organization. His writing includes more than three hundred publications including books, chapters in books, articles, and reports primarily in the field of medical and health law, including *Bioethics in Canada* (1993, with D. Roy and J. Williams). In 1990–91 he was President of the American Society of Law, Medicine and Ethics, and from 1994 has been on the Board of Governors of the World Association for Medical Law and became a Vice President in 1996. He is a Fellow of the Royal Society of Medicine (London), Chairman of the Human Subjects Ethics Review Committee of the University of Toronto, and immediate past Chairperson of the Human Subjects Research Ethics Committee of the National Research Council of Canada, in Ottawa.

DALIA DORNER completed law studies at the Hebrew University, Jerusalem, in 1956. From 1960, she served as a defense attorney in the military courts of the State of Israel, advancing to the position of Director of the Office of the Defender. In 1973 she was appointed President of the Military District Court. From 1974, she served as a judge in the Military Court of Appeals, leaving the military with the rank of colonel. Then, in December 1979, she was appointed a Judge of the District Court of Be'er Sheva (the appellate level of the Israeli judiciary) and served there until

1984, at which time she was appointed a Judge of the District Court of Jerusalem. In April 1994, she assumed the position of a permanent Justice of the Supreme Court of Israel.

Justice Dorner has delivered Supreme Court opinions recognizing the right of women to serve as pilots in the Israel Defense Forces and the right of homosexuals to equal treatment. She sat as a member of the panel that presided over the critical *Nachmani* case, which involved a woman's right to gain possession of her frozen fertilized eggs for *in vitro* fertilization over her husband's objections. In her opinion, Justice Dorner wrote that the mother's right to motherhood overrode the right of her husband not to be a father. Her published works in Hebrew include "Affirmative Action and Women's Equality" and "The Influence of the Basic Law: Human Dignity and Liberty on the Law of Arrest." She has also published an article entitled "Does Israel Have a Constitution?" in an American law journal.

DENI ELLIOTT, the University Professor of Ethics and Director of the Practical Ethics Center at the University of Montana, is also professor of philosophy and adjunct professor of journalism. Deni came to the University of Montana after serving as the founding director for the Ethics Institute at Dartmouth College.

Professor Elliott directs the nation's first graduate degree program and mid-career program in teaching practical ethics, programs funded by the U.S. Department of Education. The Center also provides seminars in ethics for faculty and professional and community audiences. The Center houses a Robert Wood Johnson National Program Office for Excellence in End-of-Life Care.

Deni Elliot has one coauthored and one coedited book in press relating to the ethics of scientific research. These books join two other edited volumes and three video documentaries in practical ethics, along with dozens of book chapters and articles for the lay, trade, and academic audiences.

JOAN MCIVER GIBSON is Director of the Health Sciences Ethics program at the University of New Mexico, and Medical Ethicist for the St. Joseph Healthcare System in Albuquerque, New Mexico. From 1971 to 1986 she was Associate Professor of Philosophy (tenured) at the University of Albuquerque. From 1986 to 1994 she was Senior Program Director at UNM's Institute of Public Law. Her areas of expertise are values and decision making, ethics committees and ethics consultation, issues surrounding life-support treatment, applied ethics in industry and business, and mediation applied to ethical issues. She was a member of the Clinton Administration's Health Policy Task Force (Ethics Working Group), and is involved in training judges around the country in issues of bioethics.

Professor Gibson is Principal Investigator on a proposal to the NIH, "Navajo and Hispanic Perspectives on Informed Consent" (a study of informed consent for genetic research in these communities). She received an A.B. in Philosophy from Mount Holyoke College, and an M.A. and Ph.D. in Philosophy from the University of California at San Diego.

GERSHON H. GROWE is a hematologist whose particular medical practice led him to become interested in certain philosophical aspects of patient care. He was involved in the early development of the palliative care program at the Vancouver General Hospital and was a founding member of the hospital's ethics committee. Another of his interests related to the ethics of the introduction of anti-HIV medications in the early days, as this involved many of the hemophilia patients in his clinic. At present he is actively involved in the undergraduate, graduate, and interdisciplinary ethics programs at the University of British Columbia.

JOHN HARRIS, B.A. Hons. University of Kent, Philosophy and English and American Literature (1969); D.Phil., Oxford University, Philosophy (1976). In 1986 John Harris jointly founded the Centre for Social Ethics and Policy of the University of Manchester, where he is the Sir David Alliance Chair of Bioethics. Professor Harris is Director of the International Association of Bioethics and a founding member of the Editorial Board of the *Journal of Medical Ethics*. He has acted as a consultant in ethics to national and international bodies and corporations including the European Parliament Committee on Energy, Research and Technology and the European Commission. He is also the series editor of *Social Ethics and Policy,* published by Routledge, and general editor of Oxford University Press book series entitled *Issues in Biomedical Ethics*.

Professor Harris published and edited twelve books and numerous number of essays that deal, *inter alia,* with the ethics of biotechnology, the ethical problems of human aging, the moral and political status of children, problems associated with just allocation of public resources, and ethical problems of genetic and other screening techniques.

GOVERT DEN HARTOGH, Ph.D. University of Amsterdam, Faculty of Philosophy 1985, Assistant Professor of Ethics (Faculty of Philosophy) 1976–1989, Associate Professor, Philosophy of Law (Faculty of Law) 1989–1995, Professor of Medical Ethics (Faculty of Medicine) 1992–1995, is at present Professor of Ethics in the Faculty of Philosophy, and Director of the Netherlands School for Research in Practical Philosophy, which coordinates the Ph.D. teaching in the field of ten universities.

Professor den Hartogh has published in Dutch, English, and German on conventionalist theories of social and legal norms, political obligation, the principle of neutrality, matters of distributive justice, the use of theories in applied ethics, embryo research and age criteria in health care. He is now working on a book evaluating the Dutch discussion on euthanasia and assisted suicide.

JAN C. JOERDEN, Dr. jur., Erlangen-Nuremberg (1985); Dr. jur. habil., Erlangen-Nuremberg (1987); scholarship from the Deutsche Forschungsgemeinschaft (Heisenberg-Program)(1988–1993); Visiting Professor for Criminal Law and Jurisprudence at the Universities of Erlangen-Nuremberg, Berlin (Free University), Jena, Trier, and Frankfurt (Oder)(1989–1993). Since 1993 he has been Full Professor (Chair) for Criminal Law, especially International Criminal Law and Comparative Criminal Law and Jurisprudence at the European-University Viadrina, Frankfurt (Oder); since 1994 Vice President (Prorektor) of the university; since 1995 Head of the Interdisciplinary Centre of Ethics at the European-University. In 1999 he was Visiting Professor at the University of the Western Cape, Bellville/Cape Town, S.A. His books include: *Dyadische Fallsysteme im Strafrecht* (Berlin: Duncker & Humblot, 1985); *Strukturen des strafrechtlichen Verantwortlichkeitsbegriffs* (Berlin: Duncker & Humblot, 1988); *Jahrbuch fuer Recht und Ethik/Annual Review of Law and Ethics* (Ed.) (Berlin: Duncker & Humblot, 1993); et seq. *Diskriminierung-Antidiskriminierung* (Ed.) (Heidelberg: Springer, 1996); *Der Mensch und seine Behandlung in der Medizin* (Ed.) (Heidelberg: Springer, 1999); *Tiere ohne Rechte?* (Ed.)

(Heidelberg: Springer, 1999); *Medizinethik, Studien zur Ethik in Ostmitteleuropa* (Ed.) (Frankfurt am Main: Peter Lang, 2000).

GERRIT KIMSMA has degrees in philosophy and medicine. He works as a general practitioner and part-time senior staff member in the Departments both of Philosophy and of Medical Ethics at the Vrije Universiteit in Amsterdam and at the Department of Family, Nursing Home and Social Medicine. He teaches the ethical and legal issues of medical practice to postgraduate fellows in family medicine. Since 1998 he functions also as physician member of the Euthanasia Evaluation Committee of the provinces of South-Holland and Zeeland. Professor Kimsma is a member of the IRB of the Vrije Universiteit's Academic Hopsital. He is co-founder and treasurer of the European Society of Philosophy and Health Care, co-editor of *Theoretical Medicine and Bioethics,* board member of *Cambridge Quarterly of Health Care Ethics* and of *Medicine, Health Care and Philosophy: A European Journal.* He has published widely on issues of death and dying, especially in relation to his experience both as a physician and as a philosopher on the subject of physician-assisted death.

EIKE-HENNER W. KLUGE, was educated in Canada (Honours B.A. *cum laude* 1965, University of Calgary) and the United States (A.M. and Ph.D., University of Michigan, in philosophy) and received a General Motors Scholarship; he was also a Woodrow Wilson Fellow and Canada Council Fellow, and is a member of Phi Kappa Phi. He taught at the University of California (Irvine) before returning to Canada in 1971, and currently is Professor and Chair, Department of Philosophy, University of Victoria. In 1989, at the request of the Canadian Medical Association, he founded the latter's Department of Ethics and Legal Affairs and was its Director until his resignation in 1991. During that time, he presented the CMA's position on various ethical issues to Parliamentary Committees. He also developed a code of ethics for the relationship between Canadian physicians and the pharmaceutical industry, and was instrumental in the formulation of the CMA's position on the new reproductive technologies (*The New Reproductive Technologies: A Preliminary Perspective of the Canadian Medical Association* (Ottawa: CMA, 1991). Dr. Kluge also coordinated the development of the CMA's position on resuscitation, and spearheaded the CMA's analysis of the status of the human fetus. In 1996 he wrote a study on ethical and legal issues in human tissue banking for Health Canada, Health Protection Branch. He is active as ethics consultant to the British Columbia Ministry of Health, and is ethics consultant to the BC Police Complaint Commissioner. He was the first expert witness in medical ethics recognized by Canadian courts. Published works include five books in medical ethics [*The Practice of Death* (Yale, 1975); *The Ethics of Deliberate Death* (Prometheus, 1982); *Withholding Treatment from Defective Newborn Children* (coauthored with J. Magnet, Yvon Blais, 1985); *Biomedical Ethics in a Canadian Context* (Prentice Hall, 1992); *Readings in Biomedical Ethics* (Prentice Hall, 1993, 1999)] and more than sixty articles.

JOHN LANTOS, M.D., studied semiotics at Brown University, medicine at the University of Pittsburgh, and completed a pediatrics residency at the Children's Hospital National Medical Center in Washington D.C. After two years as a primary care pediatrician, he accepted a fellowship in Clinical Medical Ethics at the University of Chicago. He is currently Chief of General Pediatrics and Associate Director of the MacLean Center for Clinical Medical Ethics at the University of Chicago. He has written extensively on many areas of ethics and public policy, including neonatal intensive care, bone marrow and liver transplantation, growth hormone therapy, child abuse, informed consent, medical futility, and resource allocation. His books include *Do We Still Need Doctors?* (Routledge, 1997) and *The Last Physician: Walker Percy and the Moral Life of Medicine* (Durham, NC: Duke University Press, 1999).

EVERT VAN LEEUWEN studied philosophy and mathematics at the Free University of Amsterdam. He has been a member of the IRB since 1989, and chairperson of the IRB of 17 institutions in psychiatry, care of mentally handicapped, and nursing homes since 1993. In 1994 he was appointed as chair of the Department of Metamedicine, section Philosophy and Medical Ethics. In 1996 Professor van Leeuwen became a board member of the Institute of Ethics at the Free University. In 1998 he was appointed as (ethicist) member of the Regional Euthanasia Committee in North-Holland. Since 1999 he has been a member of the Ethics Committee of the RDMA.

Evert finished his Ph.D. thesis in philosophy in 1986 on Descartes' epistemology in the Regulae (*cum laude*) and has published in philosophy, philosophy of medicine and medical ethics in *Theoretical Medicine*, the *Journal of Medicine and Philosophy*, *Cambridge Quarterly of Health Care Ethics* and several Dutch and English books. At present he is coeditor of *Theoretical Medicine* and European editor of *Cambridge Quarterly*.

Evert is Director of the Medical Ethics Program at the Free University, in which philosophy, ethics and anthropology are contained. The program has an interface with the clinical departments and combines clinical ethics, moral argumentation and philosophical studies of key concepts. His department concentrates on empirically oriented research in medical ethics, regarding issues like the moral framework for terminal care in institutions for psychiatry; psycho-geriatrics; the self-image and narrative experience of people with chronic diseases; and DNR rules and the concept of competence in relation to patients suffering from Alzheimer's disease.

FREDERICK H. LOWY was appointed Rector and Vice-Chancellor of Concordia University on August 15, 1995. Dr. Lowy is a former Dean of the University of Toronto's Faculty of Medicine and Director of the University of Toronto's Centre for Bioethics. He graduated from McGill University (B.A. 1955; M.D., C.M. 1959), interned at the Royal Victoria Hospital, and later taught at McGill as an Assistant Professor of Psychiatry. He received his training in Psychiatry at the University of Cincinnati and in Psychoanalysis at Montreal's Canadian Institute of Psychoanalysis.

Dr. Lowy has lectured and published widely. In addition to teaching at the University of Toronto and McGill University, he has also taught at the University of Ottawa, the Kennedy Institute of Ethics at Georgetown University in Washington, D.C., Italy's Università degli Studi di Siena, and Sultan Qaboos University in Oman.

JOHN A. ROBERTSON, holds the Vinson and Elkins Chair at the University of Texas School of Law at Austin. A graduate of Dartmouth College and Harvard Law School, he has written widely on law and bioethics issues, including the book, *The Rights of the Critically Ill* and numerous articles on reproductive rights, organ transplantation, and human experimentation. A Fellow of the Hastings Center, he has served on a federal Task Force on Organ Transplantation, on the National Institutes of Health Panel on Fetal Tissue Transplantation Research, and on the Ethics Committee of the American Society for Reproductive Medicine. He is the author of *Chil-*

dren of Choice: Freedom and the New Reproductive Technologies (Princeton, 1994), and serves as co-chair of the ethics committee of the American Society for Reproductive Medicine.

ANTONELLA SURBONE, Maturità Classica (1975), Turin; M.D. (1982), *cum laude,* School of Medicine, University of Turin; Ph.D. in Philosophy, New York. Her postdoctoral training was in medical oncology, clinical research, and internal medicine in Milan, Turin, and Bethesda, Maryland. Her previous appointments were at the National Cancer Institute, Milan, and at the Department of Oncology, University of Pisa. Currently she is Associate Attending Physician at the Department of Medicine at the Memorial Hospital for Cancer and Allied Diseases, New York; Associate Clinical Member at Memorial Sloan-Kettering Cancer Center, New York; Associate Professor of Clinical Medicine at Cornell University Medical College; she is also board-certified in Oncology and in Infectious Diseases.

Professor Surbone has published a numerous number of essays on various issues including the side-effects of chemotherapy, breast cancer during pregnancy, the ethical implications of BRCA1 testing, informed consent, truth-telling, and the ethics of genetic screening. She also coedited another volume of the *Annals* entitled *Communication with the Cancer Patient: Information and Truth.*

ROBERT D. TRUOG is Professor of Anaesthesia and Medical Ethics at Harvard Medical School and Director of the Multidisciplinary Intensive Care Unit at Children's Hospital in Boston. He received both his undergraduate and medical school education at UCLA. After completing a residency and chief residency in pediatrics at the University of Colorado in Denver, he returned to UCLA for a residency in anesthesiology. He then underwent fellowship training in pediatric anesthesia and critical care at Boston Children's Hospital, where he joined the faculty in 1987. After developing an interest in medical ethics, Dr. Truog undertook a two-year sabbatical to complete a master's degree in Philosophy from Brown University and the Program in Ethics and the Professions at Harvard University. In addition to his clinial and administrative responsibilities, Dr. Truog co-chairs the Children's Hospital Ethics Advisory Committee and is Associate Director of Clinical Programs in the Division of Medical Ethics. His academic work has focused primarily on the ethical issues that arise in the contexts of anesthesia and clinical care.

Index of Contributors

Beauchamp, T.L., 111–126
Berghmans, R., 105–110

Cohen-Almagor, R., vii, 1–22, 127–149
Cook, R.J., 74–87

den Hartogh, G., 174–187
Dickens, B.M., 88–104
Dorner, D., 188–197

Elliott, D., 240–247

Gibson, J.M., 218–228

Harris, J., 209–217

Joerden, J.C., 150–156

Kimsma, G., 157–173
Kluge, E.-H.W., 23–31

Lantos, J., 41–51
Lowy, F.L., 32–40

Robertson, J.A., 198–208

Surbone, A., 52–62

Truog, R.D., 229–239

Van Leeuwen, E., 157–173

Subject Index

Abortion, 88–103 (*passim*)
  and Peter Singer's theories in Germany, 150–156
  criminal legislation on, 75–79
  Dutch experience with, 95–96
  early laws on, 74–75
  illegal, conseqences of, 78–79
  related to PAS, 88–104
  relative to medically assisted death, 88–104
  religious arguments against, 89–93
  selective, and genetic testing, 243–246
  tolerance of, 93–97
  vs. assisted death, resolution of conflict between, 101–102
  vs. medically assisted death, contradictions in tolerance towards, 97–101
Abortion law, developments in, 74–87
Abortion law, reform of, 7, 79–81
Abortion law, relative to PAS, 7–8
Abortion rights, 74–86
Adkins (Janet) case, 135
Advance medical directives (*see also* DNR orders; Living will), 8, 97
Agreements for Carrying Fetuses Act (Israel), 194
Aid-in-dying, valid requests and refusals of, 119–120
Airedale N.H.S. Trust v. Bland, 91, 92
Alport's syndrome, genetic testing for, 241, 244
Amerindians, DNA research in, 226
Anglo-Saxon Common law on abortion, 74–75
Assisted reproduction: questions raised by, 14
Assisted suicide (see Euthanasia; Medically assisted death; Physician-assisted death)
Autonomy, 12
  and PAS, 111–126
  and *Volenti* principle, 180–183
  as principle in euthanasia debate, 175
  drawbacks of notion of , in communication, 219
  patient, and nondirective counseling, 240–247
  prospective (*see also* Advance directives), 105–110
Autonomy principle, 3
Autonomy principle in funding, 26
Autonomy rights, 19

Baby M case, 193–194
Beijing meeting on women, 81–82
Bioethics and medicine, tension between. 50
Biomedical ethics and education, 70–71
Biotechnology
  advances and legal issues in, 13
  jurisprudence in age of, 188–197
Bolivia, abortion rights in, 78,79, 85
Brain death
  and human dignity, 130
  and organ donation at VGH, 70
  and organ procurement, 17
  critique of criteria for, 231–235
  Japanese debate on, 236
  organ transplant without, 229–239
Brazil, abortion rights in, 79

Cairo Programme on reproductive health, 81
Canada
  abortion/assisted death laws in, 88, 89, 92–97, 100
  and abortion law, 75, 79, 82, 85
  code for human research in, 226
  Supreme Court of, and abortion rights, 82
Canadian Medical Association, resuscitation policy of, 68
Carder (Angela) case appeal, 98

Cardiopulmonary resuscitation (see CPR; Resuscitation)
Causation of death, philosophic issues of, 114–119
Chabot case, 165, 185–186
Chile, abortion laws in, 77, 86
Choice, moral issues concerning, 8
Cloning, 14–15
  initial response to, 209
Cloning, human
  and reproductive liberty, 198–208
  as organ tissue source, 204, ethics commissions on, 206–207
  ethics of, 209–217
Columbia, abortion laws in, 76,78
Committee on the Elimination of Discrimination against Women, 83
Committees, regional Dutch, to review PAS, 157–158
Communication
  metaphors for, 220
  problems with, in obtaining informed consent, 218–228
  with patients and family, 72
Competence, mental
  and advance directives, 105–110
  and decision making, 179
Confidentiality, right to, in abortion, 78
Counseling, nondirective, and genetic screening, 240–247
Council on Ethics and Judicial Affairs (AMA), resolution concerning organ harvest, 236
CPR, debate about, 67–70
Criminal code, Dutch, and euthanasia, 177
Criminal law and abortions
Cross-cultural view of medicine, 45–46
Cruzan v. Director, Missouri Dept. of Health (see also Cruzan case), 112, 123 [note]
Cultural differences and truth telling, 6
Cystic fibrosis, genetic screening for, 243

Dead donor rule, 235
Death with Dignity Act (Oregon), 124 [note], 140, 142

Death
  causation of, 114–119
  definition of, 16–17
  medically assisted (see also Euthanasia, Medically assisted death; Physician-assisted suicide)
  with dignity, 127
Dementia advance directives, 8
  ethical problems raised by, 105–110
"Democratic spirit": and medical decisions, 4
Diagnosis
  of death, history of, 229–230
  vs. prognosis, safety measures in, 131–132
Dialogue vs. monologue in informed consent, 220–222
Dignity, human (see Human dignity)
Disease
  genetic, screening for, 242–243
  reification of, 54
DNA, parental, in human reproduction, 204
DNR orders in context of terminal care, 70
Doctor, epistemic responsibility of, 55
Doctor-patient contractual bond, 163–164
Doctor-patient relationship, and disease reification, 54
Doctors' conflict in decision making, 172
Doctors' reports on PAS, 159–160
Doctor's role in euthanasia, 130–131
Doctrine, dominant, as influence on euthanasia debate, 178–179
Dolly, birth of, 209
Do-not-resuscitate orders (see DNR orders)
Dor Yeshorim and genetic screening for Tay Sachs, 243
Double-effect doctrine, 9, 91, 129–130, 133–134
Down's syndrome, genetic testing for, 243
Dresser, Rebecca, 107–108
Dutch (see also Netherlands)

Dutch experience of euthanasia, 174–187
Dutch law on death and dying, 163
Dutch Society for Voluntary Euthanasia, 175
Dworkin, Ronald, comments of, 16–17, 18
  on individual right to die, 170–171
  on procreative autonomy, 214–216
Dying, medical assistance in (*see* Euthanasia; Medically assisted death; Physician-assisted suicide)

Education, medical, in applied ethics, 70–71
Educators as ethical role models, 4
Effectiveness coefficients in resource allocation, 23–40
Epistemic dimension of truth telling, 52–53
Ethical dimension of truth telling, 56–57
Ethical directives for doctors, 132
Ethical issues viewed in fiction, 5
Ethical models
  for resource allocation, 23–40
  traditional benefits vs. rights-driven, 45
Ethical problems raised by advanced directive and dementia, 105–110
Ethical role models, educators as, 4
Ethicists, need for, on staff, 71–72
Ethics
  and medical school education, 70–71
  eduation, postgraduate, 71
  education, undergraduate, 70
  Kantian (*see* Kantian ethics)
  medical (*see* Medical ethics)
European Parliament, judgment of, on cloning, 210
Euthanasia (*see also* Medically assisted death; Physician-assisted suicide), 12, 88–103 (*passim*), 127
  and autonomy, 9
  and Peter Singer's theories in Germany, 150–156
  active and passive, 9
  active, performed by J. Kevorkian, 139
  active vs. passive, 167–168
  compassion as justification for, 176, 179, 186
  dementia as reason for, 183–186
  doctor's role in, 130-131
  Dutch experience of, 11-12, 96, 174–187
  involuntary, 143
  loss of integrity as a justification for, 175–180
  reformation of views about, 111–126
  role of doctor in, 181–182
Eyal (Benjamin) case, 128–130

Faith in healing [note], 60
Feinberg, J., 107
Fiction illuminating medical ethics, 41–51
Forgoing treatment, discussion of, 115–116
Fragmentation of medical treatment, 5
Free speech issues and Peter Singer, 11
Freedom and truth, 58

Gender as factor in life-and-death decisions, 98–99
"Genethics," 17
Genetic disease, 242–243
Genetic research and informed consent across cultures, 218–228
Genetic screening, organ transplantation, and counseling, 240–47
Genetic selection
  as part of procreative liberty, 199–207
  right to, 14
Genetic variability and cloning, 210–211
Genome research
  marshalling public support for, 227
  public involvement in, 16
Genomic engineering of offspring, philosophic issues surrounding, 199–207

Germany
  Peter Singer debate in, 10
  reception of Peter Singer's theories in, 150–156
Germline gene theory, 14
Guidelines for assisted suicide, 10

Halachic law and autonomy, 128–129
Harvard Committee on brain death, 229–239 (*passim*)
Health care resources and the role of doctors, 2–7
HIV testing at VGH and informed consent, 69
Hospital ethics committees: evolution of, 6,7, 63–73
Human dignity
  and cloning, 211–212
  and Kantian ethics, 15
Human Genome Diversity Project, 225–226
Human Genome Project, informed consent in, 222–225
Human rights, 75-86 (*passim*), 90, 95
Humphry, Derek, comments on J. Kevorkian, 138–139

Identity
  continuity in, 108–109
  human, protection of individuality of, 205
  personal, and dementia, 107
  unique, and cloning, 211
In re AC, 98
In re Quinlan (*see also* Quinlan case), 112
In vitro fertilization, legal questions posed by, 188–197
Individualism, notion of, and difficulty in communication, 219
Infanticide, 151–155
Informed consent
  and HIV testing, 69
  and incompetent patients, 68
  communications problems in, 218–222

to genetic research, 218–228
Integrity of life in euthanasia debate, 183–186
Ireland (Northern), abortion/assisted death laws in, 100
Ireland, reform of abortion laws in, 85

Jurisprudence in age of biotechnology, 188–197
Justice vs. law in Nachmani case, 190

Kahn, Axel, comment of, on cloning, 211–213
Kantian ethics
  and cloning, 212–213
  and human dignity, 15
Kevorkian, Jack
  challenges of, to legal system, 135–140
  critique of, 127–134
  legal judgment rendered on, 139
Killing vs. letting-die, 114–119
Knowledge, theory of, and truth telling, 52–53

Language and the slippery slope, 133,
Law
  and medical practice of euthanasia, 176–178
  compared with medical morality, 164–166
  concerning assisted death, 88
  Dutch, on death and dying, 163
Legal actions against PAS, 137
Legalization of PAS, 162
Letting-die, conceptual problems in, 114–119
Liberal perspectives on ethical questions, 1–2
Life, opposing views on beginning and end, 7–11
Living wills, 97
  at VGH, 66
Long-term care at VGH and cessation of treatment, 70

SUBJECT INDEX

Maternal mortality, 75, 80–83
Medical ethics
  future development in, 18–19
  illuminated by fiction and autobiography, 41–51
Medical information, imparting of, 54–55
Medically assisted death (*see also* Euthanasia; Physician-assisted suicide)
Medically assisted death,
  moral justification of, 157–173
  relative to abortion, 7–8, 88–104
  tolerance of, 93–97
  vs. abortion, contradictions in tolerance towards, 97–101
  vs. abortion, resolution of conflict between, 101–102
Medicine
  and bioethics, tension between, 50
  cross-cultural view of, 45–46
  limitations of, 49
  truth in, 52-62
Mental competence and advance directives, 105–110
Mental suffering and euthanasia, 185–186
Mercitron, 127, 134
Mexico, abortion rights in, 78
Monologue vs. dialogue in informed consent, 220–222
Morality, medical, compared with law, 164–166
Morgentaler, Smoling and Scott v. The Queen, 79–82, 88, 95, 97
Morocco, abortion rights in, 83
Motherhood, 75–76, 80, 191–192
Murder, 91, 92, 95

Nachmani case (Israel), 13–14
Nachmani v. Nachmani, 188–197
Narrative theory and informed consent, 221
Narrative unity of life in euthanasia debate, 183–186
Navajo Nation, obtaining DNA samples from, 222

Nepal, abortion laws in, 77
Netherlands (*see also* Dutch *entries*)
  abortion/assisted death laws in, 88, 89, 95, 96, 98
  developments in PAS in, 157–173
  law on advance directives in dementia, 109
Nietzsche's views on human life, 168–169

Objectivity, pure, 53
Open Heart [*Shiva M'Hodu*] (A.B. Yehoshua), 41–51
Operation Wandering Soul (R. Powers), 44
Oregon Death with Dignity Act, 124 [note], 140, 142
Oregon, PAS in, 113
Organ donation
  and human cloning, 204
  and brain death, 17, 234–238
  and PAS, 138
Organ transplantation
  and genetic screening, 240–247
  drawbacks with, 241
  ntersection of, 240–242
  without brain death, 229–239

Pakistan, abortion laws in, 77
Palliation, duty of, 29, 30
Palliative care, 19
  vs. euthanasia, 141
Parenthood (*see also* Reproduction)
  right to, 191–192
Parfit, Derek, 107
Paternalism, 12
  and euthanasia, 130–131
  indirect, 181–182
"Patholysis," 136
Patient autonomy and resuscitation, 67, 68
Personhood in Peter Singer's arguments, 154
Peru, UN recommendations for abortion rights in, 82
Peter Singer debate in Germany, 10

Physician-assisted suicide (*see also* Euthanasia; Medically assisted death)
  and autonomy, 111-126
  and organ harvest, 138
  constitutional (U.S.) right to, 113
  debate on, influenced by reigning doctrine, 178-179
  ethical guidelines for, 140-143
  fears concerning, 121-122
  guidelines for, 10
  legalization of, 162, 176-178
  moral justification of, 157-173
  overzealousness in, 134-140
  philosophical problems in, 120-122, 166-171
  physicians reporting on, 159-160
  societal objections to, 132-134
  TV broadcast of, 138-139
  voluntary, circumscribed plea for, 127-149
Planned Parenthood of Southeastern Pennsylvania v. Casey, 88, 90
Platonic view of knowledge, 52-53
Poland, abortion laws in, 75,76
Pregnancy, 74-86 (*passim*)
Prevention rather than transplantation, 240-243
Procreation (*see* Reproduction)
Prognosis vs. diagnosis, 56-57
  safety measures in, 131-132
Prosecution, criminal, for abortion, 75-79
Psychiatric suffering and euthanasia, 185-186
Public involvement in genome research, 16
Public support for genome research, 227

Quality of life vs. sanctity of life, 88-104
Quality-of-life concept. 9
Quill, Timothy [note], 147

R. *v. Bourne*, 74
Rape, 76-80 (*passim*), 82, 84, 85

Remmelink Commission, 11, 96
Reproductive autonomy, 214-216
  and cloning, 209-217
Reproductive health, 76, 80, 81, 83, 84
  UN goals towards,81-82
Reproductive liberty and cloning, 198-208
Reproductive rights, 13-15
Resource allocation
  ethical model for, 23-40
  model for, 2-4
Resuscitation policy at VGH, 66-69
Right to life and Peter Singer's views, 155-156
Right to Life argument, 90
Right to parenthood, 191-192
Rights
  concept of, 3
  human (*see also* Human rights)
  inalienable, 181-182
  vs. commodity approach to health care delivery, 23
Rodriguez v. British Columbia (Attorney-General), 88, 94-96
Romania
  abortion law in, 80, 86
  maternal mortality in, 94

Saint Vincent and the Grenadines, abortion rights in, 83
Sanctity of body speciments in DNA research, 226
Sanctity of life
  principle of, 128
  vs. quality of life, 88-104
Scheffer v. The State of Israel, 144
Screening genetics and reproductive liberty, 202-203
Self-determination (*see* Advance directives; Autonomy)
Should the Baby Live? (H. Kuhse and P. Singer), 150-151
Singer, Peter, reception in German of theories of, 150-156
60 Minutes broadcast of PAS, 138-139
"Slippery slope" arguments
  against PAS, 132-134
  and Peter Singer's theories, 152

SUBJECT INDEX

Societal objections to PAS, 132–134
Societal obligation, theories of, 24–25
Societal values in resource allocation, 26, 27
Society vs. individual in right-to-die, 170–171
South Africa, abortion rights in, 83–86
Speciesism argument by Peter Singer, 153–154
Spiritual values, loss of, by doctors, 44–51
States (U.S.) rights to PAS, 113
Suffering
  perception of, 177–178
  unbearable, 177, 185–186
Suicide, assisted (*see* Euthanasia; Medically assisted death; Physican-assisted suicide)
  religious argument against 89–93

Tay Sachs disease, genetic screeing for, 243
Technology, negative possibilities with, 41–51
Termination of pregnancy (*see* Abortion)
Terminology
  for end-of-life states, 9
  misuse of, by Peter Singer, 10
Testing, genetic (*see* Genetic screening)
The Cunning Man (R. Davies), 51
The Spirit Catches You and You Fall Down (A. Fadiman), 45–46
Traditional beneficence model of medical ethics, 4
Transplantation (*see also* Organ procurement)
  in genetic disease, prevention as alternative to, 17–18
  organ (*see also* Organ procurement)
  organ, drawbacks with, 241
Treatment, forgoing, 115–116
Truth telling
  as result of process, 6
  between patient and doctor, 52–62
Truth
  dynamic aspect of, 5–-55, 58
  pragmatic dimension of, 55–56

Turkey, abortion rights in, 83

U.S. Supreme Court rulings on reproduction, 200
UN agencies, judments against cloning of, 209–210
UN Fourth World Conference on Women (Beijing), 81–82
UN Human Rights Committee, 82
UN Programme of Action on reproductive health, 81
United Kingdom, abortion/assisted death laws in, 88, 89, 100
United States, abortion/assisted death laws in, 88, 90, 93, 97, 100, 101

Values, societal, in allocation of resources, 26, 27
Vancouver General Hospital (VGH)
  ethics committee at: policy development at, 66–70
  ethics committee at: structure and function of, 65
  neonatal problems at, 64
Venezuela, abortion rights in, 83
Volenti principle, 180–183
Voluntary active euthanasia (VAE), 11

Washington (state), aid-in-dying legislation, 113
Washington v. Glucksberg, 88, 90, 101
Well-being. subjective criteria of, 177–178, 184
Women's Convention, 83
Women's health, 75, 76, 79, 80, 83–86
Women's health and abortion law reform, 75, 79–80

Youk (Thomas) case, 138

Zeal, danger of, in PAS, 134–140